AF207987

Air Fryer

275+

RECIPES TO ABSOLUTELY NAIL IT

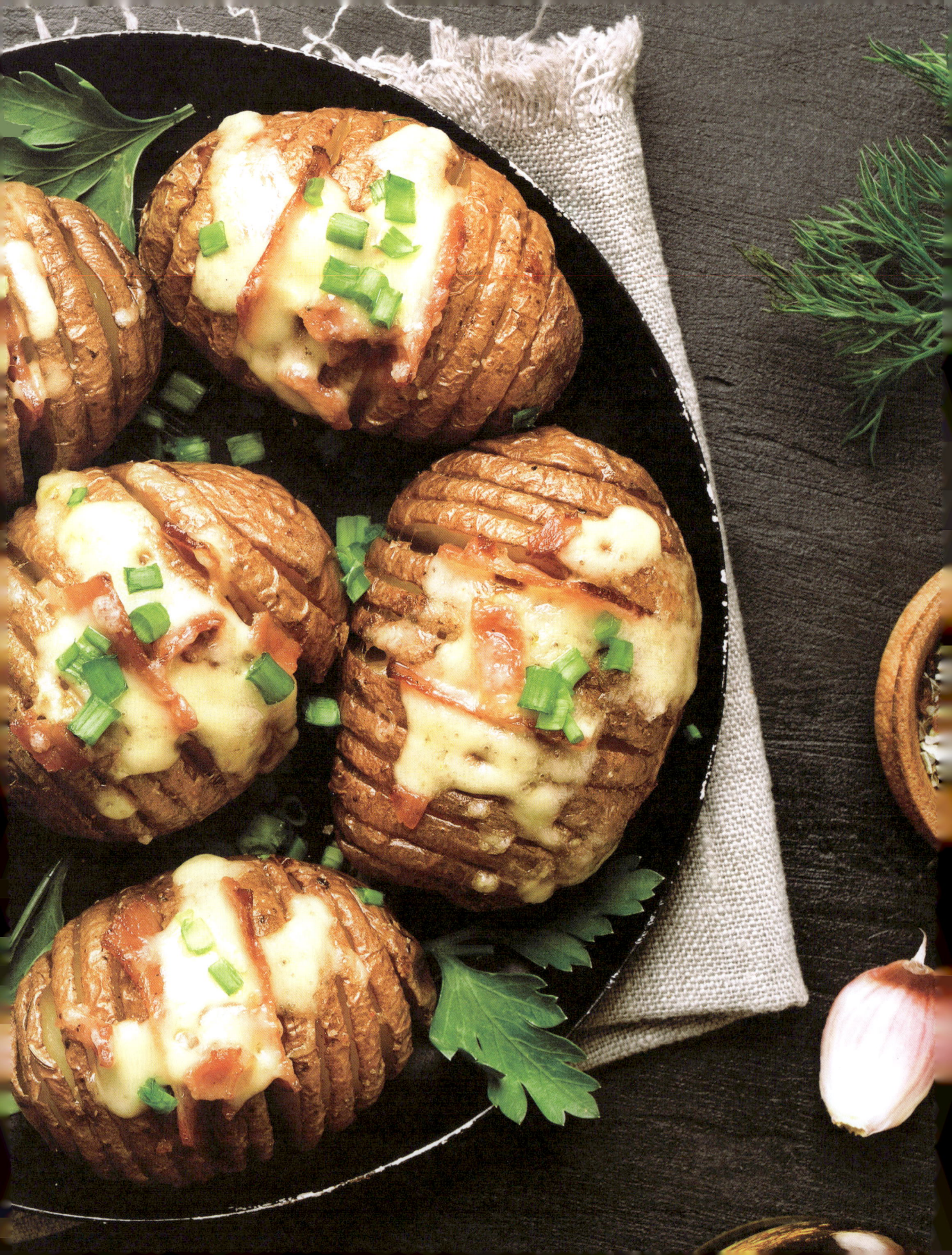

Contents

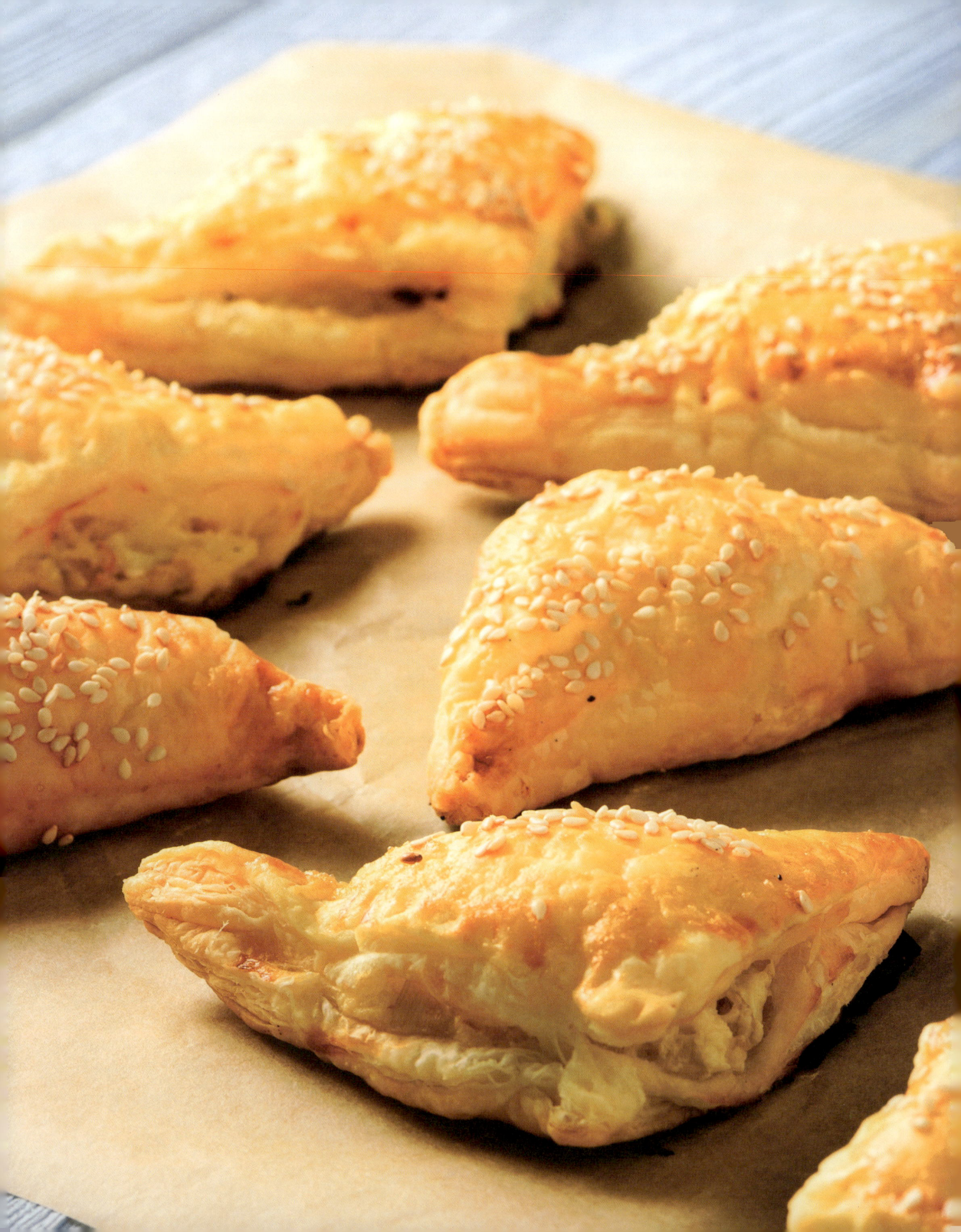

Welcome to the Air Fryer cookbook.

With recipes for every meal of the day, plus snacks and sweets, here you'll find everything you need to know to get the most out of your air fryer appliance.

WHY AIR FRY?

Air fryers are well known for providing a healthier alternative to deep-frying food, but with similar (some say even better) results. That's why they are such a hit with families who want to keep on eating their favourite crispy chips and nuggets (whether homemade or pre-packaged) but with little or no fat. The health benefit of an air fryer is number one for many people, especially those looking to conserve calories or make the shift to a healthier diet, but there are other worthwhile benefits too.

For busy people, the air fryer delivers the benefit of speed. Ready-made food can be cooked in about half the time a conventional oven would take. Food can be cooked from frozen too, so you save on defrosting time (and you don't have to remember to get it out of the freezer in advance). It's so easy as well, and you'll find lots of ideas and tips for cooking ready-made food in chapter two of this book.

It's called a 'fryer', but this machine can grill, bake and roast foods as well so it's definitely not limited to chicken nuggets and chips. It is extremely versatile and should be viewed like a conventional oven in terms of its capability to cook different foods. You can bake a cake in it, roast a chicken, poach an egg, cook a quiche or make sausage rolls. And that's just five ideas from over 275 recipes in this book.

Last but certainly not least for busy people, is the ease of clean up. Traditional fryers and even ovens tend to use a lot of oil and make a splashy mess around the place. The air fryer, by contrast, uses little oil and all 'mess' is contained within the appliance. Most have been designed to be very easy to clean, with removable non-stick parts that are dishwasher friendly.

Give the air fryer a go. It has the capacity to transform your cooking, making it easier and faster to get healthier food on the table. With the recipes in this book, we guarantee you'll absolutely nail it.

Choosing an air fryer

The two factors to consider when choosing the best air fryer for you are size (capacity) and wattage (power).

Size is measured by litre capacity. Air fryers come in three main sizes - small, medium and large. The small sizes range between 3L and 3.5L, the medium between 4L and 5L and large sizes range from 7L to 12L in capacity. These larger versions take up more bench space, but they often come with extra features such as a rotisserie or dehydrator.

If you have a large family to cook for, you will probably want to opt for a medium or large air fryer, or maybe even more than one. For couples or small families, a small air fryer may be enough. Do your homework and decide what's best for you.

Power is an important consideration during your research too. Power is measured by wattage. A higher wattage means greater power which means food will cook more quickly. If this is a priority, look for an air fryer with a high wattage.

Cooking times and temperatures

If you want to experiment with recipes beyond those in this book, you can find excellent tools online to assist with converting conventional oven temperatures to air fryer temperatures. Just google 'air fryer calculator'. A good rule of thumb to bear in mind though is the 20:20 rule: that you will generally reduce the temperature by approximately 20°C and reduce the cook time by 20%.

As with conventional cooking, the size of an ingredient, such as a potato, will influence the cooking time. Likewise, the extent to which you fill muffin trays or the size of your pies will influence cooking times. Check regularly until you are very familiar with your machine.

Air fryer cooking tips

PREHEAT

If a recipe specifies preheating, you can use the preheat setting on your air fryer or, if it doesn't have one, simply set to the desired temperature and let it run for 3 minutes.

PAT DRY

Use paper towel to pat foods dry before cooking to avoid splattering and excess smoke.

SPRITZ

Lightly spritz foods with cooking spray or toss in a small amount of oil to minimise the chance of sticking to the basket and to maximise results.

SPRITZ AGAIN DURING COOKING

You don't need to do this on fatty foods, such as steak, but for anything that's coated in breadcrumbs give an extra spritz with oil during cooking, especially on any dry, floury areas, for a crispier result.

DON'T OVERCROWD THE BASKET

Give food plenty of space so that the air can circulate. This will deliver the best and crispiest results. Cook in batches or use a double layer accessory to maximise available space.

SHAKE THE BASKET

For best results, shake the basket and/or rotate food every 5-10 minutes. This will allow the air to circulate better and will result in more uniform cooking.

Accessories

The great news is that you don't have to make a big investment in air fryer accessories up front. You can use any existing dish, ramekin, cake tin, bowl or other utensil in your air fryer so long as it is made from an ovenproof material such as glass, ceramic, metal or silicone, and fits in your air fryer basket. Likewise you can use baking paper, patty pans (paper or silicone) and aluminium foil in your air fryer, just as long as this does not completely cover the bottom of the basket, which would disrupt air flow.

However, you might decide to invest in extras designed specifically for the air fryer that you feel would be helpful. Experiment with the recipes in this book and see what you most need. We have provided a list of the basics opposite. Or, if you are a complete beginner, you might prefer to invest in a starter pack, which will generally include a cake tin with a convenient handle, a double layer accessory (to expand your cooking surfaces), a pizza pan, a cooking rack with skewer holders, and a silicone mat to protect cooking surfaces. You can also buy accessory kits to suit your cooking interests, such as baking accessory kits or grilling accessory kits.

Note: One of the best things about appliances made specifically for the air fryer is their shape and size. They are designed to fit in the air fryer, whereas utensils designed for the oven tend to be bigger.

COMMON AIR FRYER ACCESSORIES

Baking pan

Cake tin

Pizza pan

Ramekins

Grill pan

Double layer accessory (or metal rack)

Bread rack

Silicone cupcake moulds

Silicone mat

The double layer accessory is especially useful because it doubles the space you have available to cook in. As the air fryer is small compared to the conventional oven, it will enable you to create food for the family without having to cook in batches.

Note: For the purposes of this book, we have assumed that you don't have any special air fryer accessories. Where a utensil is required, we have listed it in the ingredients. You will need to ensure that it fits in your air fryer and is ovenproof.

COOKING WITH PANS AND TINS

When placing a pan or tin in the air fryer basket, leave a little space around it so that the air can circulate. For the same reason, always put the pan into the air fryer basket and never directly into the air fryer. Use oven mitts when removing pans and tins from the air fryer.

COOKING SPRAY

Not exactly an accessory, cooking oil spray is nonetheless an essential ingredient for cooking in an air fryer. Invest in a sprayer bottle (or two) that you can refill. Depending on how and what you cook, you might like to have one filled with a non-stick cooking oil and the other with olive oil (for flavour as well as its non-stick properties).

A pastry brush is also handy for applying oil to food and glaze or egg wash to pies and pastries.

Note: We have not included cooking spray in the ingredients lists for recipes, but have assumed it is a kitchen staple.

THERMOMETER

A great investment if you are serious about cooking in an air fryer is an instant-read kitchen thermometer. This will be particularly helpful for cooking meat, helping you achieve the best (and safest) results with the least fuss.

Sometimes meat and fish are simply cooked to preference, such as rare or well done (see below), but some meat, such as chicken, needs to reach a certain temperature to be safe. Chicken is cooked when the internal temperature reaches 74°C, but note that a thicker piece of meat might require a few more minutes' cooking.

Practice makes perfect, but a good rule of thumb for cooking red meat is:

For rare meat: 50°C

For medium meat: 55°C

For well-done meat: 60°C

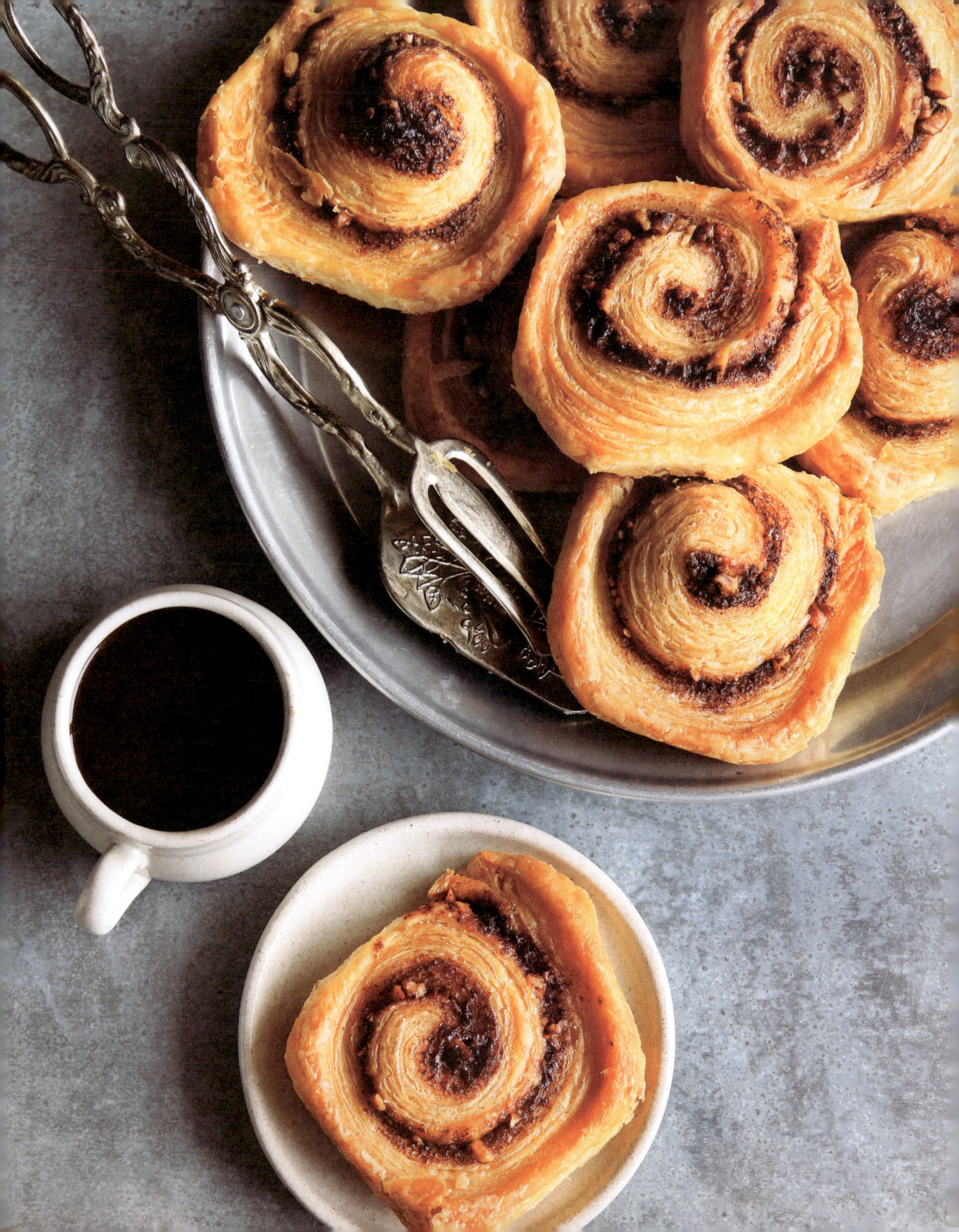

Breakfast

Fried Eggs

2 eggs

2 tbsps butter

Salt and pepper

Baking pan

Place butter in the baking pan and insert the pan into the air fryer. Heat butter until just melted (approximately 1 minute).

Remove the pan and crack both eggs into it.

Return to the air fryer and cook at 160°C.

For soft yolks, cook for 4 minutes.

For hard yolks, cook for 8 minutes.

Check occasionally during cooking to ensure eggs are cooked to your preference.

SERVES 1

Eggs in Shell

4 eggs

Don't prick the eggs.

Place the eggs in the air fryer basket.

Cook the eggs at 160°C.

For soft yolks, cook for 6 minutes.

For medium eggs, cook for 8 minutes.

For hard-boiled eggs, cook for 10 minutes.

When cooked place immediately into cold water to stop further cooking.

SERVES 4

Scrambled Eggs

4-5 eggs

Knob of butter

Baking pan

Preheat the air fryer to 220°C.

Whisk the eggs until fully combined.

Place butter in the baking pan and insert the pan into the air fryer. Heat butter until just melted (approximately 1 minute).

Add the eggs and cook for 1 minute. Remove, stir and check the consistency. Repeat until the eggs are cooked to your liking.

SERVES 2

Poached Eggs

4 eggs

Baking pan

Place the baking pan in the air fryer basket.

Using a jug or the kettle, fill to halfway with boiling water.

Carefully crack the eggs and slide them into the water.

Cook the eggs at 200°C for 3 and a half minutes for soft yolks or longer to suit your preference.

Remove from the air fryer using a slotted spoon.

SERVES 4

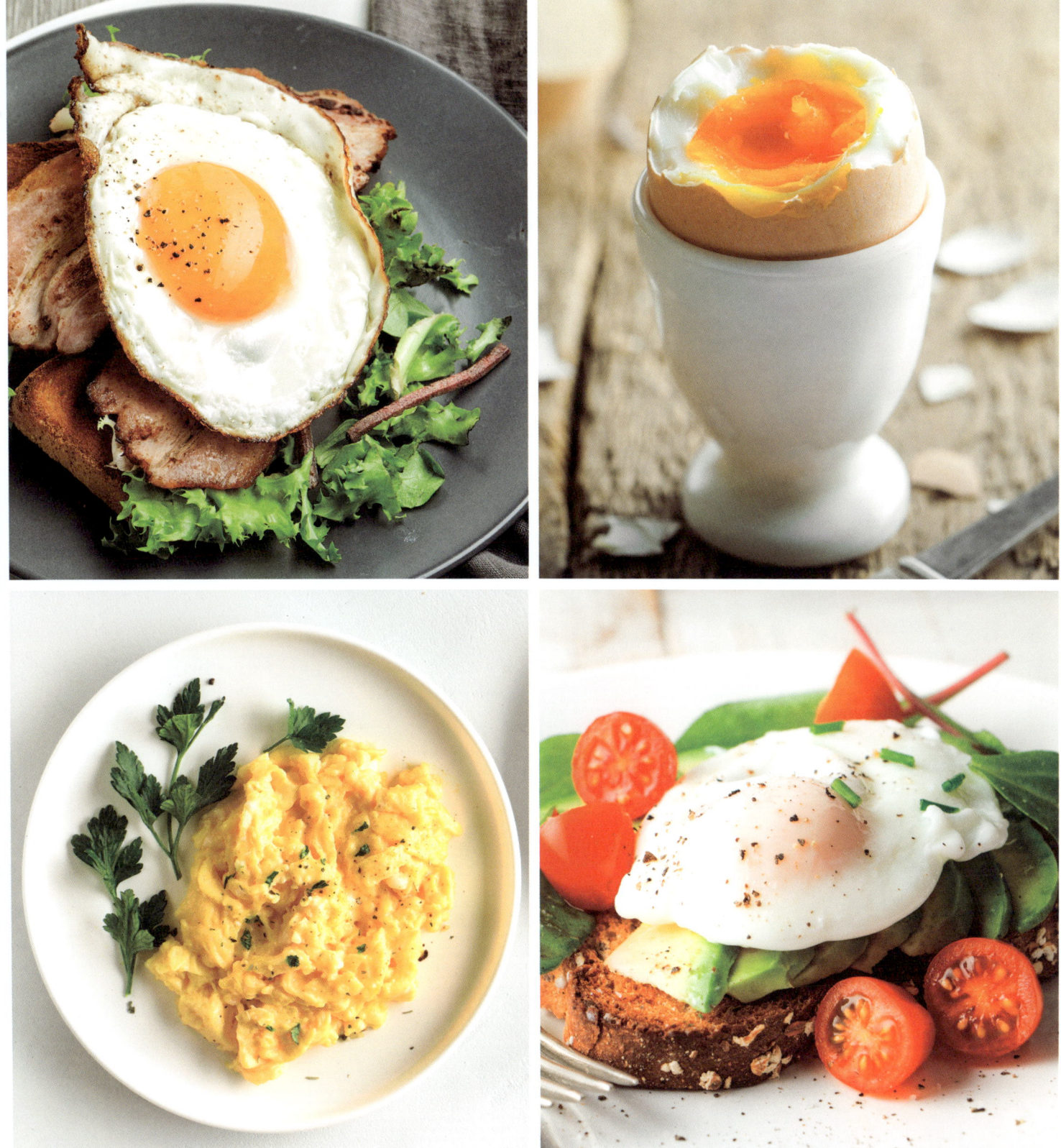

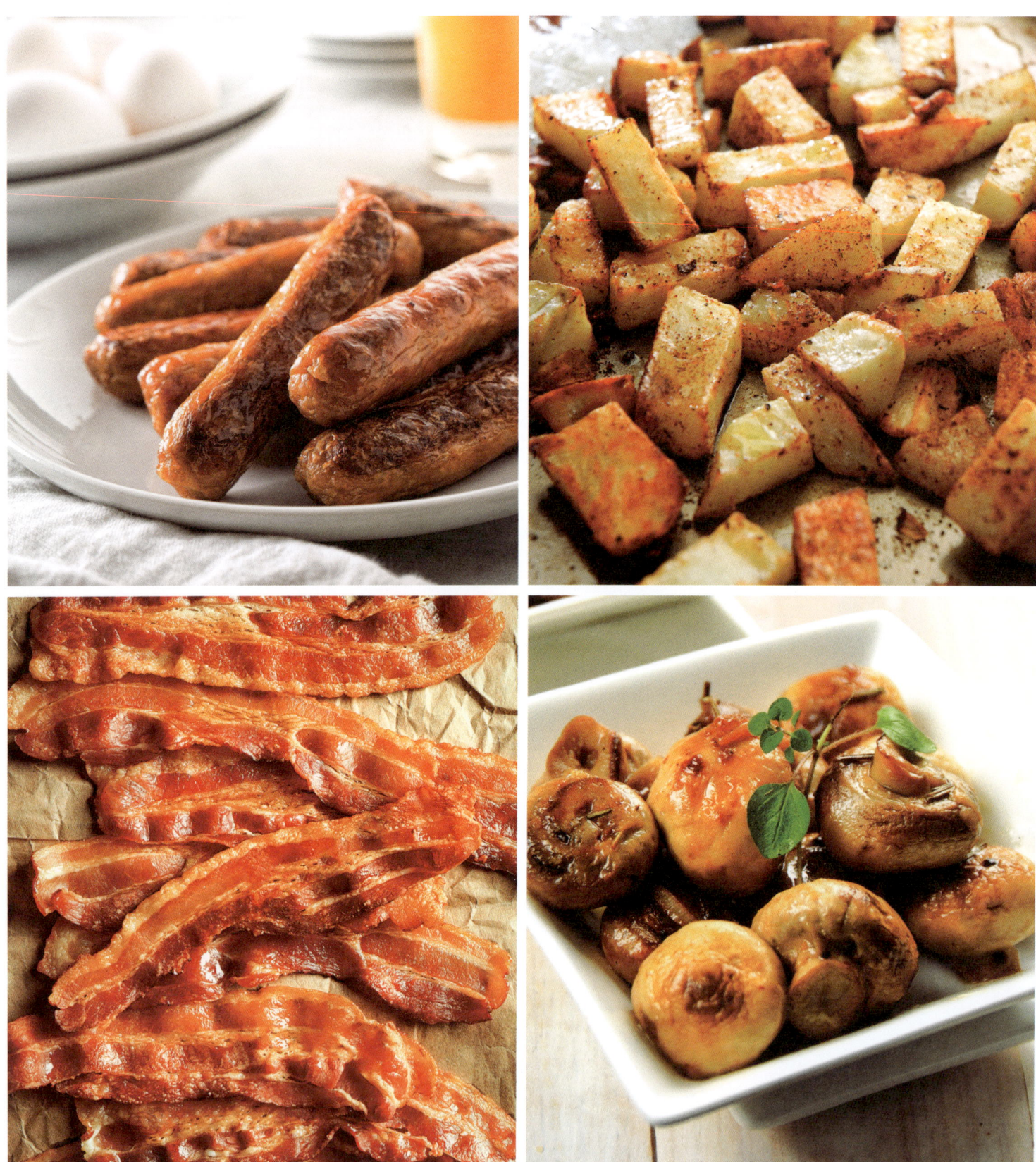

Sausages

8 sausages

Prick the sausages on one side.

Place the sausages in the air fryer basket, pricked-side down. Allow enough space between them that they don't touch. Cook in batches or use a double layer accessory if needed.

Cook for 15 minutes at 180°C.

Halfway through the cooking cycle, flip the sausages.

Remove sausages from the air fryer basket and serve.

SERVES 4

Note: Pricking the sausages allows the fat to drain out, meaning that they will 'fry' rather than 'boil'.

Paprika Potatoes

700g potatoes

1 tbsp olive oil

1 tsp garlic powder

1 tsp paprika

1 tsp salt

1 tsp pepper

Cut the potatoes into cubes of a similar size to ensure even cooking.

In a mixing bowl, coat the potatoes with oil, garlic powder, paprika, salt and pepper.

Place in the air fryer basket and cook for 20 minutes at 200°C.

Halfway through the cooking cycle, toss potatoes so they cook evenly.

Remove potatoes from the air fryer basket and serve.

SERVES 2

Note: For best results, use fresh potatoes of a floury variety such as Coliban.

Bacon

8 thin rashers bacon

Preheat the air fryer to 200°C.

Place the bacon in the air fryer basket in a single layer (you may need to cook in two batches or use a double layer accessory).

Cook for 5 minutes, checking halfway and rearranging with tongs as needed.

For thicker bacon, cook for 10 minutes.

Notes: Cook for an extra minute or two for extra crispy bacon.

If cooking in batches, drain the grease after each cook time to avoid the fat smoking.

SERVES 2

Garlic Mushrooms

200g button mushrooms, washed and dried

1 tbsp olive oil

2 cloves garlic, minced (or ½ tsp garlic powder)

1 tsp soy sauce

½ tsp pepper

1 tsp dried rosemary

Lemon juice, to serve

Wash the mushrooms and rub dry with paper towel.

Place mushrooms in a bowl with the other ingredients and toss to coat them.

Cook for 10 minutes at 190°C, removing and shaking the basket halfway through cooking.

Squeeze over fresh lemon juice to serve.

SERVES 2

Breakfast Burritos

6 flour tortillas

6 eggs, scrambled (see p 12)

4 cooked sausages, chopped (see p 15)

½ cup (60g) Cheddar cheese, grated

1 cup (270g) tomato salsa

Fresh parsley, to serve

Preheat the air fryer to 180°C. Spray the air fryer basket with olive oil spray.

Combine the egg, sausage, cheese and salsa in a mixing bowl.

Spoon ½ cup of the mixture into the centre of a flour tortilla. Fold in the sides and then roll to form a burrito.

Repeat with the remaining ingredients.

Place the burritos into the air fryer basket and cook for 5 minutes.

Serve garnished with fresh parsley, if desired.

SERVES 3

Homemade Hash Browns

4 large potatoes, peeled and finely grated

2 tbsps cornflour

½ tsp salt

2 tsps olive oil

Place the grated potatoes in a bowl of cold water and soak for 30 minutes. Drain and then pat dry with a paper towel. Transfer to a clean, dry bowl.

Add the cornflour, salt and oil and mix together. Form into small patties and transfer to the fridge for 10 minutes.

Preheat the air fryer to 200°C.

Lightly spray the air fryer basket. Place the patties in the basket and cook for 15 minutes, flipping halfway through cooking.

SERVES 2

Note: Don't skip the soaking stage as this will remove the starch from the potatoes, making the hash browns crispier.

Polenta Fries

1½ cups (250g) polenta

⅓ cup (30g) Parmesan cheese, grated

Pinch of salt

1 tbsp fresh rosemary leaves

Heat two cups of water in a large saucepan over high heat. Add the polenta in a steady stream, stirring constantly. Reduce heat to low and cook for 3 minutes, until thickened. Remove from the heat and stir in the cheese. Pour into a greased square pan, cover with plastic wrap and transfer to the fridge to chill for a minimum of 3 hours and up to 24 hours.

Remove polenta from the pan and place on a chopping board. Cut into fries of the desired size.

Preheat the air fryer to 190°C and spritz the air fryer basket with cooking spray.

Transfer fries to the air fryer basket, leaving a little space around them. (You may need to cook in batches).

Cook for 20 minutes, turning halfway, until crispy. Sprinkle with rosemary to serve.

SERVES 2

Ham and Cheese Puffs

2 sheets frozen puff pastry, thawed

1 ham steak, diced

1⅔ cups (200g) Cheddar cheese, grated

Milk, to glaze

Preheat the air fryer to 200°C.

Mix the ham and cheese together in a mixing bowl.

Roll and cut the pastry into squares of 5 x 5cm and scoop a heaped teaspoon of filling onto each square.

Fold over the corners of squares so that they almost meet in the centre.

Place the parcels in the air fryer basket and brush the pastry with milk. Be careful not to overcrowd the basket. Cook in batches or use a double layer accessory if needed.

Slide the basket into the air fryer and cook for 10 minutes until crispy and golden.

SERVES 2

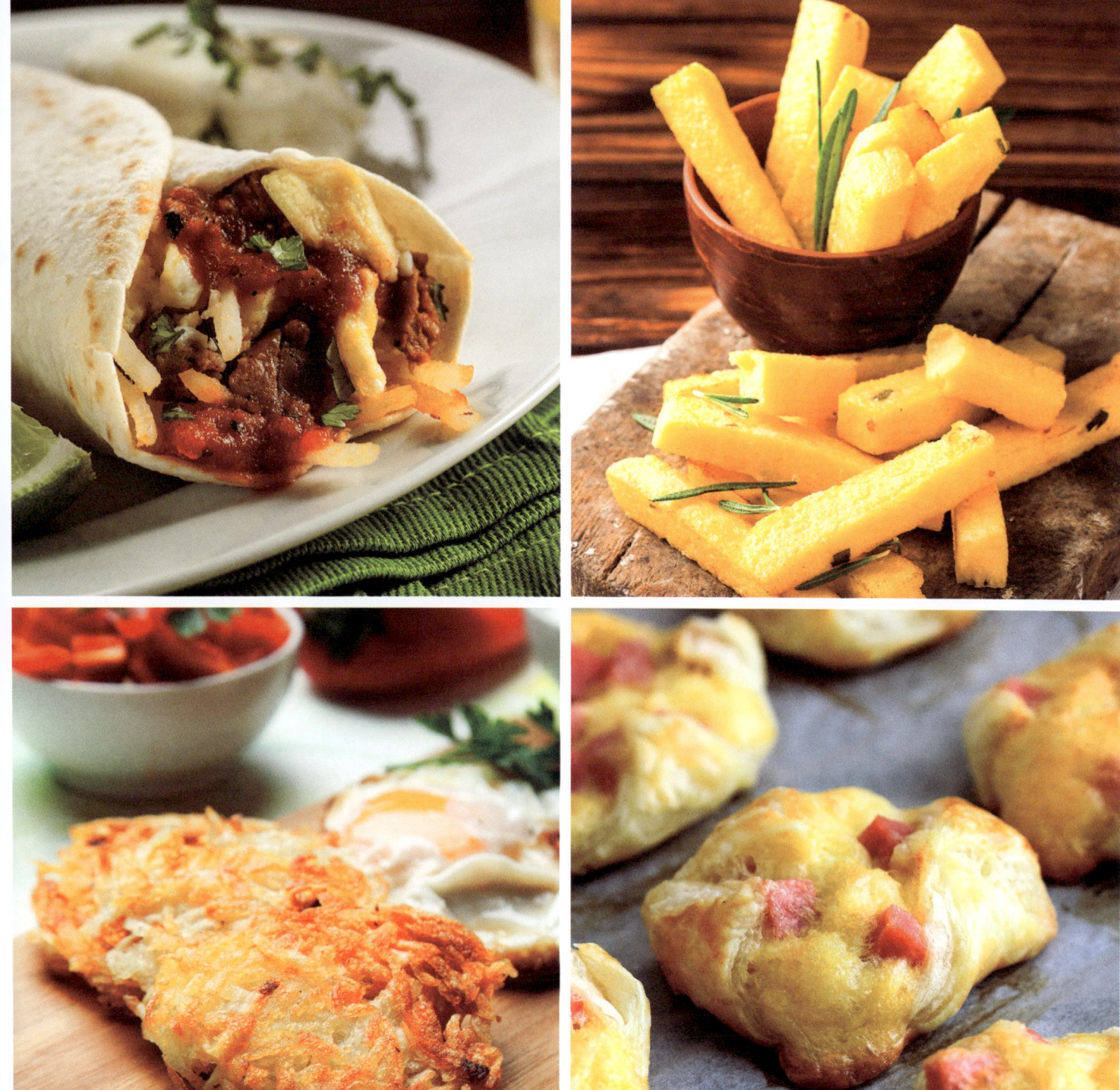

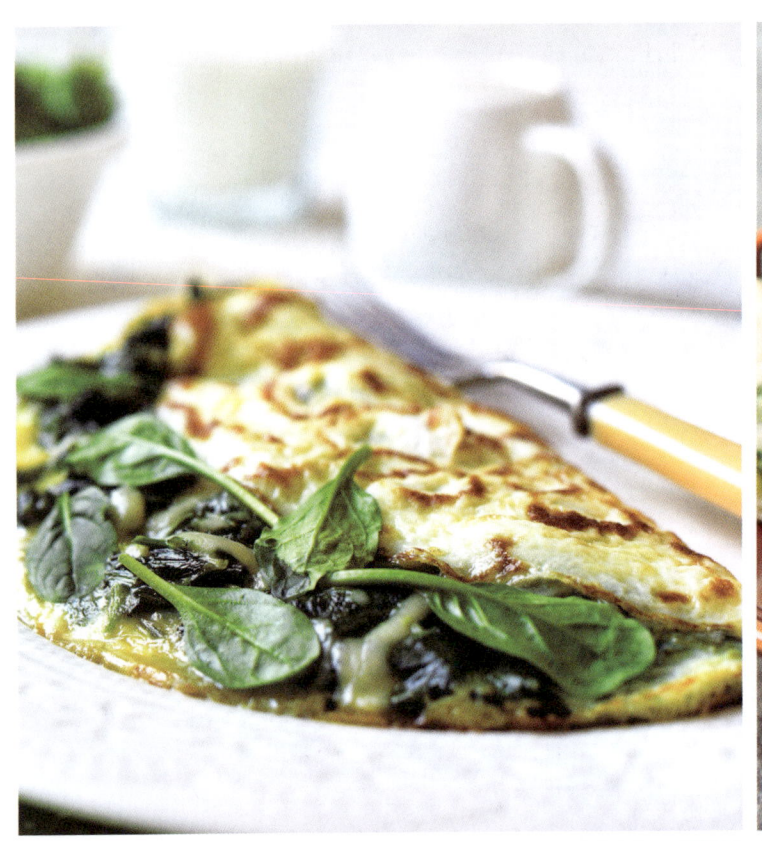

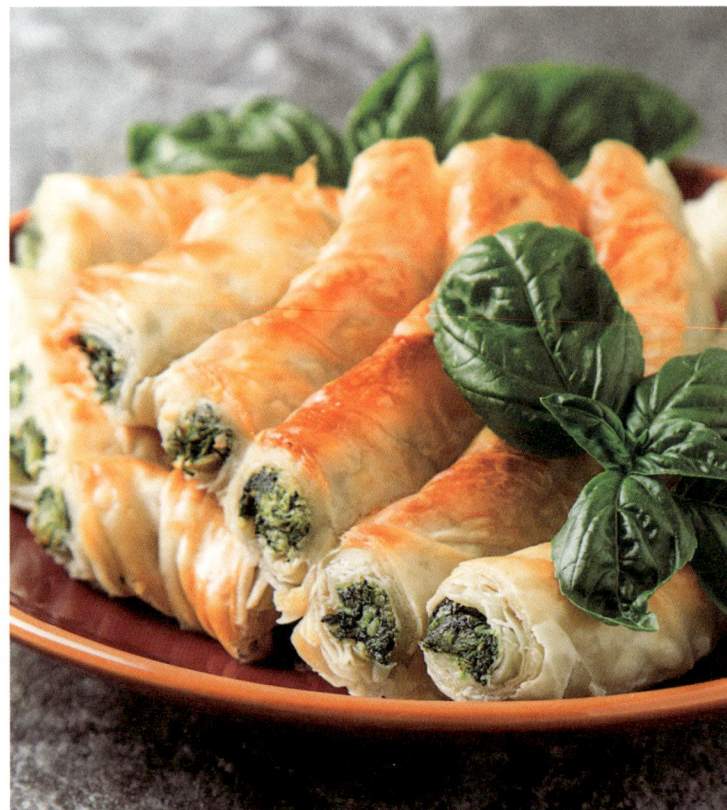

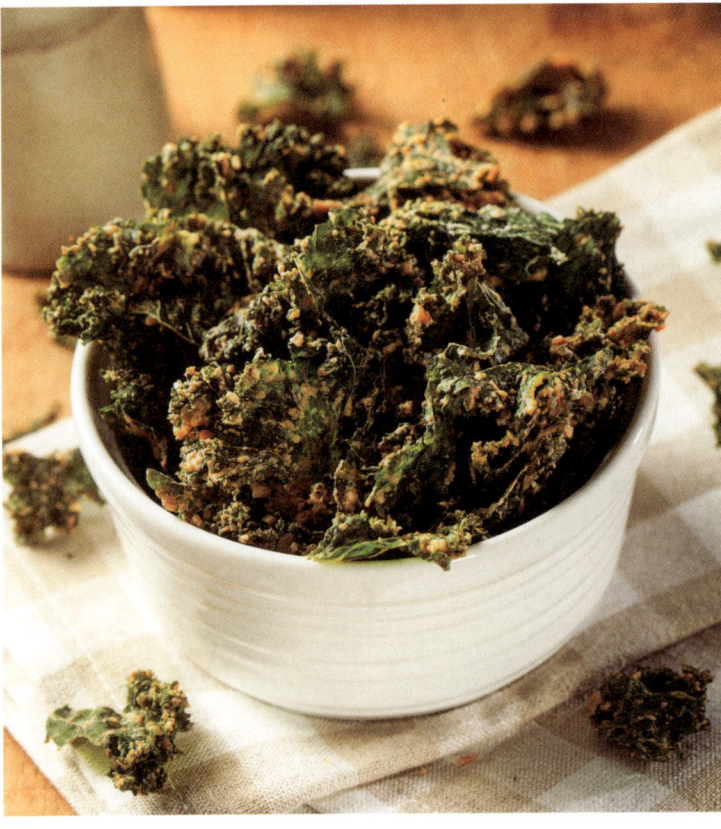

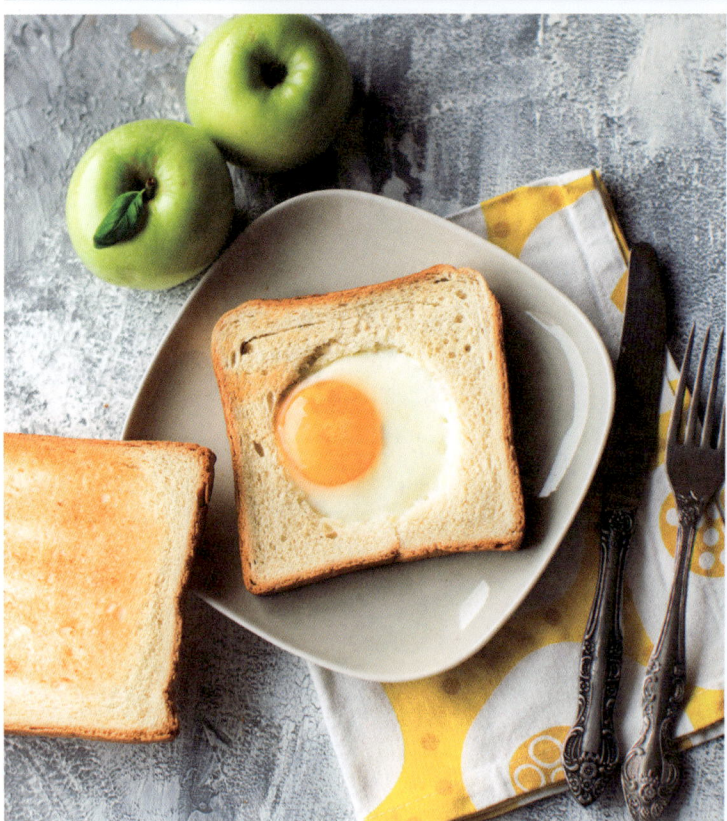

Spinach Omelette

2 eggs

¼ cup (60ml) milk

Pinch of salt

100g baby spinach

¼ cup (30g) Cheddar cheese, grated

Baking pan

Whisk the eggs, milk and salt in a small bowl until well combined. Add the spinach and loosely combine.

Pour the mixture into a well-greased baking pan.

Place the pan into the air fryer basket and cook for 4 minutes at 180°C. Sprinkle the cheese over the top and return to cook for a further 4 minutes.

Use a thin spatula to loosen the omelette from the sides of the pan and transfer to a plate. Flip one half of the omelette over.

SERVES 1

Spinach and Cheese Rolls

2 cups (500g) ricotta

¾ cup (75g) Parmesan cheese, finely grated

250g feta, broken into small pieces

125g baby spinach, finely chopped

1 egg + 1 egg, beaten

4 sheets puff pastry, just thawed

1 tsp nutmeg

Salt and pepper

Preheat the air fryer to 180°C.

Place all ingredients except the pastry and the beaten egg into a large bowl and mix until combined.

Cut pastry sheets in half lengthways. Brush one edge with the beaten egg, then add a spoonful of mixture in a line down the centre. Roll the pastry (starting from the edge without the egg) and gently press to seal. Repeat process until all the pastry and mixture has been used up.

Place the into the air fryer basket and brush with the beaten egg. Cook for 12 minutes until golden.

SERVES 4

Kale Chips with Vegan Cheese

2 tbsps olive oil

1 small bunch kale, leaves picked

1 tbsp nutritional yeast flakes

¼ tsp salt

Place all the ingredients in a mixing bowl and toss to fully coat.

Transfer to the air fryer basket and slide into the air fryer. Cook for 5 minutes on 190°C.

Check regularly after 2 minutes cooking as they can burn quickly.

Serve immediately.

SERVES 3

Notes: Use the leaves of the kale only and discard the stems, as the stems will not cook without the leaves burning.

Use grated Parmesan instead of yeast flakes if you prefer (and are not vegan).

Egg in Hole

1 slice of bread

1 egg

Pinch of salt and pepper

Baking pan

Lightly spray the inside of the baking pan and set aside.

Place the piece of bread on a bread board and make a hole, using the rim of a cup or a cookie cutter.

Place the piece of bread in the prepared baking pan and crack the egg into the hole.

Transfer to air fryer and cook at 160°C for 5-7 minutes, depending on how you like your yolk cooked (longer for a firmer yolk).

SERVES 1

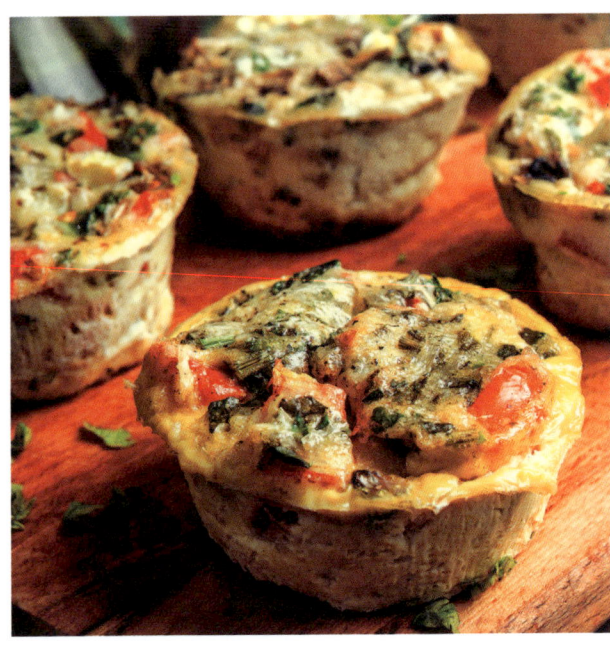

Egg and Veggie Cups

6 eggs

2 tbsps milk

Pinch of salt and pepper

½ cup (15g) fresh spinach, finely chopped

¼ cup (45g) red capsicum, finely diced

¼ cup (35g) onion, finely diced

½ cup (60g) Cheddar cheese, grated

¼ cup (30g) mozzarella cheese, grated

6 silicone moulds

Lightly spray the moulds with oil and transfer to the air fryer.

Place the eggs, milk, salt and pepper in a large mixing bowl and whisk to combine.

Sprinkle in spinach, capsicum, onion and Cheddar cheese and stir to combine.

Pour the egg mixture into the silicone moulds. Sprinkle the mozzarella cheese over the top.

Cook for 15 minutes at 160°C.

MAKES 6

Bacon and Egg Cups

6 large eggs

2 tbsps cream

Pinch of salt and pepper

½ red capsicum, diced

¼ small onion, diced

½ cup (60g) Cheddar cheese, grated

3 rashers bacon, cooked and chopped

¼ cup (30g) mozzarella cheese, grated

1 tbsp chopped fresh chives, to garnish

6 silicone moulds

Lightly spray the moulds with oil and transfer to the air fryer.

Place the eggs, milk, salt and pepper in a large mixing bowl and whisk to combine.

Sprinkle in the capsicum, onion, Cheddar cheese and bacon and stir to combine.

Pour the egg mixture into the silicone moulds. Sprinkle the mozzarella cheese over the top.

Cook for 15 minutes at 160°C. Garnish with chives, if desired.

MAKES 6

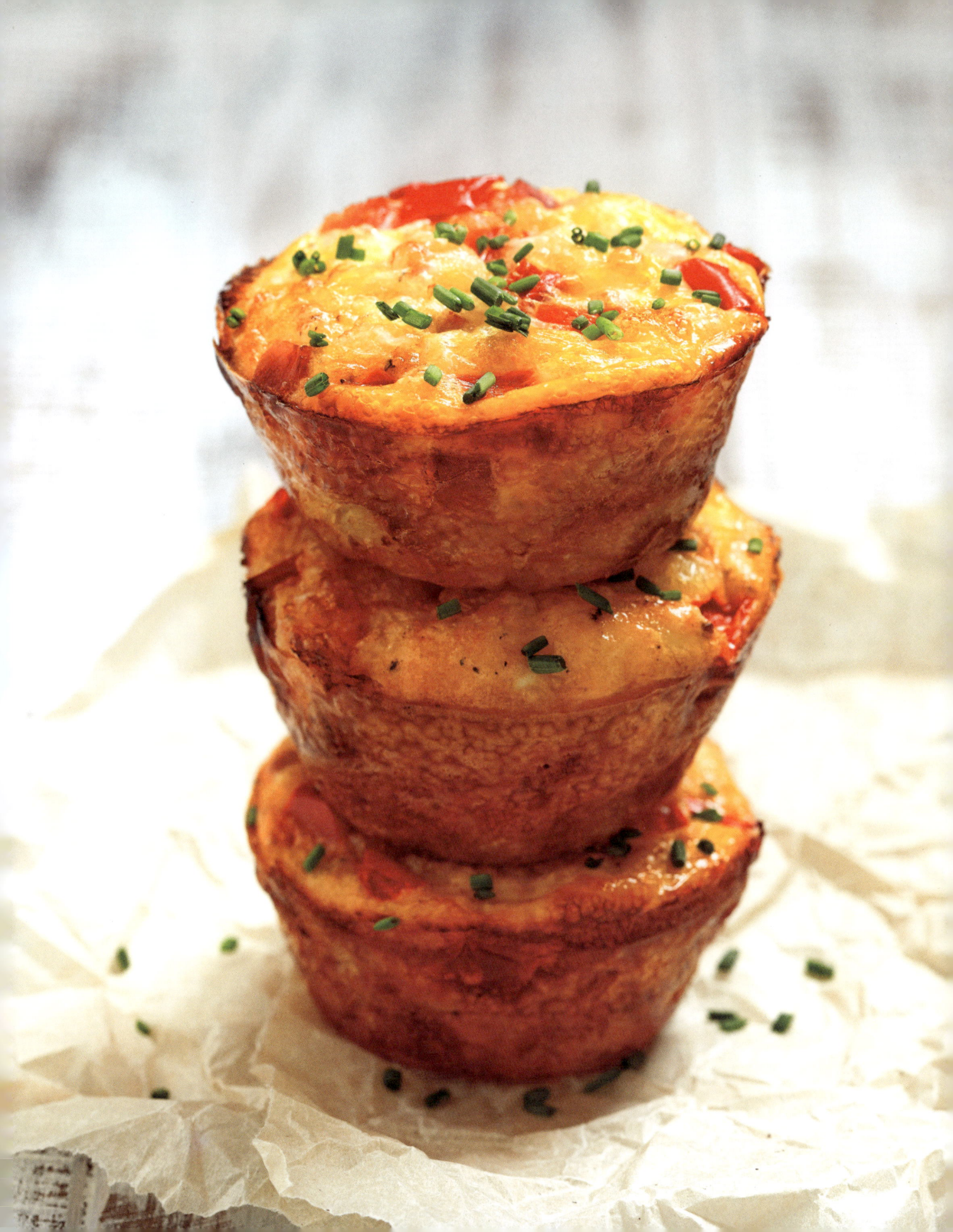

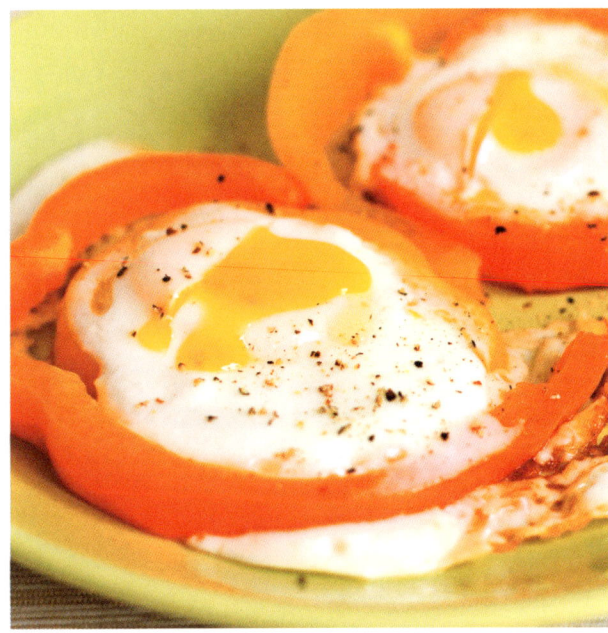

Eggs in a Capsicum Ring

1 large capsicum, deseeded

4 eggs

Pinch of salt and pepper

4 ramekins

Lightly grease or spray each ramekin with oil and place the ramekins in the air fryer basket.

Slice the capsicum into thick (approximately 2cm) rings.

Place a capsicum ring in each ramekin and then crack an egg inside each. Season with salt and pepper.

Cook for 5 minutes at 180°C. For a firm yolk cook for a further 2 minutes.

SERVES 2

Egg, Tomato and Thyme Tarts

Plain flour, for dusting

1 sheet frozen puff pastry, just thawed

¾ cup (90g) Cheddar cheese, grated

4 large eggs

8 cherry tomatoes, halved

1 tbsp fresh thyme leaves

Preheat the air fryer to 200°C.

Place the pastry sheet on a floured workbench and cut into four squares. Place one or two squares (depending on space) in the air fryer basket, spacing them apart so they do not touch. Cook for 10 minutes or until pastry is golden brown.

Remove the basket from the air fryer. Using a spoon, press down in the centre of the pastry to make an indentation. Sprinkle cheese into each indentation and then crack an egg into it. Dot the cherry tomato halves around the corners of each and sprinkle with thyme leaves.

Return to the air fryer and cook for a further 6-8 minutes or until cooked to your preference. Transfer to a wire rack and allow to cool for 5 minutes. Serve warm.

Repeat steps with the remaining ingredients until you have made four tarts.

MAKES 4

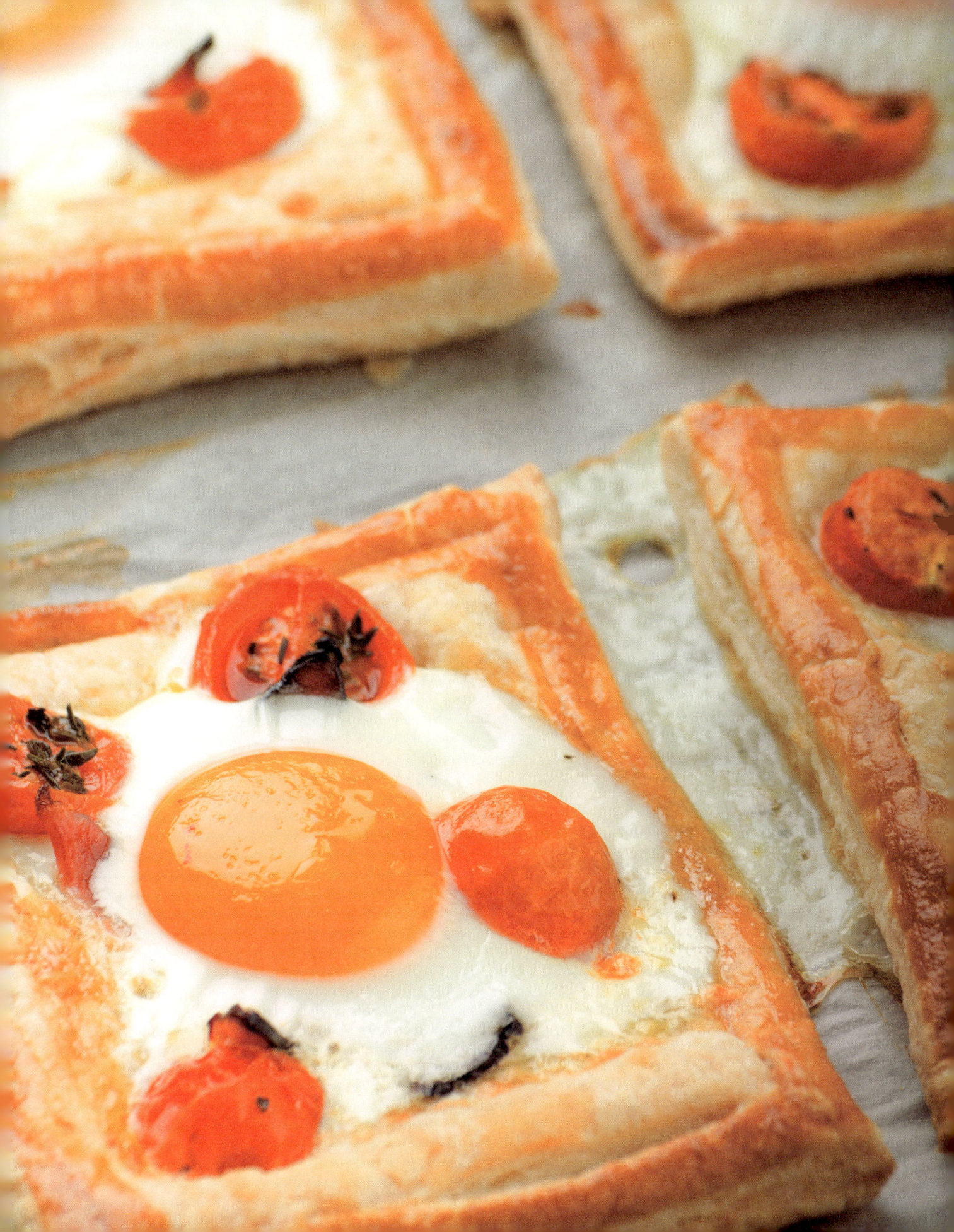

Bacon Avocado Wedges

12 rashers bacon

2 ripe avocados, cut into 12 wedges

Pinch of salt and pepper

Lightly spray the avocado with olive oil spray and season with salt and pepper.

Wrap each avocado wedge in bacon and place in the air fryer basket.

Cook on 180°C for 10 minutes.

Serve warm.

MAKES 12

Smoky Slow-Roasted Tomatoes

500g ripe cherry tomatoes on the vine

Baking pan

Place tomatoes in the baking pan and insert the pan into the air fryer basket. Cook at 115°C for 45 minutes, checking and shaking the basket occasionally.

Continue to cook in 15-minute intervals for approximately 1 hour or until tomatoes reduce to half their original size.

Increase the air fryer temperature to 200°C and cook for a further 5 minutes, checking regularly as the tomatoes will char quickly at this stage.

When lightly charred, remove with a spoon, being sure to retain any juices.

Notes: Perfect for use in salads, sandwiches or on pizza.

Store in an airtight container in the fridge for up to five days.

Chilli and Bacon Asparagus Spears

2 tsps olive oil

Pinch of salt and pepper

½ tsp chilli flakes

12 rashers bacon

12 spears of asparagus, trimmed

Drizzle the olive oil over the asparagus spears. Season with salt, pepper, and chilli flakes. Toss to coat evenly.

Wrap each asparagus spear in a rasher of bacon.

Cook in the air fryer at 180°C for 10 minutes, and then turn and cook for a further 5 minutes (or longer for crispier bacon).

MAKES 12

Egg Baked in Avocado

1 large avocado

2 small eggs

Salt and pepper, to taste

1 tsp fresh parsley, chopped

Preheat air fryer to 200°C.

Cut the avocado in half and remove the seed.

Place the avocado halves face up on a chopping board.

Crack an egg into each avocado half, and sprinkle with salt and pepper.

Cook for 12 minutes, or longer for a firmer yolk.

Sprinkle with fresh parsley to serve, if desired.

SERVES 2

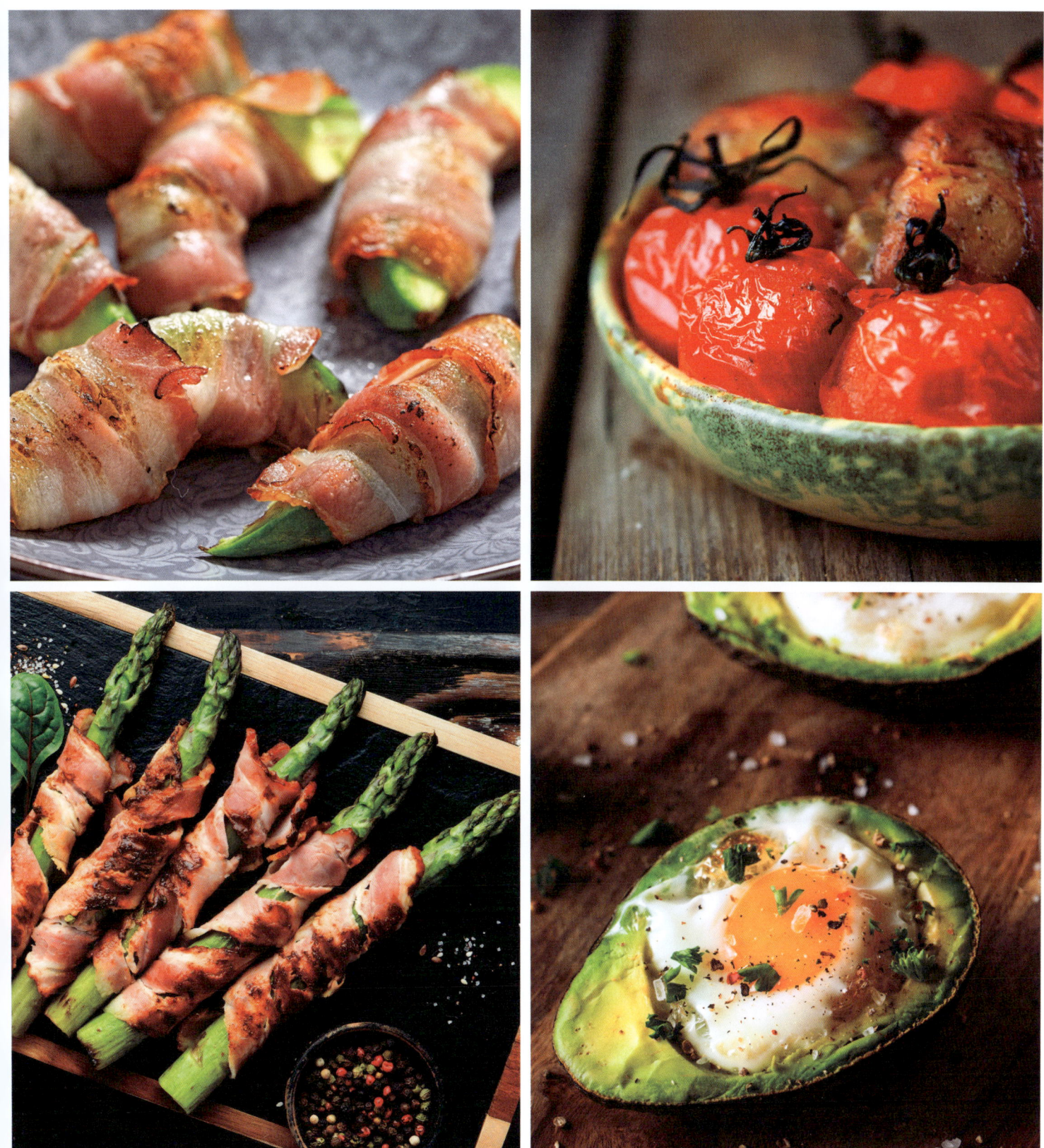

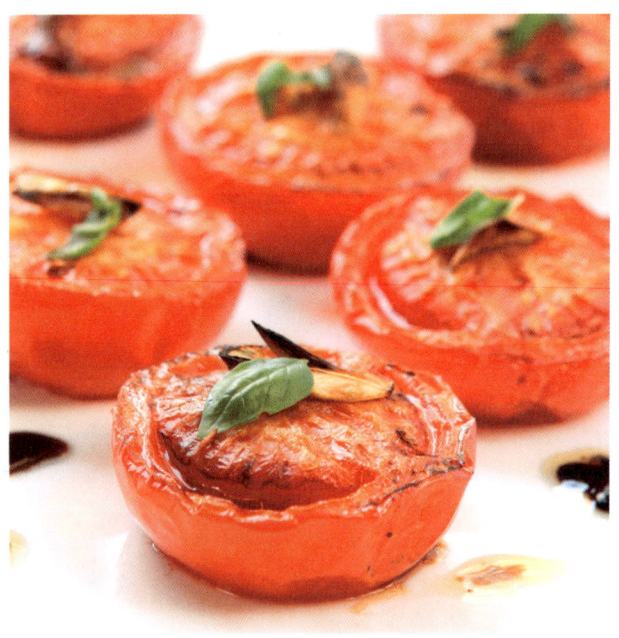

Balsamic Tomatoes

4 large tomatoes, halved

1 tbsp olive oil

1 tbsp balsamic vinegar

1 tsp fresh basil, chopped + leaves to garnish

½ tsp salt

Pinch of pepper

Preheat the air fryer to 175°C.

In a large bowl, combine the olive oil, balsamic vinegar, basil, salt and pepper.

Add the halved tomatoes and stir until fully coated.

Place the tomato halves, cut-side up, in the air fryer basket.

Cook for 25 minutes. Garnish with fresh basil to serve.

SERVES 4

Bruschetta with Roasted Tomatoes

2 large tomatoes

Pinch of salt and pepper

1 tbsp fresh basil, finely chopped + leaves to garnish

¼ small onion, finely diced

1 tbsp garlic, finely chopped (or use a puree)

3 tbsps olive oil

1 ciabatta loaf

8 slices mozzarella cheese

Grill pan

Finely dice the tomato and mix together with the salt and pepper, basil and onion in a mixing bowl.

Place the garlic and olive oil in a small mixing bowl. Stir and set aside.

Slice the ciabatta into eight medium slices and place on the grill pan. Using a pastry brush, coat one side of the bread with the garlic oil. Turn the slices of bread over so that the oil side is down on the pan. Place the slices of mozzarella and seasoned tomatoes on top.

Transfer (in batches) to the air fryer and cook for 5 minutes per batch at 180°C.

Garnish with fresh basil, if desired.

SERVES 4

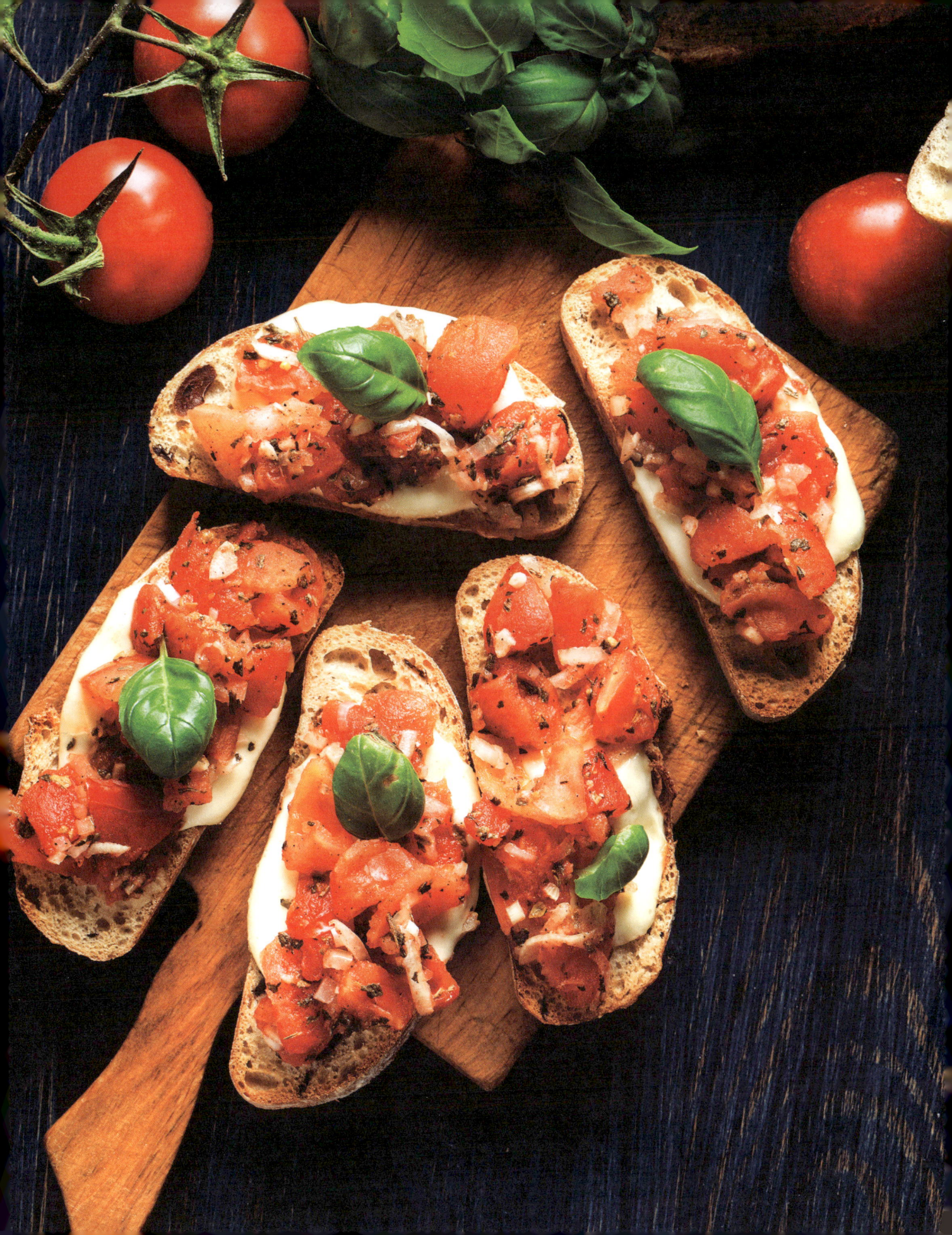

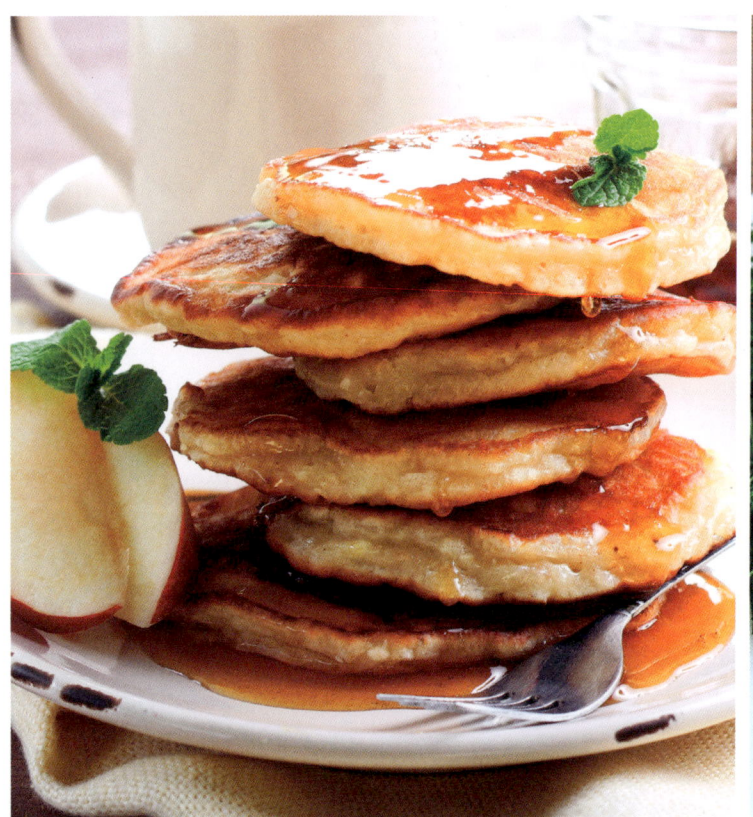

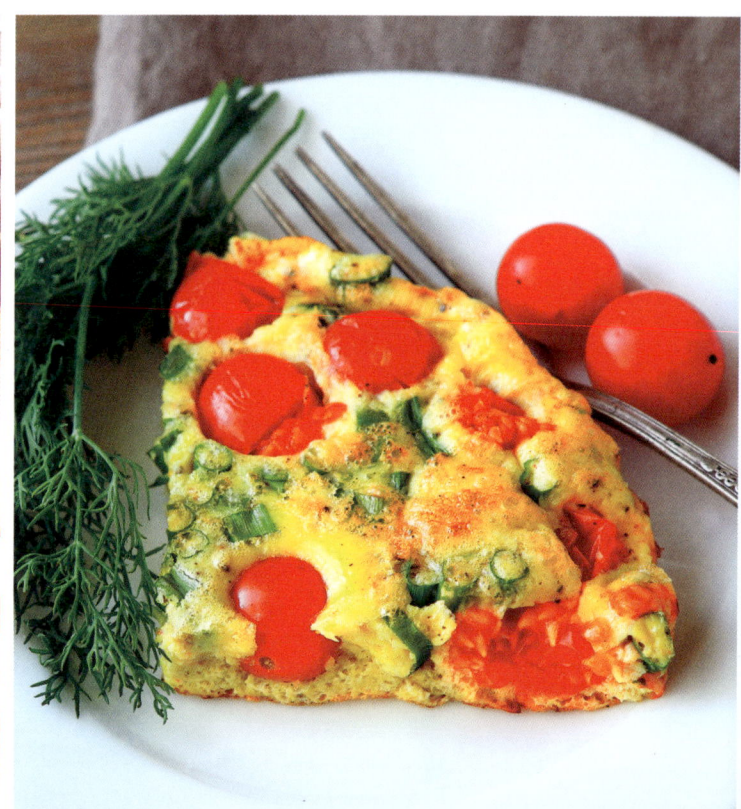

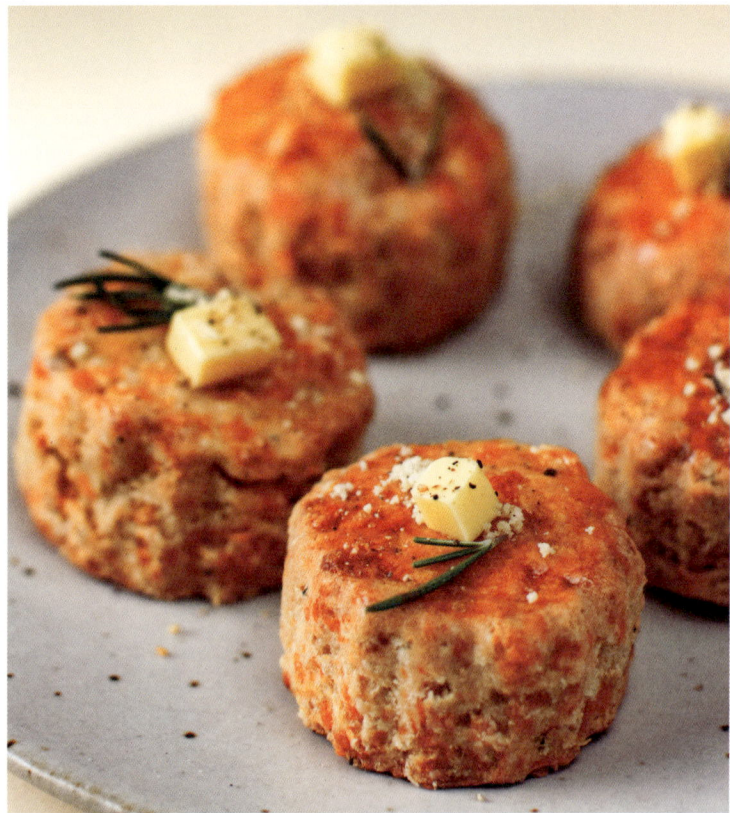

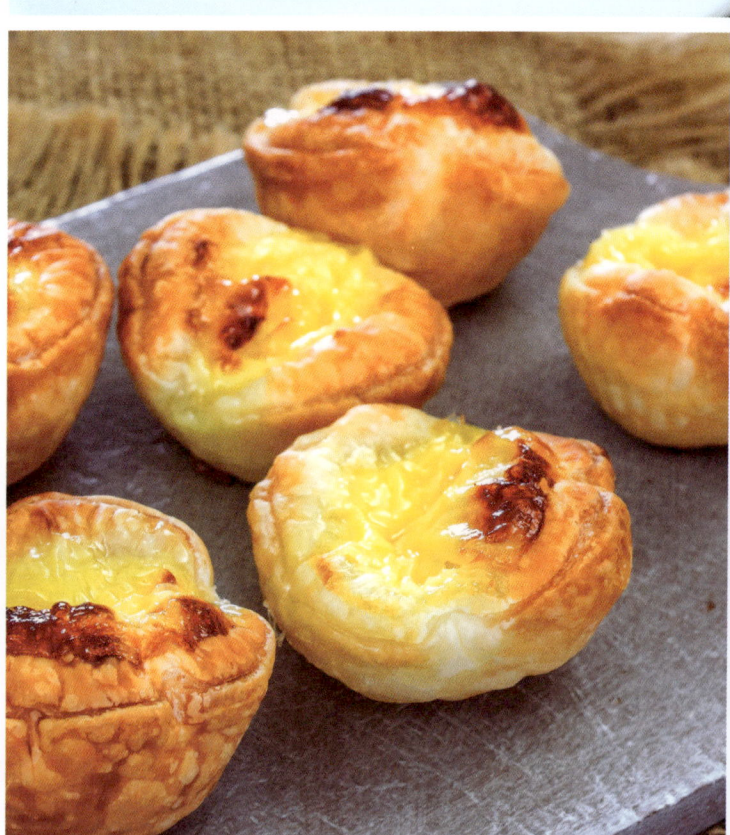

Apple Pancakes

60g butter, melted

1 egg

1 cup (250ml) milk

1¼ cups (150g) plain flour, sifted

1 tsp baking powder

Pinch of ground cinnamon

2 tbsps brown sugar

1 apple, grated

Baking pan, lightly greased

Preheat the air fryer to 180°C. Whisk together the butter, egg and milk in a large bowl. Combine the flour, baking powder, cinnamon and sugar in a separate bowl. Pour the wet ingredients into the dry and stir until just combined. Gently stir in the apple.

Scrape 2 heaped tablespoons of batter into the pan. Cook for 7 minutes or until golden. Repeat for remaining mixture.

SERVES 2

Note: Cook a couple of pancakes at a time depending on the size of your pan.

Breakfast Frittata

4 eggs

3 tbsps double cream

¼ cup (30g) Cheddar cheese, grated

3 cherry tomatoes, halved

1 spring onion, finely sliced

Pinch of salt

Baking pan

Preheat the air fryer to 180°C.

Lightly spray and line a baking pan with greaseproof paper and set aside.

Whisk the eggs and cream together in a mixing bowl.

Add the remaining ingredients to the bowl, and stir to combine.

Pour the mixture into the baking pan and place inside the air fryer basket.

Cook for 15 minutes, or until eggs are set. To check, insert a toothpick in the centre of the frittata. The eggs are set if it comes out clean.

SERVES 2

Mini Cheese Scones

1½ cups (175g) self-raising flour

25g butter

⅔ cup (75g) Cheddar cheese, grated

Pinch of salt and pepper

1 tbsp milk (more as needed)

1 egg

Baking pan

Preheat the air fryer to 180°C. Lightly spray and line a baking pan with greaseproof paper and set aside.

Place flour in a large mixing bowl. Add butter and rub into the flour using fingertips until it reaches a breadcrumb consistency. Add two-thirds of the cheese, salt and pepper and mix well. Add the milk and egg and stir until the mixture forms a soft dough (add more milk if needed).

Roll out the dough to a thickness of around 1½ cm and then cut out 10 rounds using a cookie cutter. Place remaining cheese into the middle and then roll into balls.

Place scones into the pan and cook for 20 minutes.

MAKES 10

Cheese Tarts

1 tsp oil

1 cup (125g) tasty cheese, grated

4 eggs

½ cup (125ml) milk

4 sheets puff pastry, thawed

6-hole muffin tray, lightly greased

Place the oil, cheese and eggs into a mixing bowl. Whisk to combine.

Preheat the air fryer to 200°C.

Cut the pastry into 12 circles (use a cookie cutter or the rim of a glass). Press six of the circles into the prepared pan. Divide half the filling between the pastry shells.

Brush the edges of the pastry with the milk.

Slide the tray into the air fryer and cook for 10 minutes until golden brown.

Repeat with the remaining pastry and filling.

MAKES 12

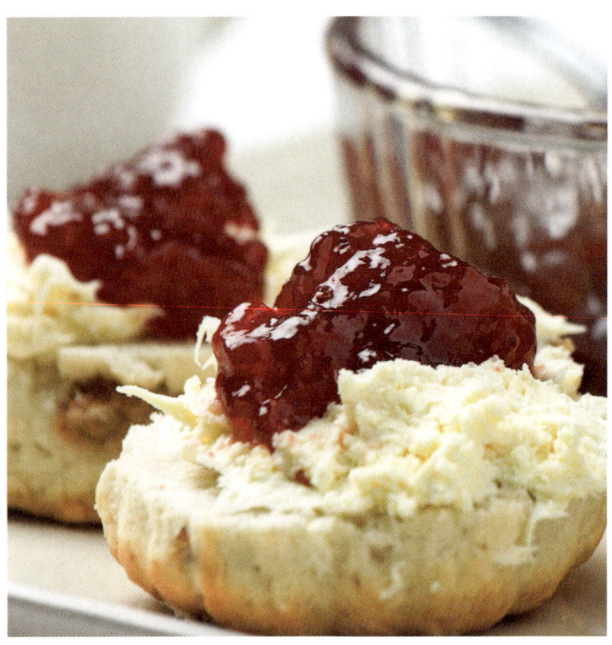

Scones with Strawberry Jam

1 cup (125g) self-raising flour, sifted

¼ cup (55g) caster sugar

30g chilled butter, cut into pieces

⅓ cup (80ml) milk

Jam and whipped cream, to serve

Baking pan

Lightly spray and line the baking pan with greaseproof paper and set aside.

Combine the flour and sugar in a large mixing bowl. Add the butter and rub it into the flour using fingertips until it reaches a breadcrumb consistency.

Make a well in the centre and pour in the milk. Stir until well combined.

Turn the mixture out onto a floured workbench and gently knead the dough until it comes together. Roll out the dough to a thickness of around 1½ cm and then cut out six rounds using a cookie cutter.

Place the rounds into the prepared pan and cook for 12 minutes at 200°C.

Serve with jam and cream.

MAKES 6

Cinnamon Scrolls

1 cup (250ml) milk

3 tbsps butter + 2 tbsps butter, melted

2¼ tsps instant yeast

¼ tsp salt

¼ cup (55g) firmly packed brown sugar

5⅓ cups (660g) plain flour, sifted

2 tsps ground cinnamon

¾ cup (100g) pecans, toasted and roughly chopped

Cake tin, greased

Gently heat the milk and 3 tablespoons of butter in a saucepan over medium heat. Stir until butter has melted. Do not allow to boil. Remove from the heat and allow to cool until the mixture is warm to the touch. Transfer to a large mixing bowl.

Sprinkle the yeast on top and set aside for 10 minutes to activate. Add salt and 1 tablespoon of the brown sugar and stir to combine.

Add the flour in thirds, stirring after each addition. When a sticky dough forms transfer this to a floured work surface. Wipe and then lightly spray the mixing bowl with oil and set aside.

Knead the dough for 1-2 minutes until workable. Place in the greased bowl and cover with plastic wrap. Transfer to a warm place for 1 hour to rise.

To make the filling, stir together the remaining brown sugar and cinnamon, breaking up any lumps with the back of the spoon. Stir in the pecan nuts.

On a lightly floured surface, roll out the dough into a thin rectangle. Brush with some of the melted butter and sprinkle evenly with the brown sugar mixture, leaving a 1cm border.

Starting at one end, roll up the dough tightly and place with the seam side down. Cut the roll into approximately 1½ cm sections and place in the prepared tin. Brush with the remaining melted butter.

Preheat air fryer to 180°C.

Bake rolls for 25-30 minutes or until slightly golden brown.

MAKES 8-10

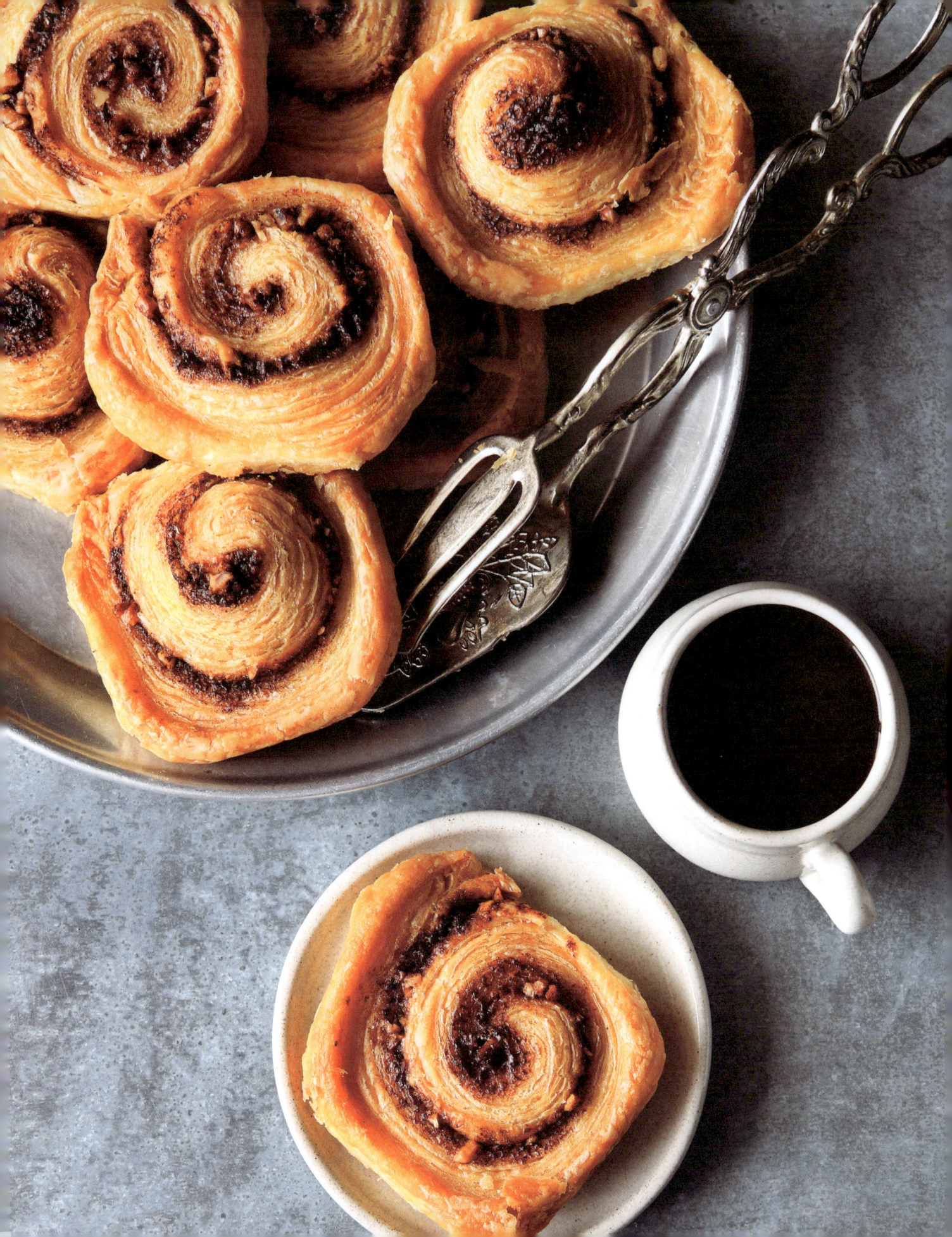

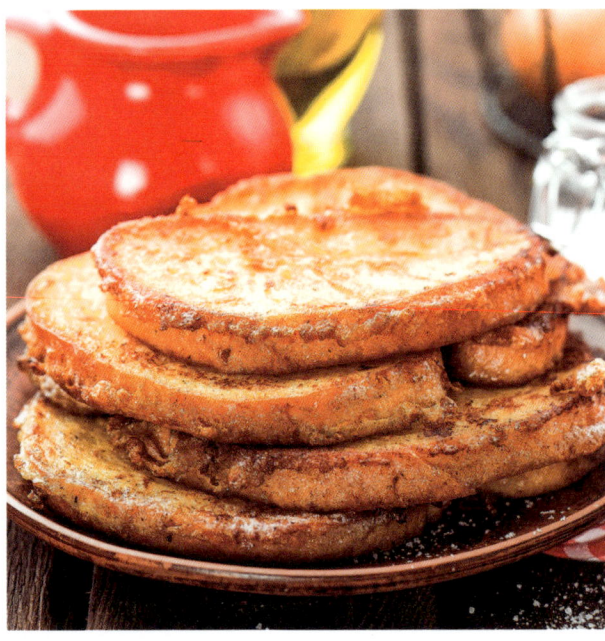

Easy French Toast

2 eggs

⅔ cup (160ml) milk

1 tsp vanilla essence (optional)

4 slices bread

Baking pan

Spray the baking pan with non-stick spray.

Combine the eggs, milk, and vanilla essence, if using, in a small bowl. Whisk together until well combined.

Dip a slice of bread into the mixture. Coat well, then shake to remove the excess. Place into the prepared pan.

Place into the air fryer and cook for 3 minutes at 175°C. Flip over and cook for a further 3 minutes.

Repeat with the remaining slices of bread.

SERVES 2

Spiced Toast Sticks

4 slices bread

2 tbsps butter, softened

2 eggs

Pinch of salt

2 tsps ground cinnamon

1 tsp ground nutmeg

½ tsp ground cloves

Icing sugar, to serve

Maple syrup, to serve

Baking pan

Preheat air fryer to 180°C and spray the baking pan with non-stick spray.

Butter both sides of the bread slices and cut into thick strips.

In a large mixing bowl, beat together the eggs, salt, cinnamon, nutmeg and cloves.

Dredge each strip in the egg mixture and arrange in a single layer in the pan. Cook in batches or use a double layer accessory with a second pan.

Cook for 2 minutes and then remove. Liberally spray the bread with cooking spray on both sides.

Return pan to the air fryer and cook for a further 4 minutes, checking a few times. Remove when nicely browned.

Sprinkle with icing sugar and serve with a small bowl of syrup for dipping.

SERVES 2

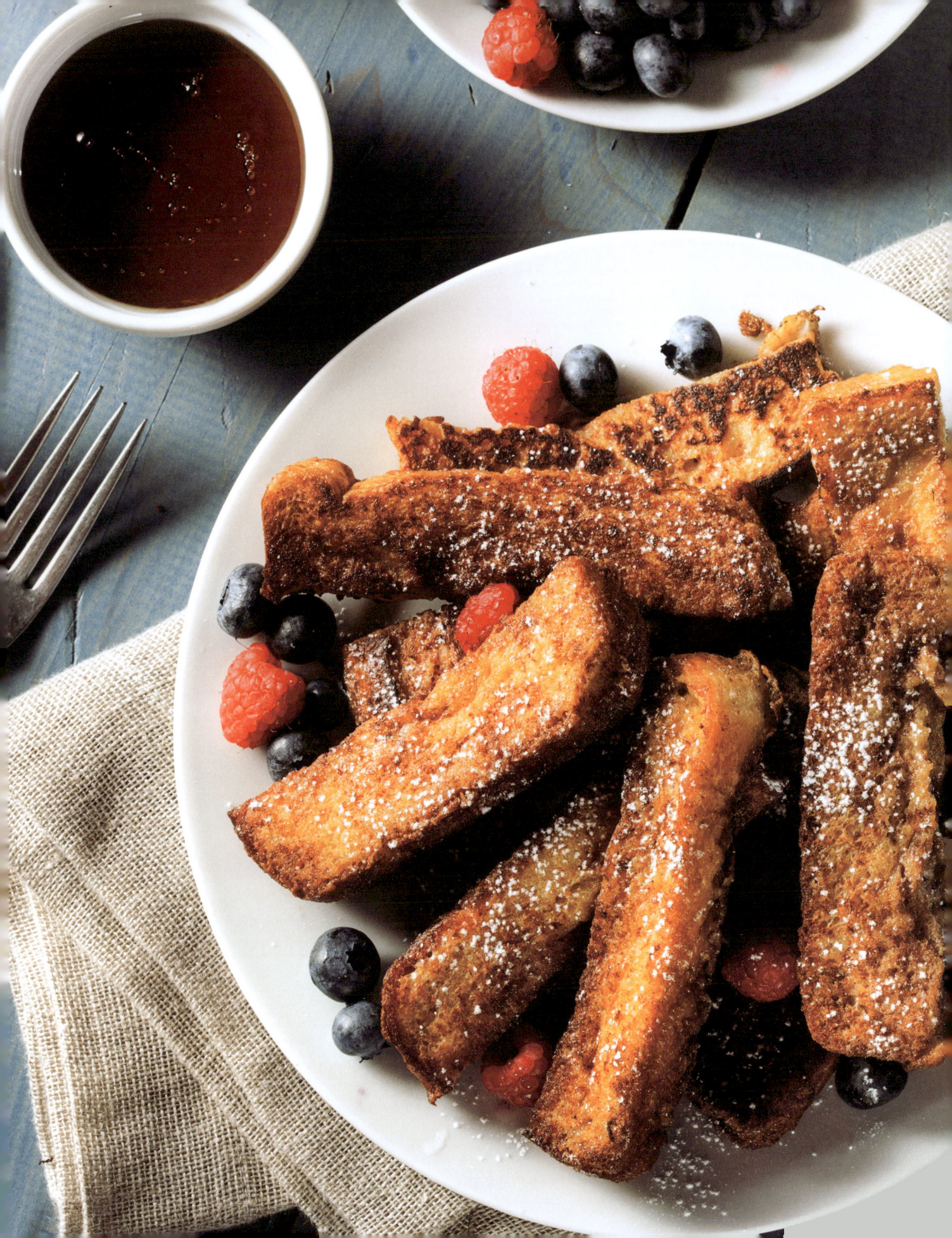

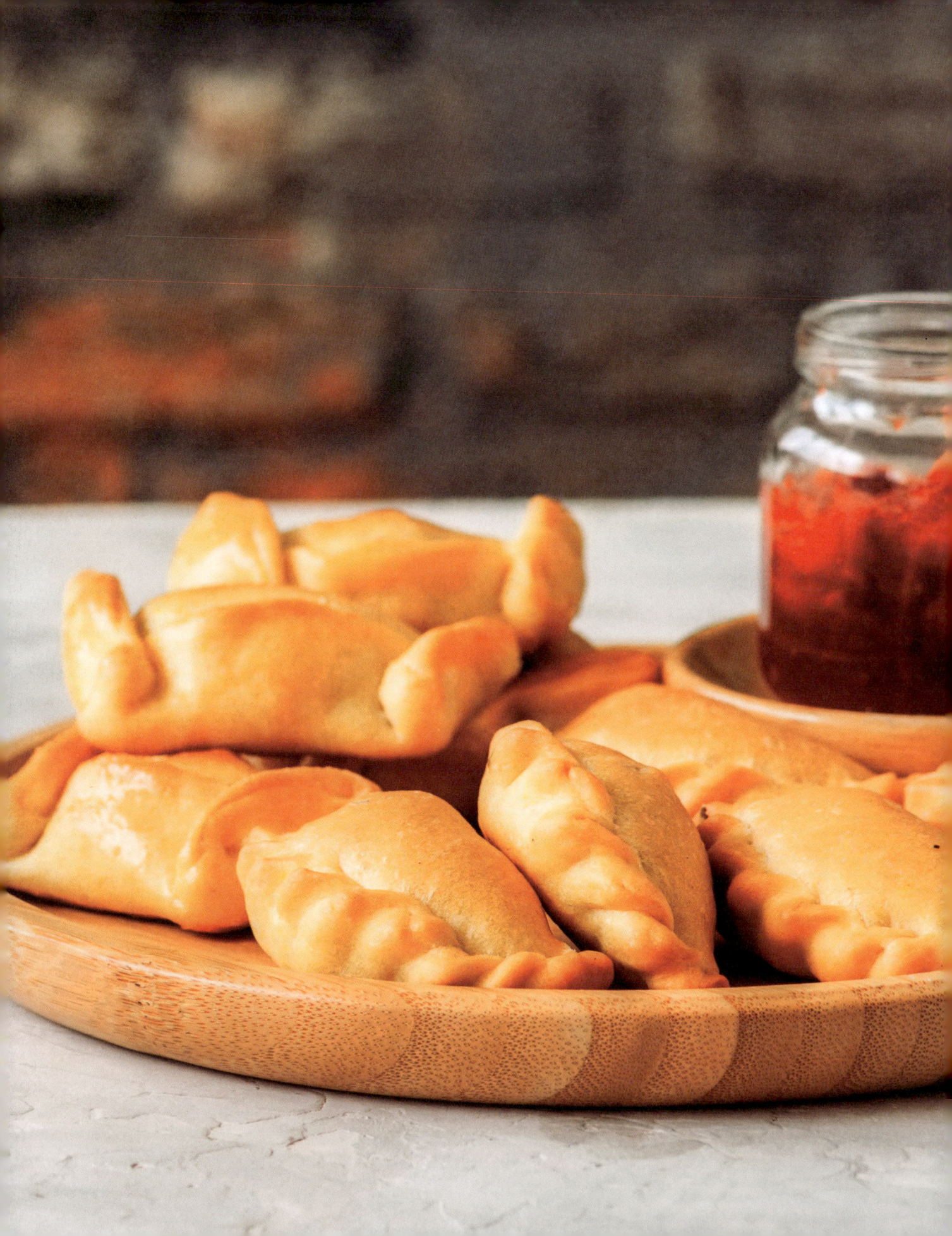

Ready-Made Food

French Fries

1kg frozen French fries

Salt, to taste

Preheat the air fryer to 200°C.

Place the frozen fries in the air fryer basket and spread evenly over the base.

Cook for 15 minutes, removing and shaking the basket a couple of times during cooking.

Continue to cook for a few extra minutes if needed to crisp up the fries.

Season with salt before serving.

SERVES 4

Cheese and Ham Croquettes

300g (8-pack) frozen cheese and ham potato croquettes

Preheat the air fryer to 180°C.

Place all the frozen potato croquettes in the air fryer basket.

Cook for 13 minutes, turning halfway.

SERVES 4

Sausage Rolls

500g (12 pieces) frozen party-size sausage rolls

Preheat the air fryer to 180°C.

Place all the frozen sausage rolls in the air fryer basket.

Cook for 13 minutes, turning halfway.

SERVES 4

Potato Gems

1kg frozen potato gems, potato royals or potato minis

Salt, to taste

Preheat the air fryer to 200°C.

Place the gems in the air fryer basket and spread evenly over the base.

Cook for 15 minutes, removing and shaking the basket a couple of times during cooking.

Continue to cook for a few extra minutes if needed to crisp up the gems.

Season with salt before serving.

SERVES 4

Note: Brands differ slightly but most take approximately 15 minutes to cook, resulting in a crispy golden outside and soft centre.

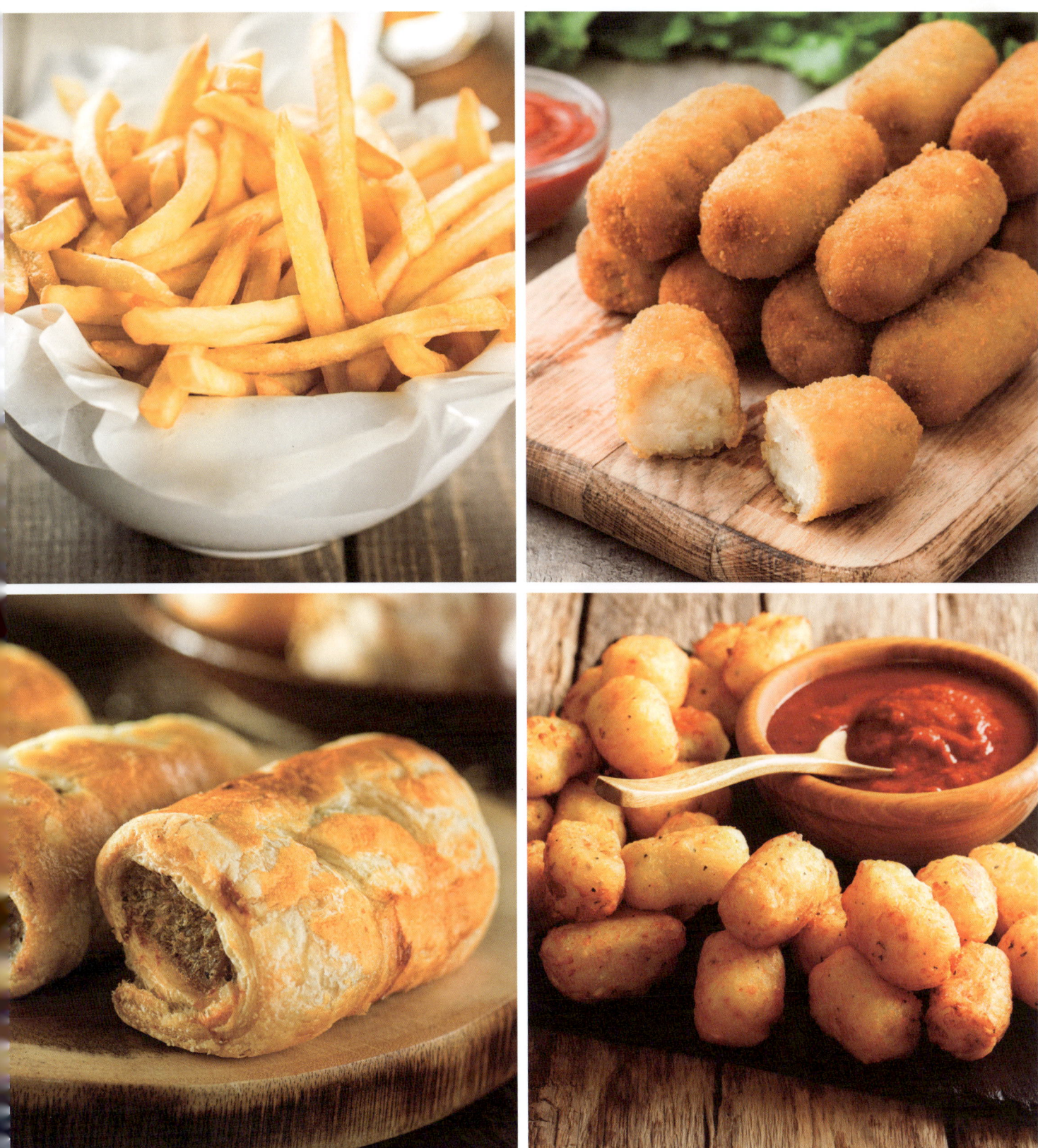

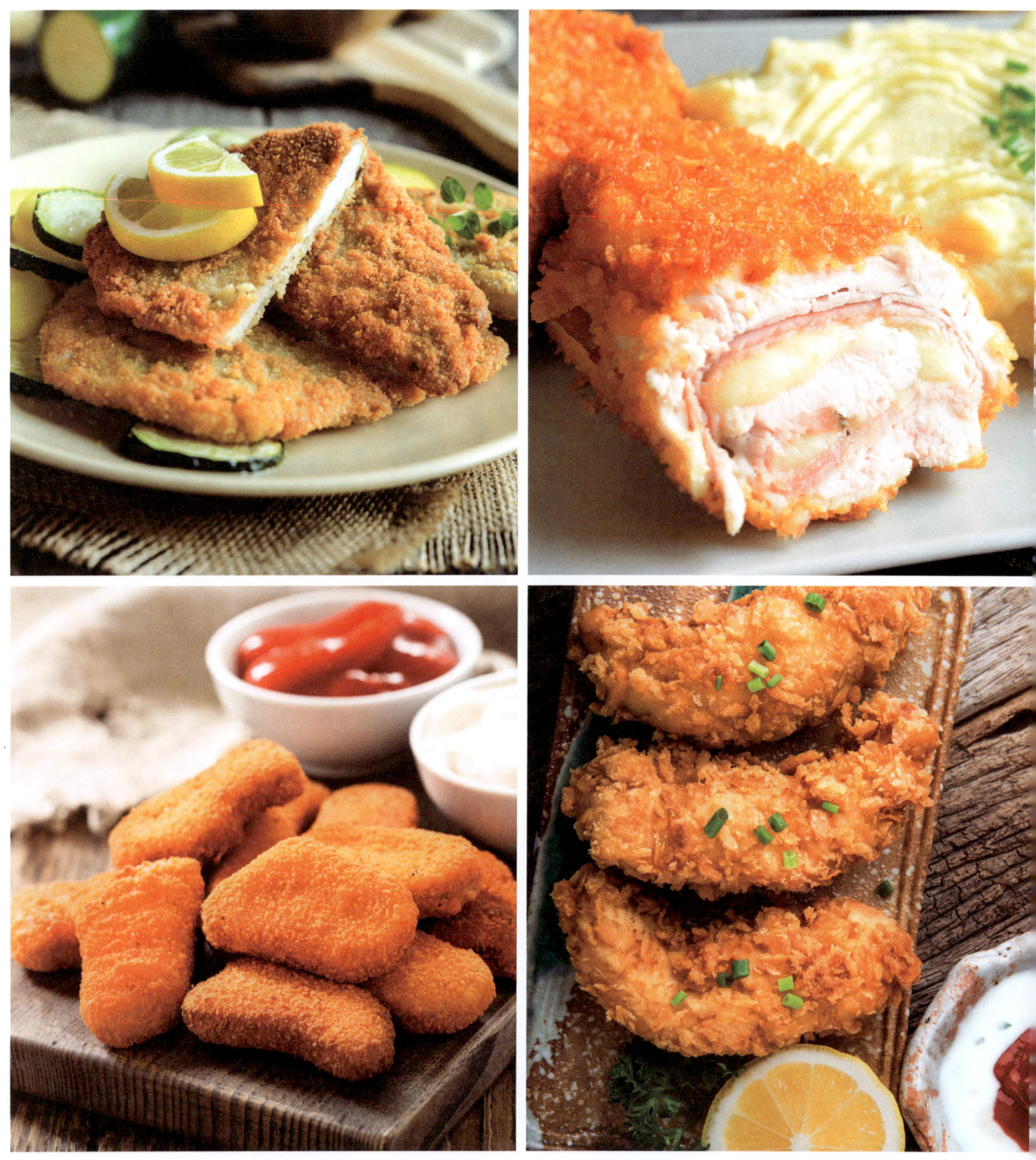

Chicken Schnitzel

400g frozen chicken schnitzel

Lemon slices, to serve

Preheat the air fryer to 200°C.

Place the chicken schnitzel in the air fryer basket and arrange evenly over the base.

Cook for 11 minutes, removing and shaking the basket halfway.

SERVES 2

Chicken Cordon Bleu

350g (2-pack) chicken cordon bleu or chicken Kiev

Preheat the air fryer to 180°C.

Place the chicken in the air fryer basket.

Cook for 20 minutes, turning halfway.

SERVES 2

Kids' Chicken Nuggets

400g frozen chicken breast nuggets

Preheat the air fryer to 200°C.

Place the nuggets in the air fryer basket and arrange evenly over the base.

Cook for 12 minutes.

Continue to cook for a few extra minutes if needed to crisp up.

SERVES 3-4

Chicken Tenders

400g frozen crumbed chicken tenders

Preheat the air fryer to 200°C.

Spritz the air fryer basket with cooking spray.

Place the tenders in the air fryer basket and arrange evenly over the base.

Cook for 12 minutes, turning halfway.

SERVES 2

Dagwood Dogs

8 dagwood dogs

Mustard, to serve

Tomato sauce, to serve

Preheat the air fryer to 200°C.

Place the hot dogs in the air fryer basket and cook for 5 minutes.

Serve with French fries, tomato sauce and mustard.

SERVES 4

Chicken Dinosaurs

400g frozen chicken breast dino snacks or nuggets

Preheat the air fryer to 200°C.

Place the chicken in the air fryer basket and arrange evenly over the base.

Cook for 11 minutes, removing and shaking the basket halfway.

SERVES 4

Onion Rings

500g frozen crumbed onion rings

Preheat the air fryer to 200°C.

Place the onion rings in the air fryer basket and cook for 8 minutes, removing the basket and flipping them over halfway through cooking.

Cook for an extra minute or two for a crispier result.

SERVES 4

Fish Fingers

12 frozen fish fingers

Preheat the air fryer to 200°C.

Place the fish fingers into the air fryer basket.

Cook for 8 minutes, removing and shaking the basket at least once during cooking.

If fish fingers are tightly packed in the basket, remove and shake the basket a few times during cooking to ensure they don't stick together.

SERVES 4

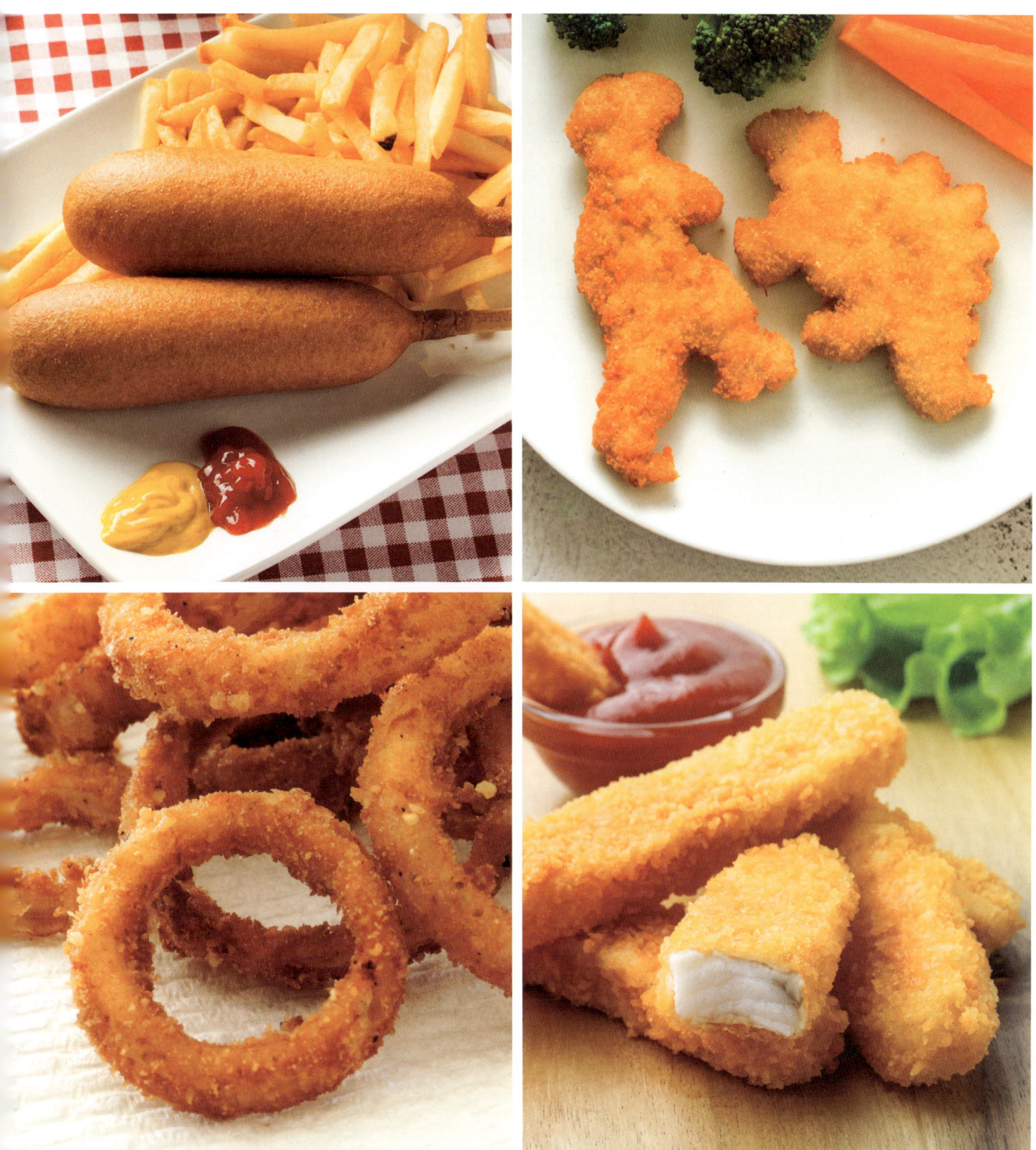

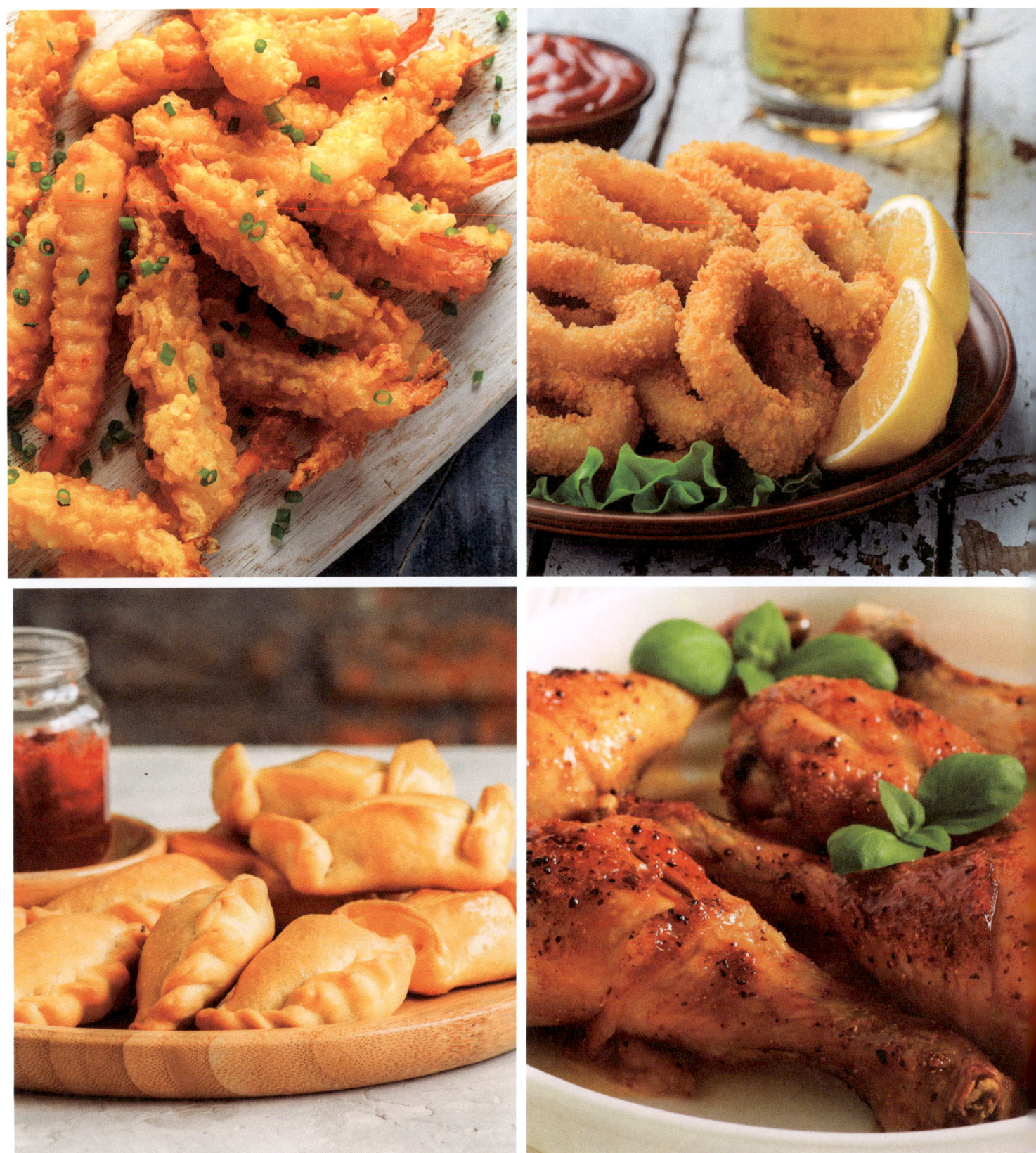

Prawn Cutlets

500g frozen crumbed prawns, prawn cutlets or tempura prawns

Preheat the air fryer to 200°C.

Place the frozen prawns into the air fryer basket.

Cook for 8 minutes, removing and shaking the basket at least once during cooking.

SERVES 4

Calamari Rings

360g frozen crumbed calamari rings or salt and pepper calamari rings

Preheat the air fryer to 200°C.

Place the calamari into the air fryer basket.

Cook for 9 minutes, removing and shaking the basket at least once during cooking.

SERVES 3

Sweet Potato and Cashew Empanadas

300g sweet potato and cashew empanadas (or try the Mexican chicken and cheese variety also available at Woolies)

Preheat the air fryer to 200°C.

Place the frozen empanadas into the air fryer basket.

Cook for 12 minutes, removing and flipping them over once during cooking.

SERVES 2

Note: If these flavours don't appeal it is easy to create your own by buying the frozen wrappers and stuffing them with the filling of your choice.

Chicken Tikka Drumsticks

8 chicken drumsticks

1 x 280g jar Tikka Masala Curry Paste Medium (such as Patak's)

Place the chicken drumsticks in a large bowl. Add the curry paste and stir to coat thoroughly and evenly. Cover with glad wrap and transfer to the fridge to marinate for 1 hour.

Preheat the air fryer to 180°C.

Remove the drumsticks from the fridge and shake off any excess marinade.

Transfer to the air fryer basket.

Cook for 30 minutes.

SERVES 4

Spring Rolls

1 egg

1kg frozen cocktail spring rolls

Grill pan

Preheat the air fryer to 160°C.

Whisk the egg in a small bowl.

Using a pastry brush, brush the tops of the frozen spring rolls with a little of the egg mixture until well coated. Place as many rolls as will comfortably fit into the grill pan.

Transfer the grill pan to the air fryer and cook for 8 minutes. Remove from the appliance and turn the rolls over using tongs. Brush the other side of the rolls with a little more egg mixture and then return to the air fryer for a further 8 minutes.

Repeat with the remaining rolls.

SERVES 10

Gyoza

10 frozen gyoza

Preheat the air fryer to 200°C.

Spritz air fryer basket with cooking spray.

Place the frozen gyoza in a single layer in the air fryer basket and lightly spray the tops with cooking spray.

Cook for 5 minutes.

Remove the basket and turn gyozas over, spray again with cooking spray and cook for another 5 minutes.

If using a double layer accessory, you should be able to cook in one batch. Otherwise, repeat the process.

SERVES 2

Cheese Balls

300g packet frozen cheese (or macaroni cheese) balls

Preheat the air fryer to 200°C.

Place the balls in the air fryer basket and spread evenly over the base.

Cook for 12 minutes, removing and shaking the basket halfway.

Continue to cook for a few extra minutes if needed to crisp up.

SERVES 4

Vegetable Samosas

10 frozen vegetable samosas

Preheat the air fryer to 190°C.

Lightly spray each frozen samosa with oil and place in the air fryer basket.

Cook for 20 minutes, removing the basket and shaking halfway. Cook a few minutes longer, if needed, until browned to your liking.

Using a double layer accessory, you should be able to cook in one batch. Otherwise, repeat the process.

SERVES 4

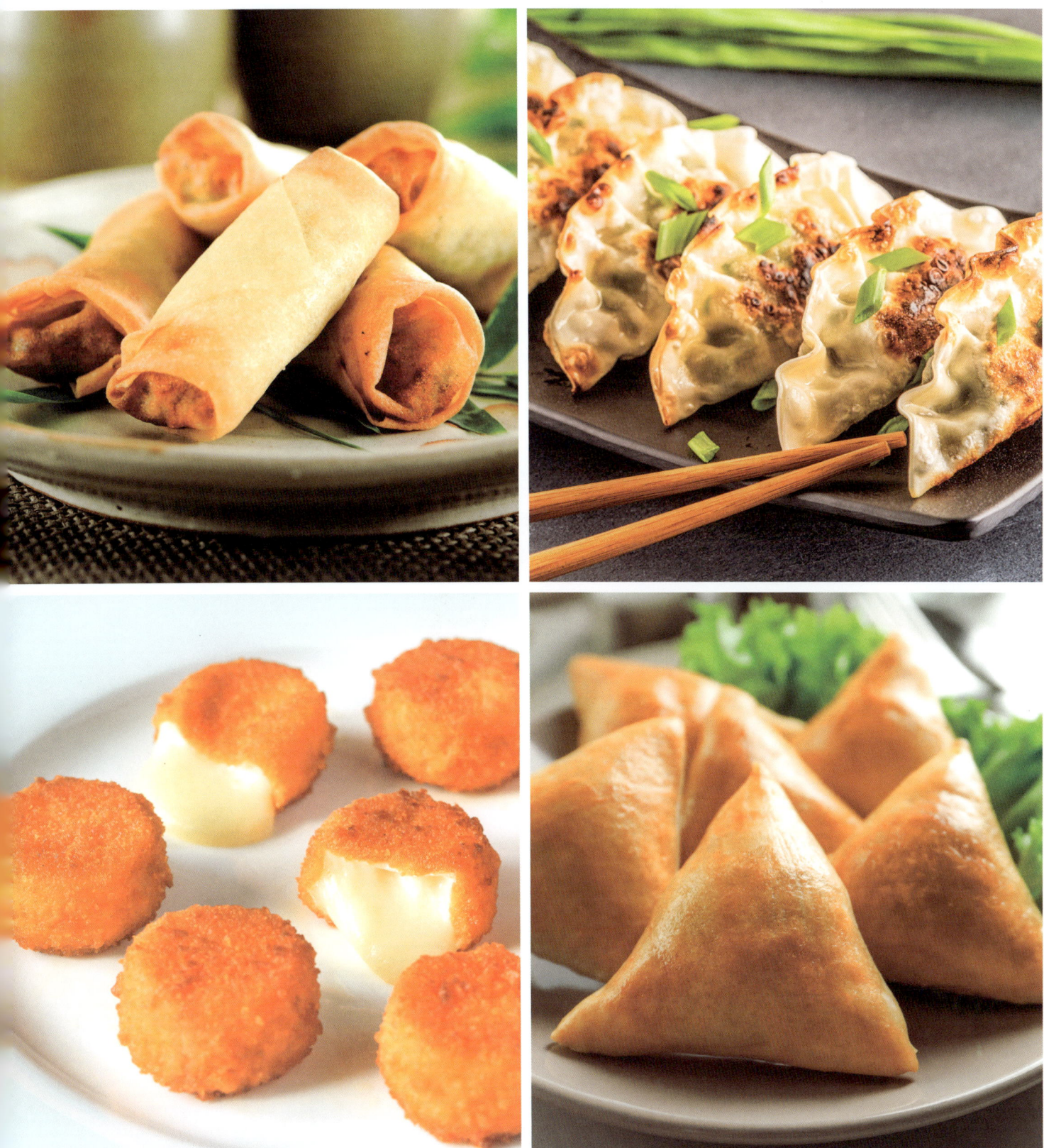

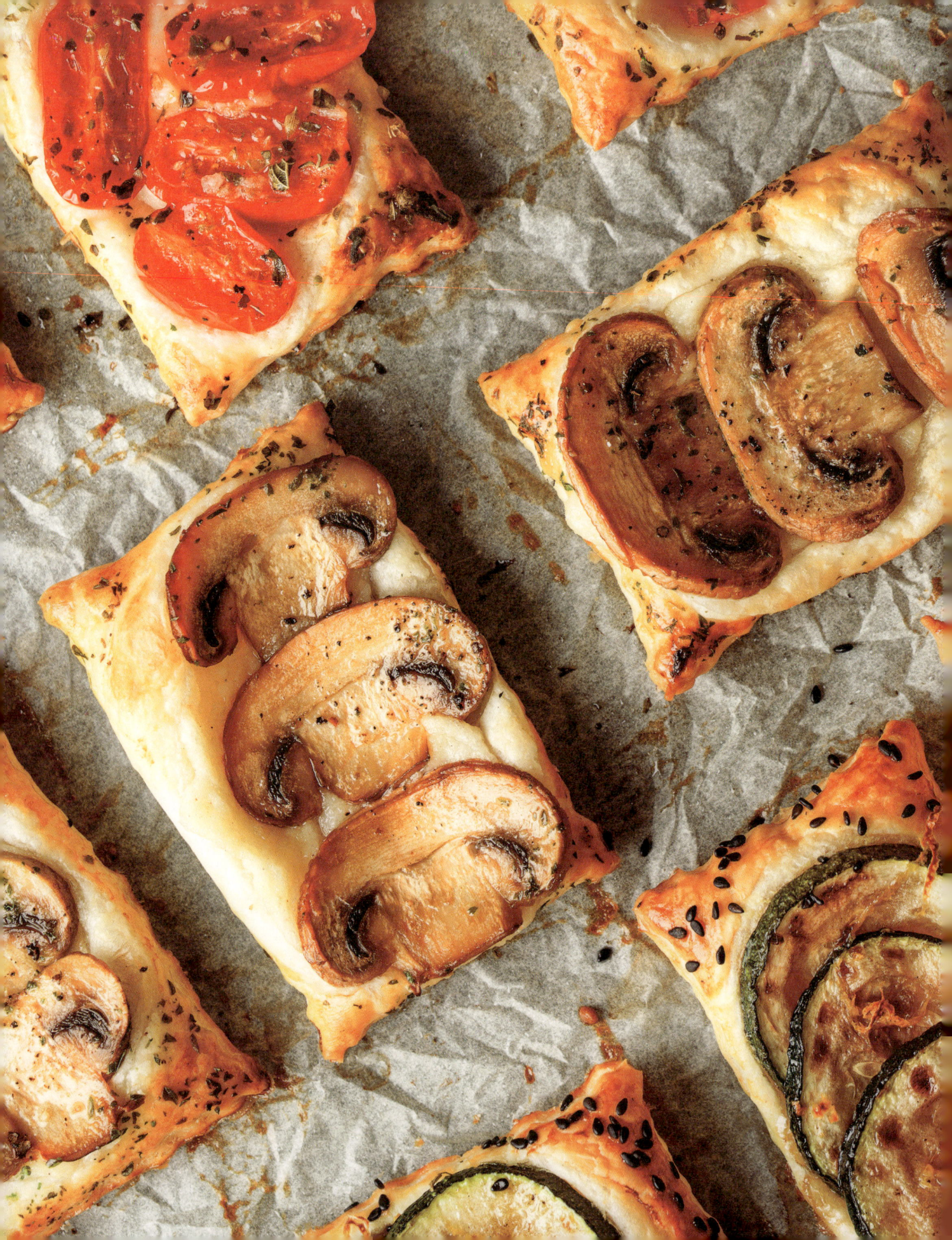

Snacks

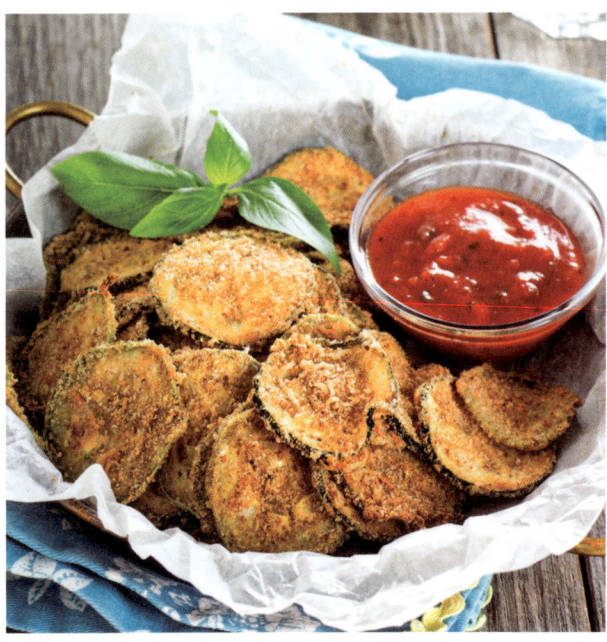

Crumbed Zucchini Chips

1 cup (125g) breadcrumbs

¾ cup (75g) Parmesan cheese, grated

Pinch of salt and pepper

1 egg

1 zucchini, thinly sliced

Skewer rack

Preheat the air fryer to 180°C.

Combine the breadcrumbs, cheese, salt and pepper on a plate.

Lightly whisk the egg in a bowl.

Dip a zucchini slice into the beaten egg and then into breadcrumb mixture, pressing to coat. Place the zucchini slice on a skewer.

Repeat with more zucchini slices until you have filled the rack with slices, without any overlapping. Lightly spray zucchini slices with cooking spray.

Cook for 10 minutes. Flip with tongs. Cook for a further 2 minutes. Remove from air fryer.

Repeat with remaining zucchini slices.

SERVES 2

Note: Use panko or rice crumbs instead of breadcrumbs for a gluten-free variation on this recipe.

Scotch Eggs

500g Devon roll

1 tbsp all-purpose seasoning

Salt and pepper, to taste

6 eggs, hard-boiled and shelled + 2 eggs, lightly beaten

⅓ cup (40g) flour

1 cup (125g) panko breadcrumbs

Place meat in a bowl. Add the seasoning, salt and pepper and mix (using clean hands) to combine.

Divide the meat into 6 even portions. Flatten each portion into a thin patty. Place a hard-boiled egg in the middle of each patty and wrap the meat around the egg, sealing all sides. Repeat with all 6 eggs and patties and set aside.

Preheat the air fryer to 200°C.

Place the flour into a small bowl and beaten eggs into another small bowl. Arrange the breadcrumbs on a plate. Make ready a clean plate.

Dip each egg patty into flour, then into beaten egg. Shake off the excess and then roll in breadcrumbs and place onto the clean plate.

Spray the basket of the air fryer with cooking spray and place crumbed egg patties into the basket.

Be careful not to overcrowd the basket. Cook in batches or use a double layer accessory if needed.

Cook for 12 minutes, removing the basket and turning eggs over halfway through. Repeat with remaining eggs, if necessary.

SERVES 3

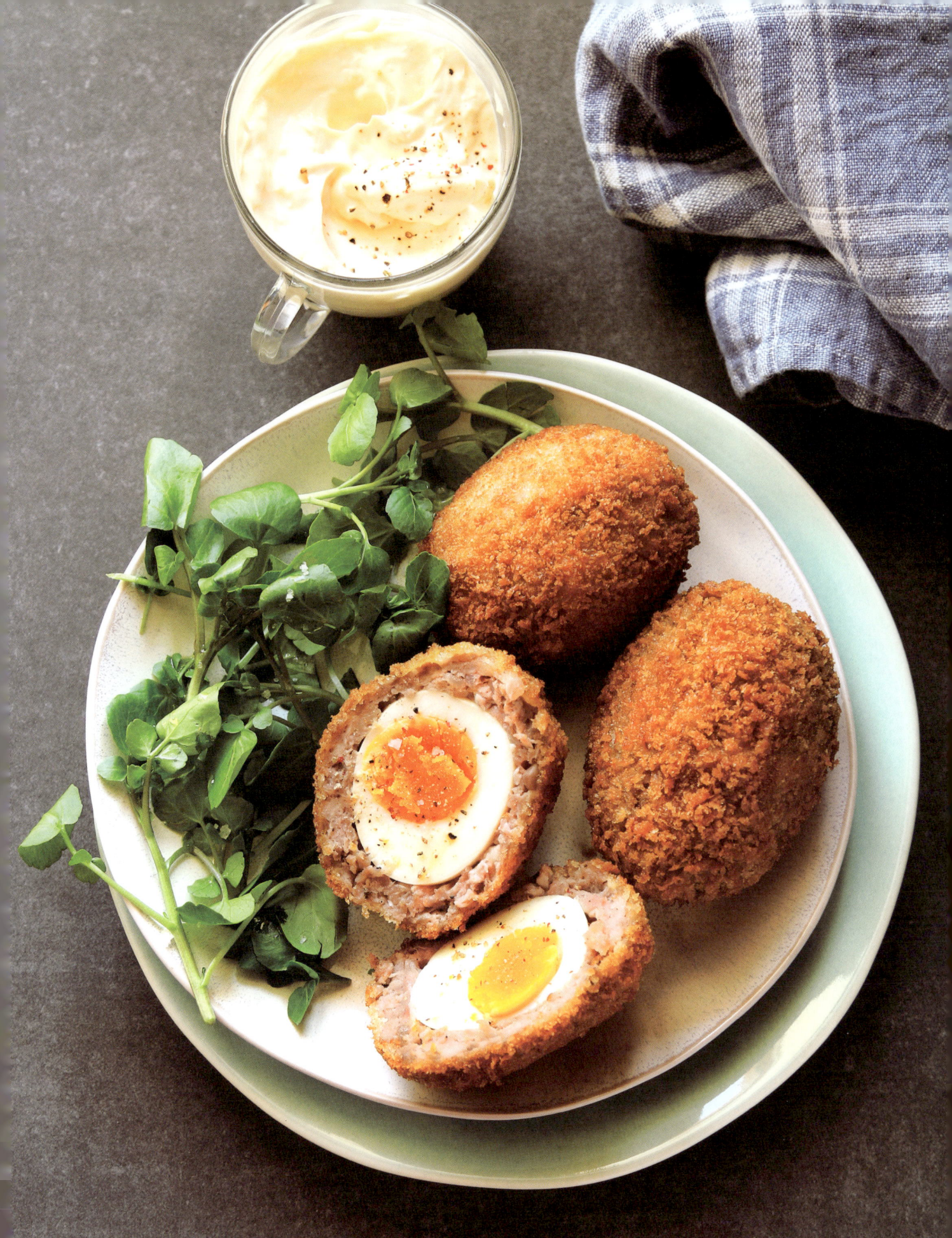

Grilled Cheese Sandwich

2 slices wholemeal bread

Butter, for spreading

4 slices tasty cheese

Preheat the air fryer to 180°C.

Butter the two slices of bread.

Place the cheese between the two unbuttered sides of the bread (the buttered sides should face out).

Place in the air fryer basket and cook for 5 minutes. Cook for another minute or two to crisp the bread up further, if desired.

SERVES 1

Cheesy Garlic Bread

1 small baguette

Butter, for spreading

1 tbsp minced garlic

1 cup (125g) mozzarella cheese, grated

Wire rack

Preheat the air fryer to 180°C.

Slice the baguette in half lengthwise, and cut in half so that the pieces fit into the air fryer.

Liberally butter both sides and then spread the minced garlic on top. Sprinkle with cheese.

Place the baguettes onto the wire rack and transfer to the air fryer.

Cook for 8 minutes until cheese is nicely browned.

SERVES 2

Cheese Cigars

1-2 filo pastry sheets

1 tbsp fresh herbs (such as parsley or thyme), chopped

60g butter, melted

125g soft goat's cheese

4 tsps honey

Cut the filo sheet to make four large rectangles. Brush the rectangles generously with butter, retaining 1 tablespoon to brush the tops.

Sprinkle some herbs along the long edge of each rectangle and fold the edge over them. Then crumble a line of goat's cheese along the same edge. Drizzle some honey over the cheese. Fold over the ends and then roll up to form a cigar shape. Repeat the process to make four cigars. Brush the tops with remaining melted butter.

Preheat the air fryer to 190°C.

Place the cheese cigars in the air fryer basket. Cook for 20 minutes, removing the basket and shaking halfway. Cook a few minutes longer, if needed, until browned to your liking.

SERVES 2

Toasted Sandwich

2 slices bread

Butter, for spreading

100g mozzarella cheese, sliced

2 slices tomato

¼ small red onion, finely sliced

Handful of baby spinach

Preheat the air fryer to 180°C.

Butter the two slices of bread. Place them on a work surface buttered-side down.

Add the cheese, tomato, onion and spinach onto one slice of bread and then close the sandwich with the remaining slice, buttered side out.

Place in the air fryer basket and cook for 5 minutes. Cook for another minute or two to crisp the bread up further, if desired.

SERVES 1

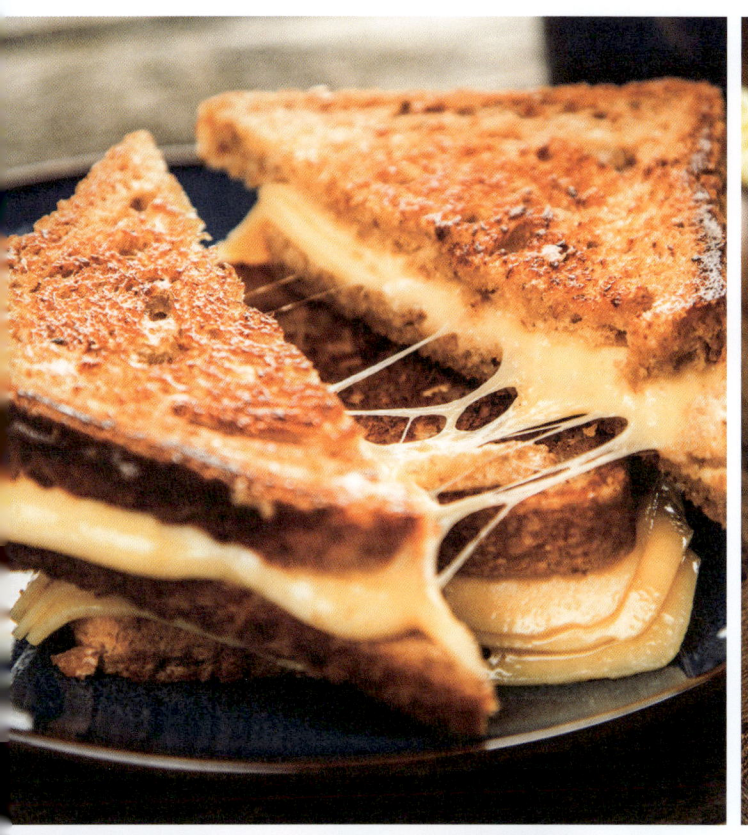

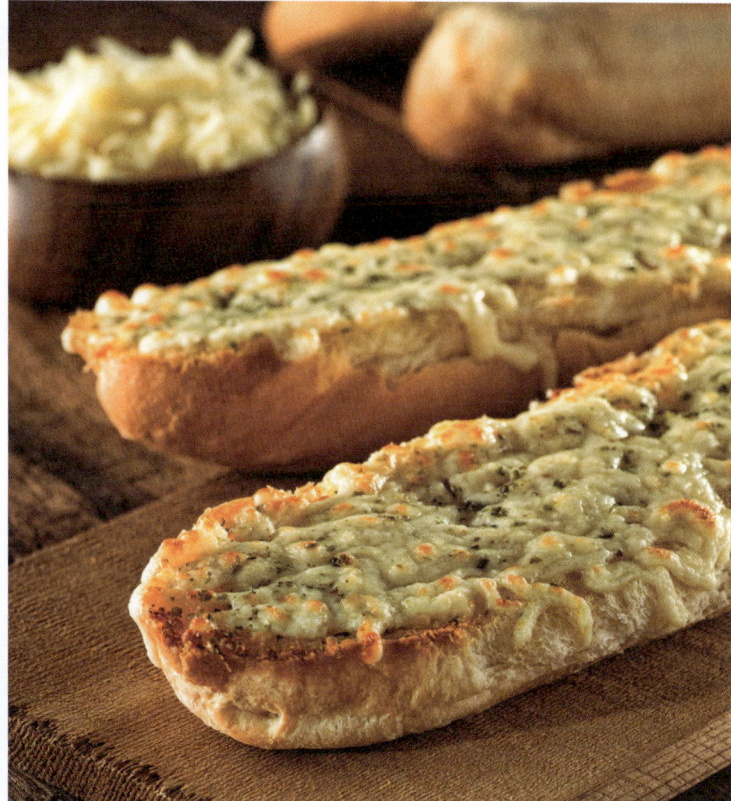

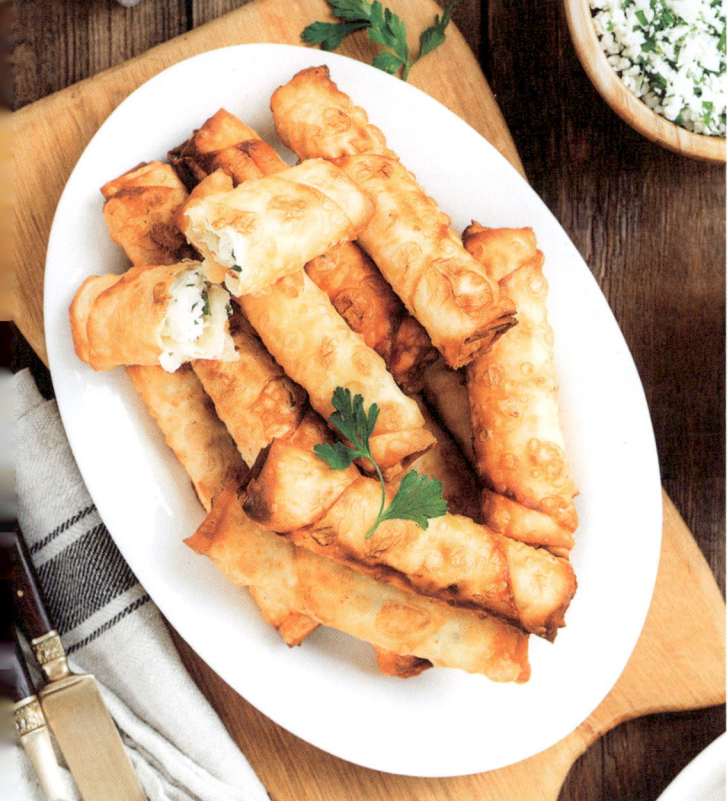

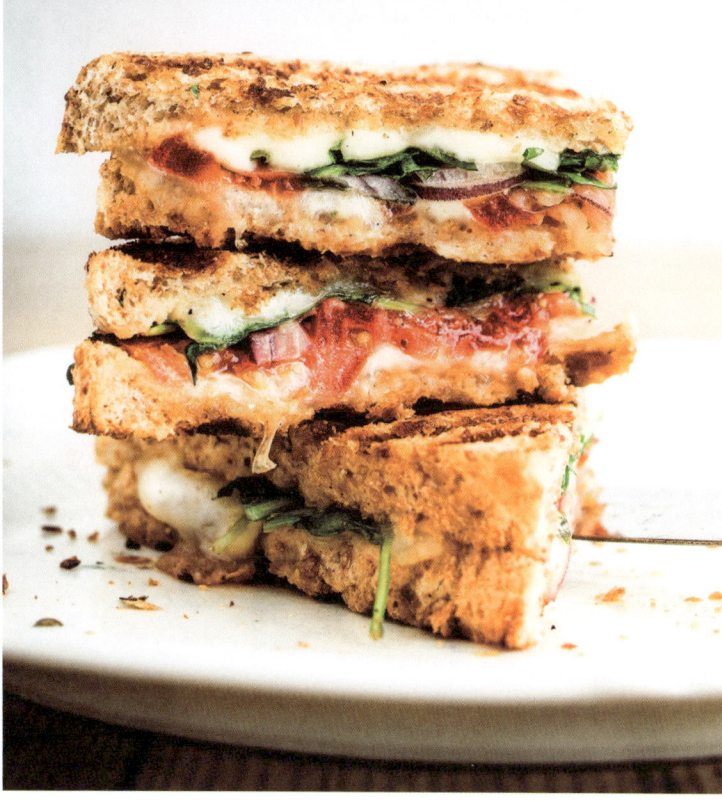

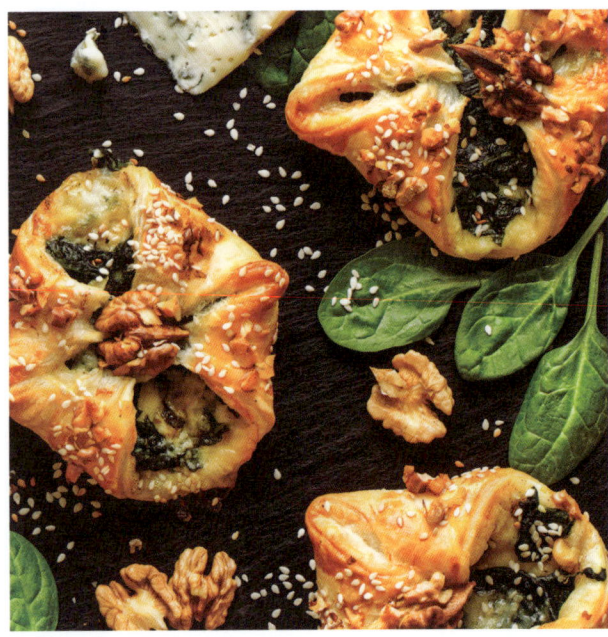

Spinach and Gorgonzola Puffs

500g baby spinach

195g gorgonzola, crumbled

⅔ cup (75g) Cheddar cheese, grated

1 egg, lightly beaten

¼ cup (30g) walnuts, chopped + 16 walnut halves

Salt and pepper, to taste

4 sheets frozen puff pastry, just thawed

2 tbsps sesame seeds

Bring a large pan of water to the boil. Add the spinach and cook for 30 seconds, until wilted.

Drain well to remove all the water. Transfer to a large bowl.

Add the gorgonzola, Cheddar, egg and chopped walnuts and roughly chop the mixture with a knife to combine. Season with salt and pepper.

Preheat the air fryer to 200°C.

Cut each pastry sheet into four squares. Place a tablespoon of the mixture onto each square. Fold the corners into the centre and seal with a walnut half. Sprinkle with sesame seeds.

Cook for 4 minutes (you may need to cook in batches or use a double layer accessory). Cook for a further minute or two, as needed, until golden brown.

MAKES 16

Salmon and Ricotta Puff Pastry Bites

¾ cup (200g) ricotta

100g smoked salmon

1 tbsp chives, finely chopped

4 sheets frozen puff pastry, just thawed

3 tbsps milk

2 tbsps sesame seeds

Preheat the air fryer to 200°C.

Combine the ricotta, smoked salmon and chives in a mixing bowl.

Cut each pastry sheet into four squares.

Place a heaped teaspoon of filling onto each square.

Fold the squares into triangles and moisten the edges with water. Press the edges firmly together using a fork.

Place four parcels in the basket and brush with half the milk. Sprinkle with half the sesame seeds.

Slide the basket into the air fryer and cook for 10 minutes, or until golden brown.

Repeat the process for the remaining parcels.

MAKES 16

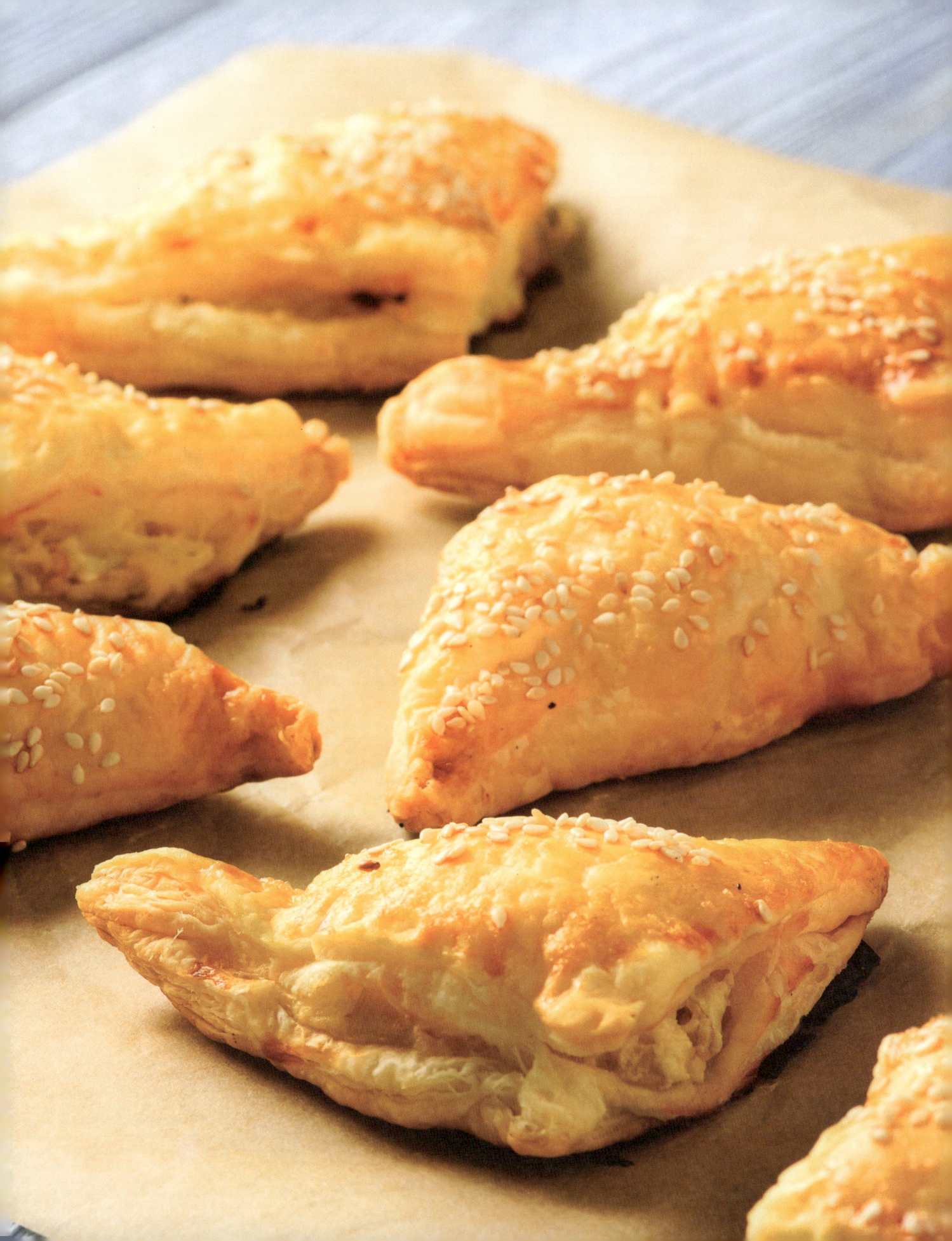

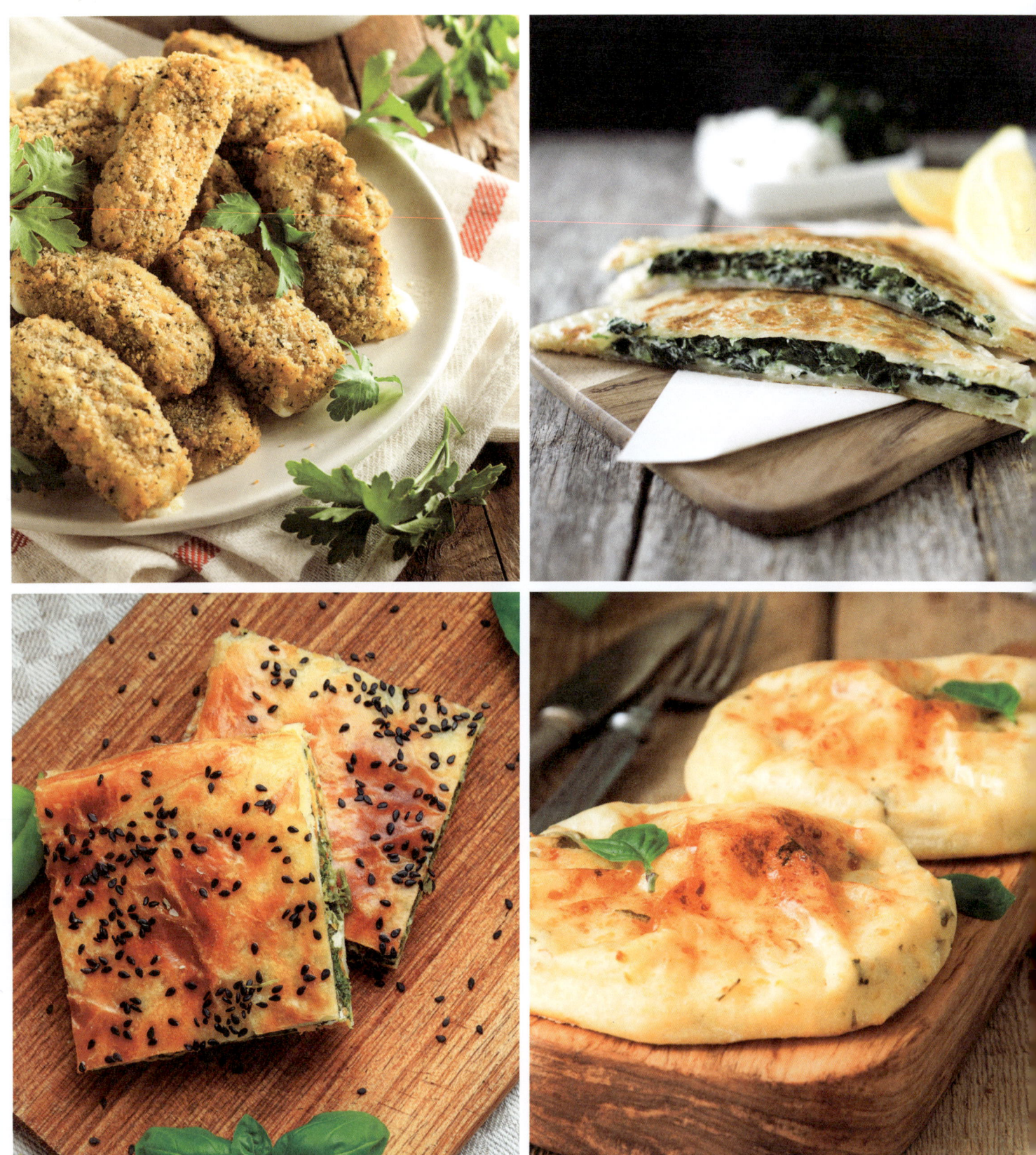

Mozzarella Sticks

500g mozzarella cheese block

¼ cup (30g) plain flour

1 cup (125g) breadcrumbs

3 tbsps milk

2 eggs

Cut cheese into sticks roughly 2cm wide and 1cm thick.

Place the flour in a small bowl. Place the breadcrumbs in another small bowl. In a third bowl, beat the milk together with the eggs.

Dip a cheese stick first in the flour, then the egg mixture and finally the breadcrumbs.

To avoid the cheese oozing out, place onto a baking tray and transfer to the freezer for 2 hours. (Skip this step if in a big hurry).

When ready to cook, preheat the air fryer to 200°C. Cook the cheese sticks in small batches for 12 minutes each or until golden, removing the basket and flipping halfway.

SERVES 4

Spinach and Mozzarella Toasted Tortilla

2 soft tortillas (large)

175g frozen spinach, thawed

Pinch of nutmeg (optional)

Pinch of salt

1 cup (125g) mozzarella cheese, grated

Lightly spray one side of the tortillas with oil and place oil-side down on a plate.

Place the spinach, nutmeg, salt and cheese in a bowl and stir to combine.

Scrape the filling into the centre of one tortilla and spread almost to the edges with a knife. Place the second tortilla on top with the oiled side facing up.

Use a shape knife to cut into four segments.

Transfer to the basket of the air fryer in an even layer (you may need to cook in two batches).

Cook for 7 minutes until golden and cheese has melted.

SERVES 1

Spinach Pie

1 egg yolk + 1 egg

100g feta

2 tbsps parsley, finely chopped

300g frozen spinach, thawed

1 spring onion, finely sliced

Pinch of pepper

2 sheets frozen filo pastry, thawed

1 tbsp black sesame seeds (optional)

Baking pan or roasting tin, lightly sprayed

Beat the egg yolk in a bowl and then mix in the feta, parsley, spinach and spring onion. Season with pepper.

Fold one sheet of filo in 4, spraying with oil at each fold. Place in the pan. Scoop the feta mixture on top. Repeat with the second sheet of pastry and place it on top.

Preheat the air fryer to 200°C.

Beat the egg in a small bowl. Brush the pastry with egg and sprinkle with black sesame seeds, if using, and slide the basket into the air fryer. Cook for 6 minutes.

SERVES 2

Cottage Cheese Potato Cakes

8 potatoes, peeled and chopped

2 tbsps milk

1 tbsp chives

Pinch of pepper

¼ cup (50g) cottage cheese

Cook the potatoes in a large saucepan of salted water. When soft, drain and transfer to a large bowl. Add the milk, chives and pepper and mash well. Add the cottage cheese and stir gently to combine.

Place the mashed potato mixture in the freezer to chill for 20 minutes.

Remove from the freezer and shape into patties.

Preheat the air fryer to 180°C and lightly spritz the air fryer basket with cooking spray. Transfer the potato cakes into the air fryer, being careful not to crowd them. You may need to cook in batches. Lightly spray the tops.

Cook for 12 minutes.

SERVES 2

Note: If you have leftover mashed potatoes in the fridge this is a great recipe for using them up.

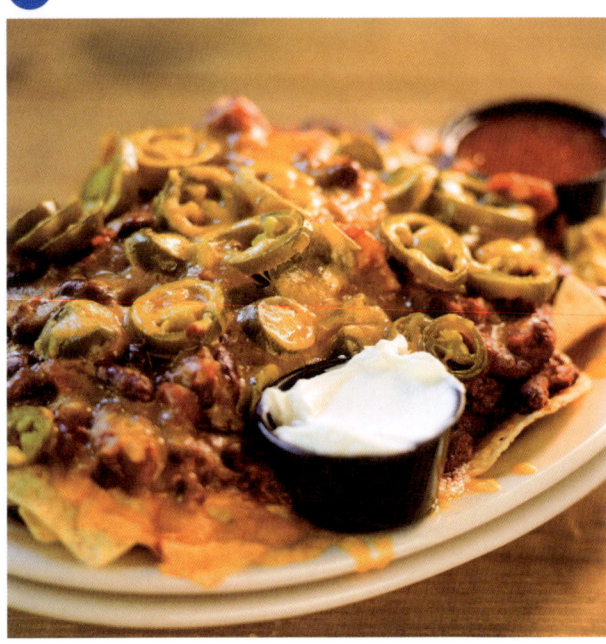

Nachos

230g tortilla chips

285g canned red kidney beans, drained and rinsed

200g jalapenos, sliced

2 cups (250g) Colby cheese, grated

Tomato salsa and sour cream, to serve

Line the basket of the air fryer with foil and lightly spritz with cooking spray.

Place the chips in first and then add beans, gherkins and cheese on top.

Cook at 180°C for 5 minutes until the cheese has melted. Serve with tomato salsa and sour cream.

SERVES 2

Note: Add your preferred ingredients such as cherry tomatoes, black beans, gherkins or spring onion.

Homemade Crispy Spring Rolls

125g cooked chicken breast, roughly shredded

1 stalk celery, sliced into strips

1 small carrot, sliced into strips

2 button mushrooms, finely diced

1 tsp ginger, finely chopped

1 tsp sugar

1 tsp chicken stock powder

1 egg

1 tsp cornflour

8 spring roll wrappers

Place the shredded chicken, celery, carrot and mushrooms into a bowl and mix together. Add the ginger, sugar and chicken stock powder and stir to combine.

In a separate bowl, whisk the egg, then add the cornflour and stir to create a paste. Set aside.

Place a spring roll wrapper on a non-stick or floured surface. Spoon on an eighth of the mixture in a line. Fold over the ends and roll up. Seal the edge with the egg paste. Brush or spray with a little oil. Repeat with the remaining ingredients.

Preheat the air fryer to 200°C.

Place the rolls into the air fryer basket and cook for 15 minutes, removing the basket and turning once or twice during cooking.

MAKES 8

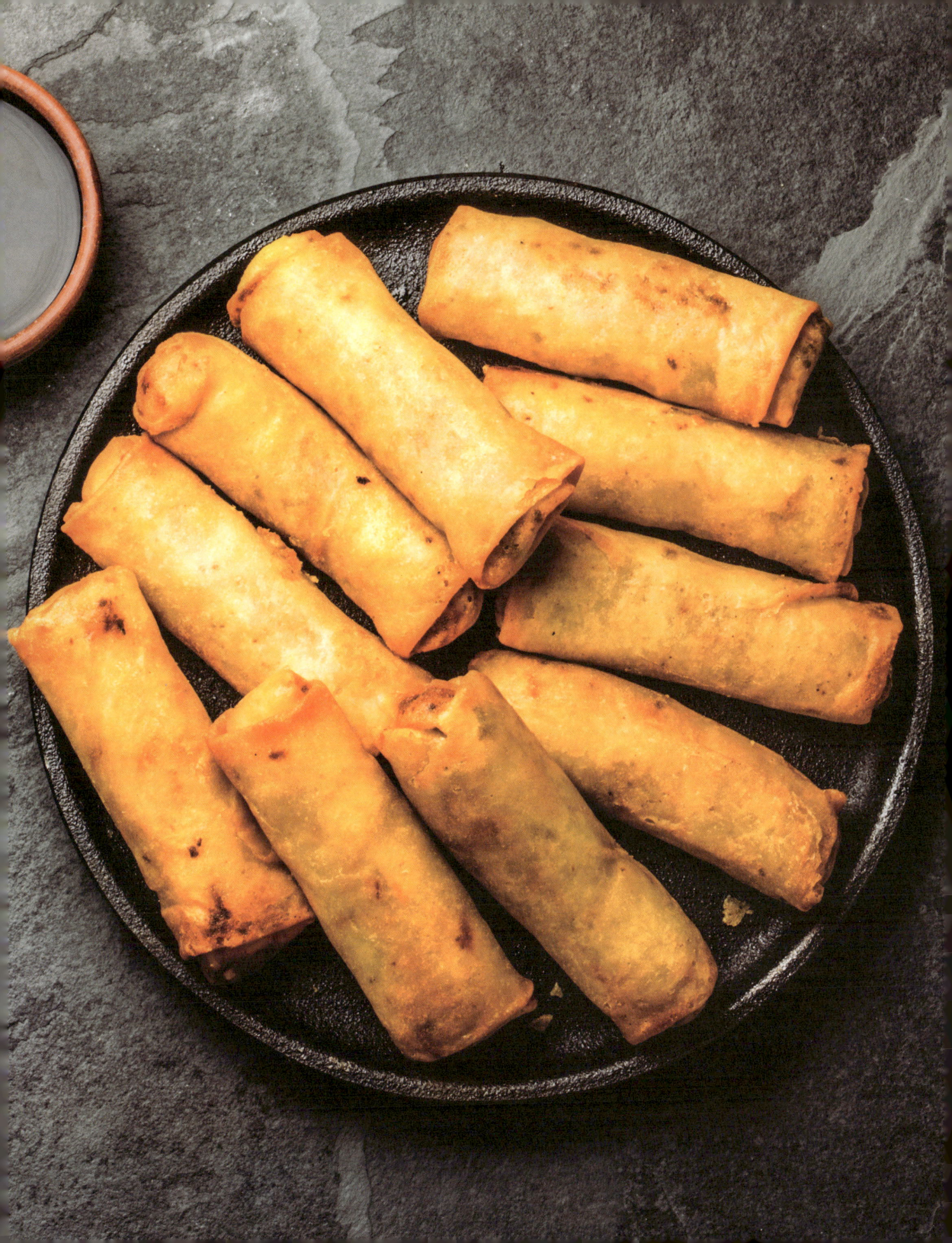

Mushroom Slices

1 sheet frozen puff pastry, just thawed

¾ cup (90g) Cheddar cheese, grated

2 button mushrooms, sliced

1 tsp dried mixed herbs

Pinch of pepper

Place pastry sheet on a floured surface and cut into four squares. Preheat the air fryer to 190°C.

Place two squares in the air fryer basket, ensuring they don't touch. Cook for 8 minutes, until pastry is golden brown.

Open basket and, using a spoon, press down the centre of each square to make an indentation. Sprinkle 2 tablespoons of cheese into it and then layer with mushroom slices. Sprinkle with mixed herbs and pepper.

Brush the edges of the pastry with melted butter.

Cook for a further 5 minutes.

Repeat with the remaining pastry squares and fillings.

SERVES 2

Homemade Sausage Rolls

½ tbsp olive oil

1 tbsp garlic, minced

1 small stalk celery, grated

1 small carrot, peeled and grated

250g pork mince (not lean)

¼ cup (30g) breadcrumbs

1 small egg + 1 egg, beaten

Pinch of salt and pepper

1½ sheets puff pastry, thawed

2 tbsps sesame seeds

Place all ingredients except for the pastry, beaten egg and sesame seeds in a bowl and mix together well.

Cut the whole pastry sheet in half. Place filling in a log shape down the side of each pastry piece. Brush edges of pastry with beaten egg. Roll up, pressing edges together. Brush top with egg and sprinkle with sesame seeds. Cut into four. Cook for 20 minutes at 160°C. Increase temperature to 200°C and cook for a further 5 minutes.

MAKES 12

Bacon-Wrapped Meatballs

500g chicken mince

1 egg

½ cup (60g) breadcrumbs

½ cup (50g) Romano (or Parmesan) cheese, grated

80g Cheddar cheese, cut into 12 cubes

6 rashers bacon, cut in half lengthways

Place the chicken mince, egg, breadcrumbs and Romano cheese into a mixing bowl and stir until well combined.

Using clean hands, shape into 10-12 small balls. Press a cheese cube into the centre of each and re-form the meatball around it.

Wrap a strip of bacon around each meatball.

Preheat the air fryer to 180°C.

Place the meatballs in a single layer in the air fryer basket.

Cook for 15 minutes.

SERVES 4

Cottage Cheese Pancakes

2 eggs

1 cup (200g) cottage cheese

½ tsp vanilla extract

1 tbsp honey

Pinch of salt

½ cup (60g) plain flour

½ tsp baking powder

Baking pan, greased

Place the eggs in a mixing bowl and whisk until combined. Add the cottage cheese, vanilla, honey and salt and stir to combine.

Mix together the flour and baking powder in a separate bowl. Pour the wet ingredients into the flour mixture and stir until just combined.

Preheat the air fryer to 180°C. Scrape a portion of batter (approximately 2 heaped tablespoons) into the pan. Cook for 7 minutes until golden. Repeat until mixture has been used up.

SERVES 2

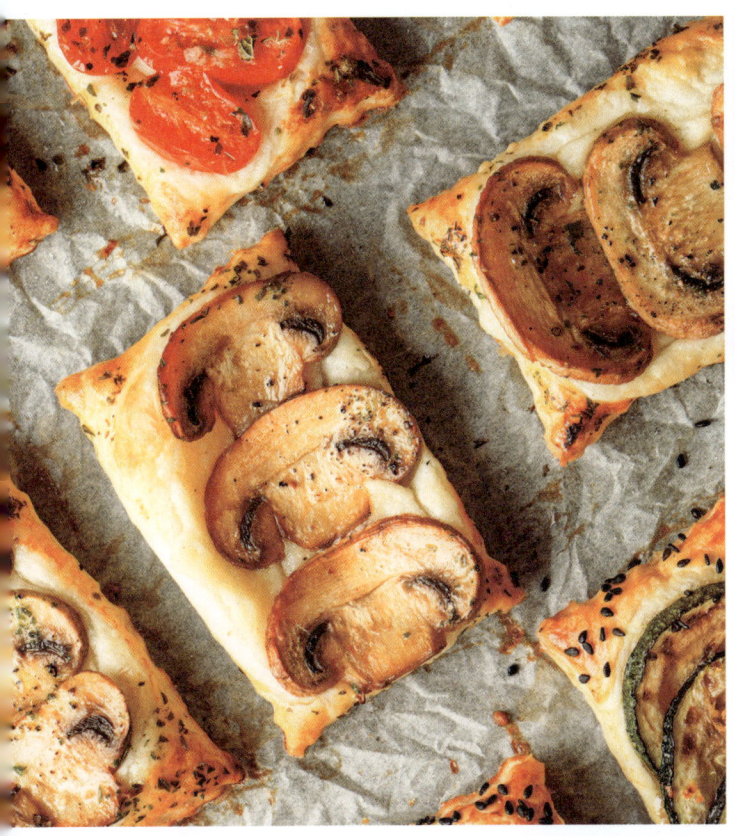

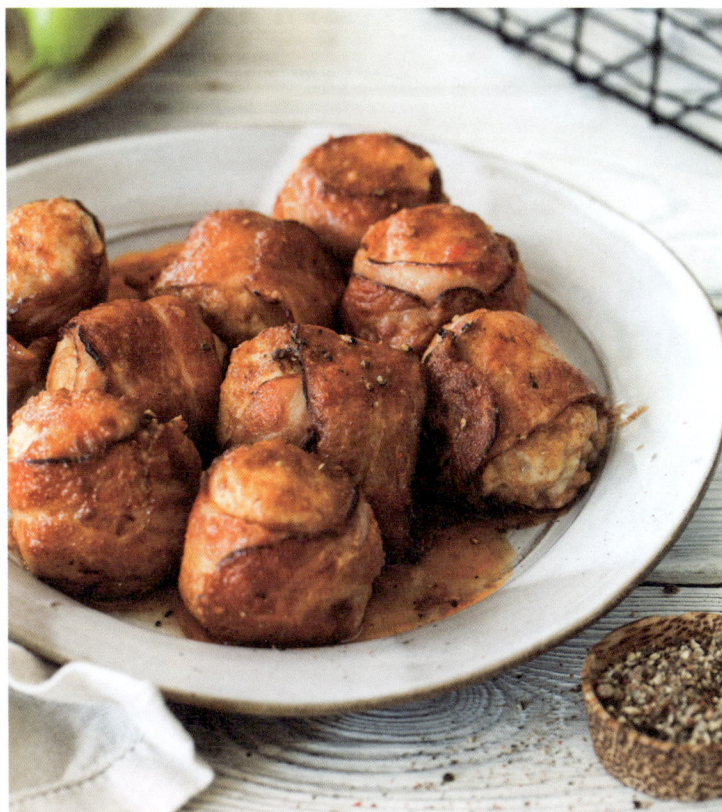

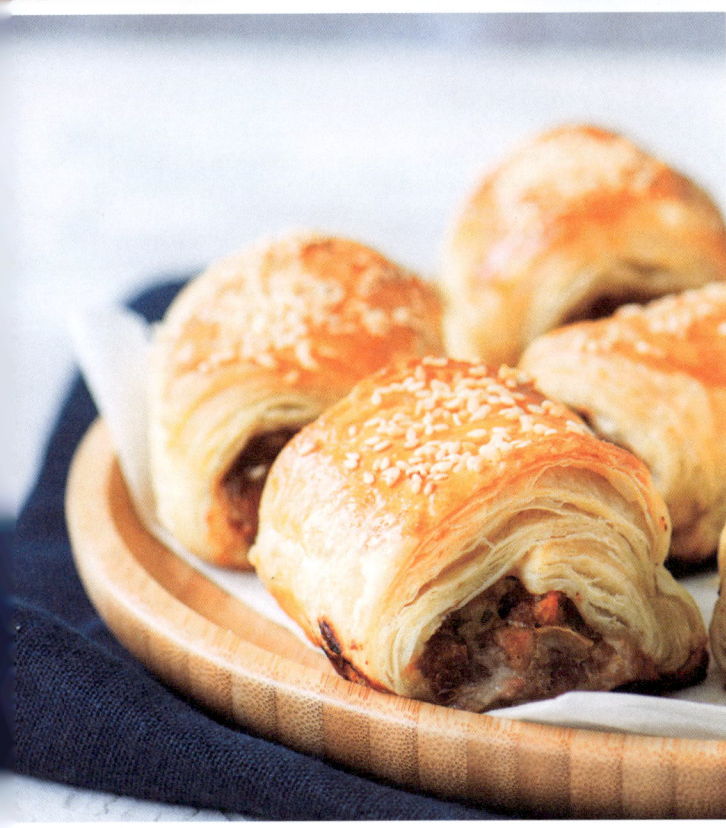

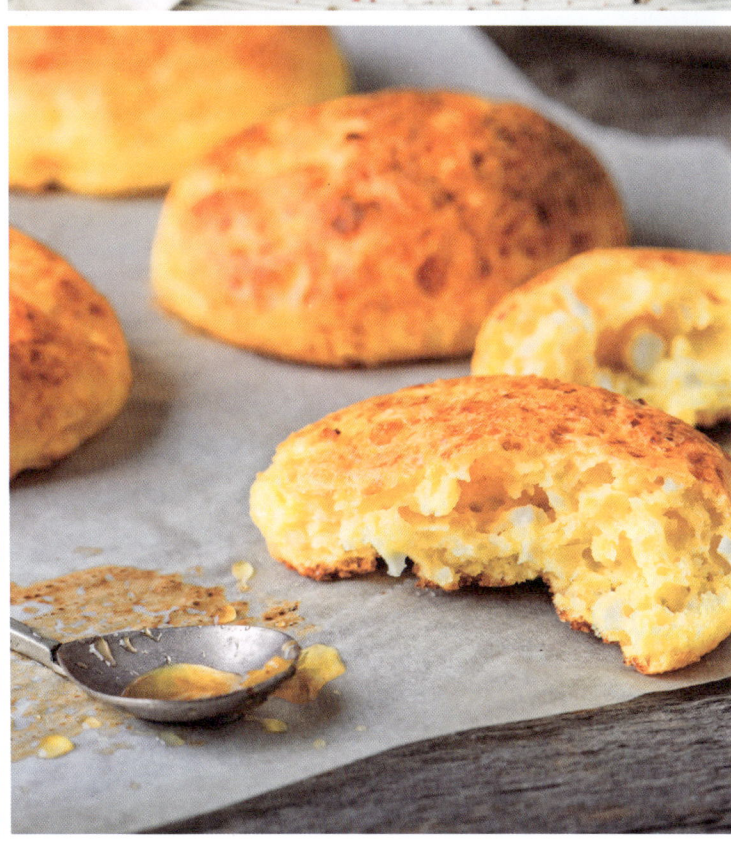

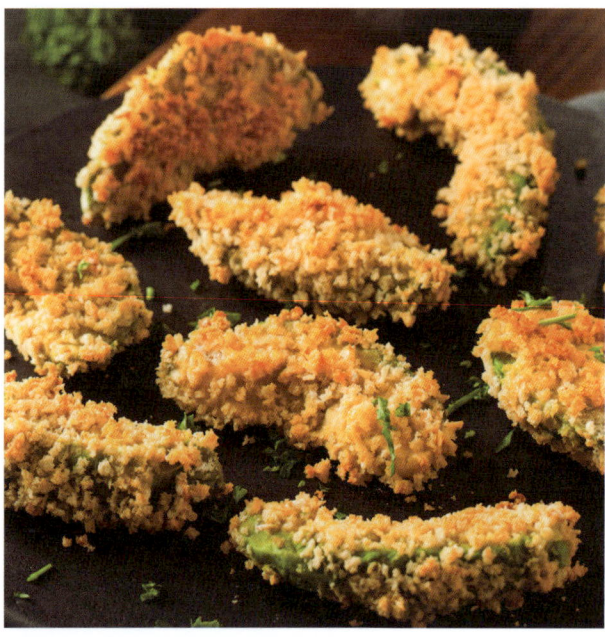

Avocado Fries

¼ cup (30g) plain flour

½ tsp pepper

¼ tsp salt

1 egg

1 tsp water

½ cup (60g) panko breadcrumbs or rice crumbs

1 ripe avocado, halved, seeded, peeled and cut into 8 slices

Preheat air fryer to 200°C.

Combine the flour, pepper and salt together in a bowl. Beat together egg and water in a second bowl. Place panko in a third bowl.

Dredge an avocado slice through the flour, shaking off any excess. Then dip it into the egg and let excess drop off. Next dip it into the panko, ensuring both sides are covered. Set on a clean plate and repeat with the remaining slices.

Spray coated avocado slices with cooking spray and arrange in the air fryer, sprayed-side down. Spray the top side of the avocado slices.

Cook for 8 minutes, removing the basket and turning the slices over halfway through cooking.

SERVES 1-2

Sweet Potato Gems

2 whole sweet potatoes, peeled

½ tsp Cajun seasoning

1 tsp salt

Bring a pot of salted water to a boil and add the sweet potatoes. Boil for 15 minutes until cooked but still firm enough to grate. Drain and set aside to cool.

Grate sweet potatoes into a bowl using a box grater. Mix in the Cajun seasoning.

Using clean hands, form mixture into gem-shapes.

Preheat the air fryer to 200°C.

Lightly spray the air fryer basket. Place gems in the basket in a single layer ensuring that they do not touch each other or the sides of the basket. (You may need to cook in batches or use a double layer accessory.) Spray with olive oil spray and sprinkle with salt.

Cook for 15 minutes. Halfway through cooking, remove the basket and shake the gems to rotate. Spray again with olive oil.

Repeat, if cooking in batches.

SERVES 3

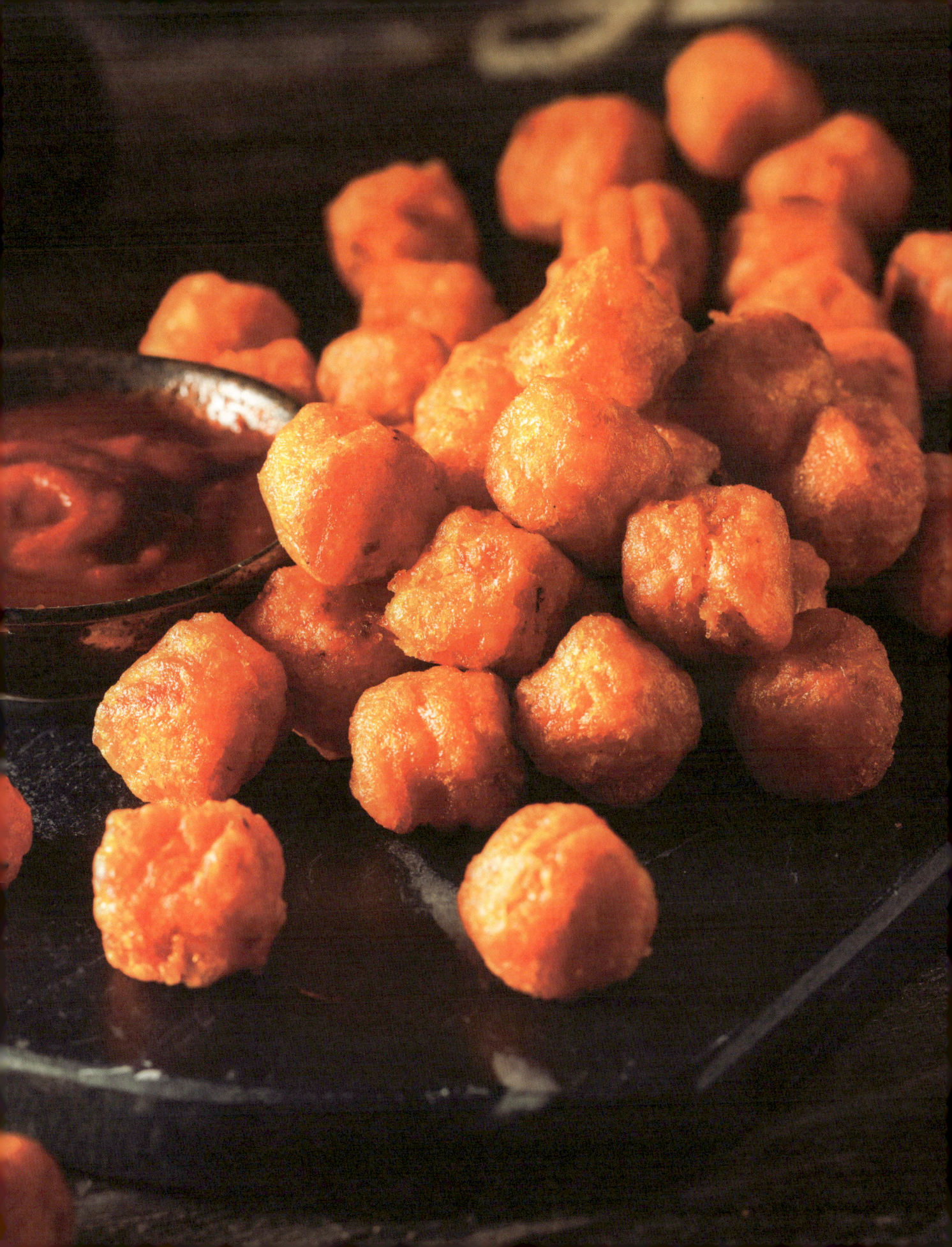

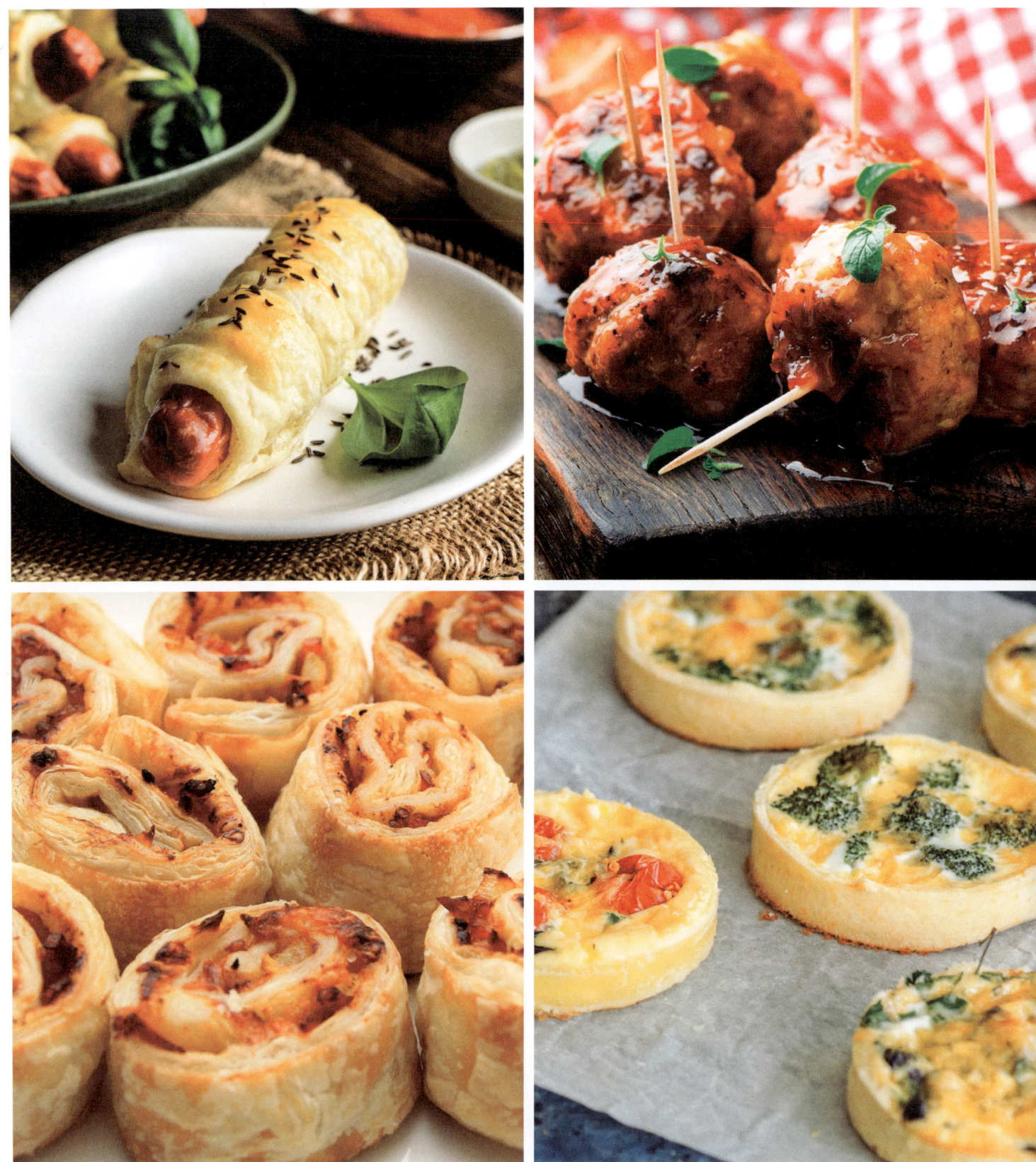

Pigs in Blankets

12 cocktail frankfurts

3 sheets frozen puff pastry, thawed

1 tbsp mustard

1 tbsp fennel seeds, to serve (optional)

Preheat the air fryer to 200°C.

Using paper towel, thoroughly dry the cocktail franks.

Lay a pastry sheet on a floured surface and cut into rectangular strips wide enough to hold the franks.

Coat the strips with a thin layer of mustard.

Roll each sausage into a strip of pastry. Seal the edge using water.

Place half the pigs in blankets into the air fryer basket and slide it into the air fryer. Cook for 10 minutes or until golden grown.

Repeat the process with the remaining pigs in blankets.

Sprinkle with fennel seeds to serve, if using.

SERVES 4

Easy Pizza Rolls

250g pizza dough

1 cup passata (or pizza sauce)

1 cup (125g) mozzarella cheese, grated

Roll out the pizza dough in a rectangle (approximately 30cm x 40 cm) to the desired thickness. Spoon passata over the dough and sprinkle with the cheese.

Roll up the dough to form a firm log. Use a sharp knife to slice the log into circular pieces.

Lightly spray the air fryer basket and carefully place each roll into the basket.

Cook at 190°C for 20 minutes.

SERVES 4

Party Meatballs

500g lean beef mince

1 clove garlic, crushed

1 tsp dried mixed herbs

1 egg, beaten

1 tbsp fresh breadcrumbs

175g Masterfoods Tuscan meatballs recipe base

Mix together all ingredients except recipe base until well combined.

Form mini meatballs (you should get about 14) using your hands.

Lightly spray the air fryer basket and carefully place meatballs into the basket.

Cook at 200°C for 7 minutes, turning halfway.

Meanwhile, prepare the Tuscan recipe base sauce per the packet instructions.

Allow meatballs to cool slightly then coat with the sauce.

Insert toothpicks to serve.

SERVES 4

Mini Quiches

1 shortcrust pastry sheet

1 egg

3 tbsps thick cream

⅓ cup (40g) tasty cheese, grated

Pinch of salt and pepper

1 cup (165g) broccoli, cooked and chopped

2 pie moulds (or use ramekins)

Preheat the air fryer to 200°C and lightly spray the moulds with oil.

Cut two rounds of approximately 7cm from the pastry sheet. Press down into the moulds. Transfer to the air fryer.

Beat the egg, cream, cheese, salt and pepper together until combined. Pour the mixture into the pastry moulds and add the broccoli.

Cook for 12 minutes until firm and golden.

Remove the quiches from the moulds before serving.

SERVES 2

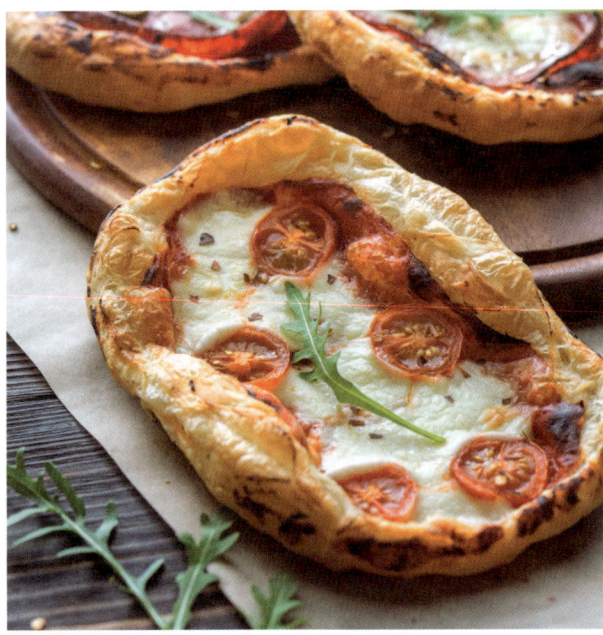

Cheese and Tomato Mini Pizza

2 sheets frozen puff pastry, just thawed

1 egg, beaten

1 cup (125g) Colby cheese, grated

8 cherry tomatoes, halved

Baking tin, lightly greased

Preheat the air fryer to 200°C.

Cut pastry sheets into two shapes corresponding to the shape of your tin. Place one piece of pastry in the fridge and press the other into the tin. Brush the edges with the beaten egg. Transfer to the air fryer basket. Cook for 10 minutes or until pastry is golden brown.

Remove the basket from the air fryer. Using a spoon, press down in the centre of the pastry to make an indentation. Sprinkle cheese into the indentation and then dot with the cherry tomato halves.

Return to the air fryer and cook for a further 6-8 minutes until cheese is gooey. Transfer to a wire rack and allow to cool for 5 minutes. Repeat for the other piece of pastry.

Serve warm.

MAKES 2

Fried Wontons

500g pork mince

2 tsps ginger, minced

2 cloves garlic, minced

1 spring onion, finely chopped

1 tbsp soy sauce

2 tbsps oyster sauce

2 cups (200g) white cabbage, finely chopped

10 wonton wrappers

1 egg

1 tbsp water

Place the pork, ginger, garlic, spring onion, soy sauce, oyster sauce and cabbage in a large bowl and stir well to combine.

Beat the egg and water together in a small bowl to make an egg wash

Place a wonton wrapper flat in the palm of your hand. Using your free hand, dip a pastry brush in the egg wash, and brush all around the edges of the wrapper with the egg wash. Place roughly 1 teaspoon of the filling into the centre of the wrapper. Fold one corner of the wrapper diagonally to the opposite corner to make triangle shapes, or pinch and twist edges together and tie with strips of pandan leaves (or string) to make pouches. Seal the wrapper tightly around the filling, squeezing out any air bubbles.

Place the wontons in the basket of the air fryer in a single layer and spray liberally with oil on both sides.

Place in the air fryer and cook at 180°C for 8 minutes, removing the basket and shaking it from time to time to turn the wontons over. Fry for an additional minute or two until golden brown, if needed.

MAKES 10

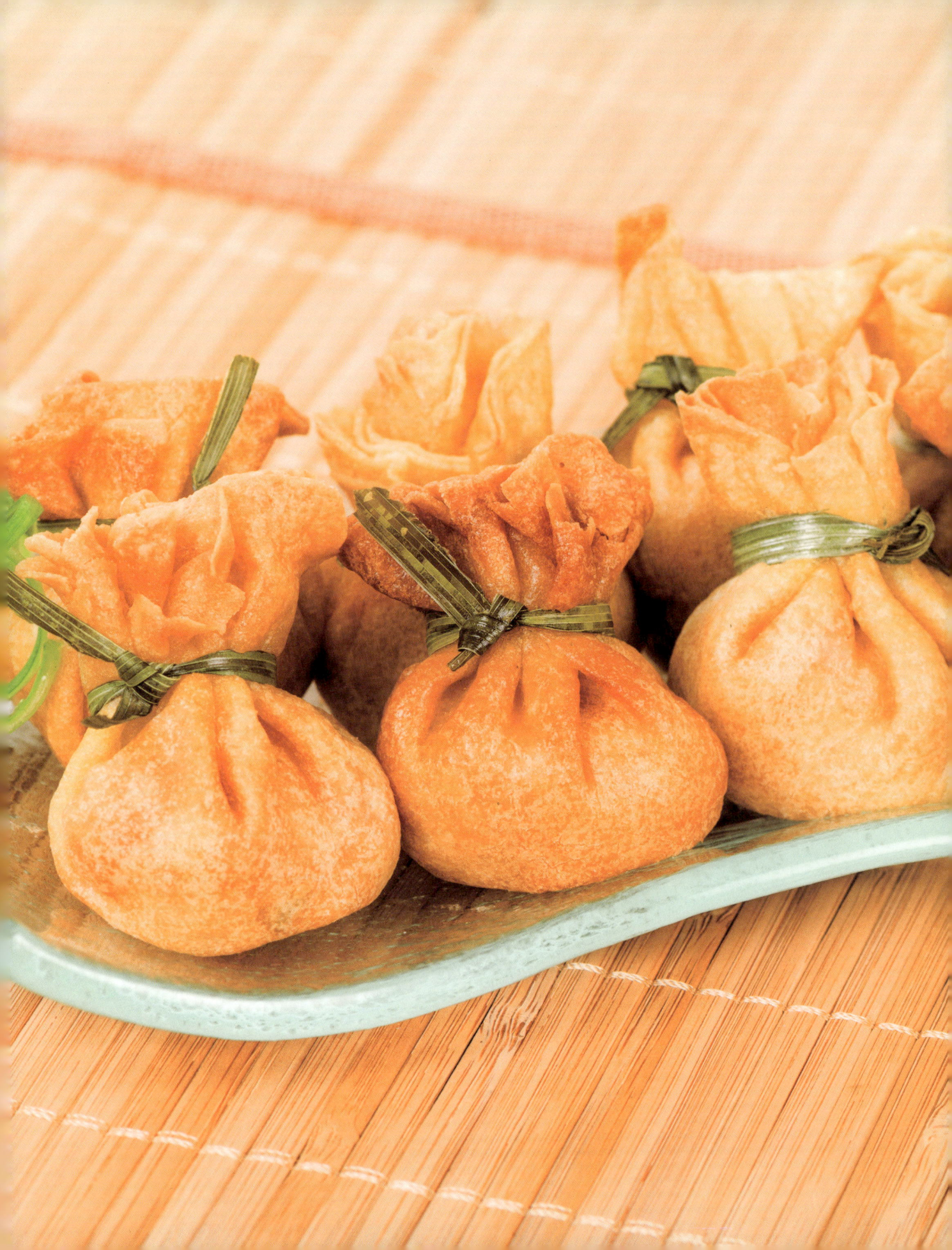

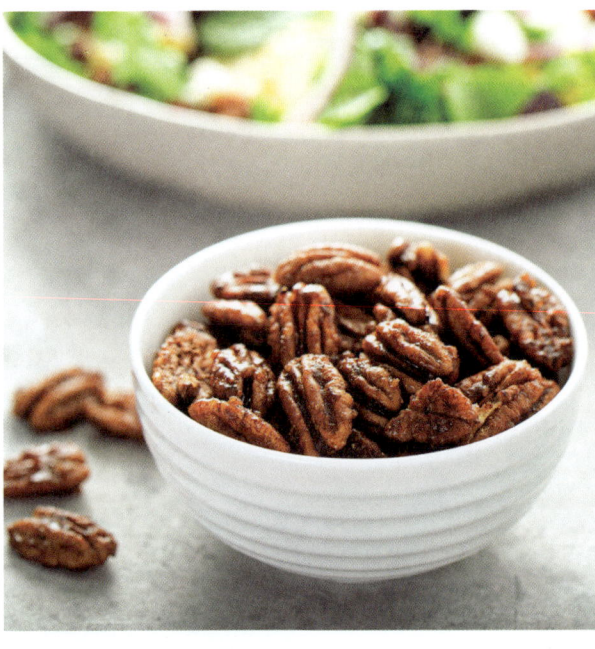

Roasted Pecans

2 cups (250g) pecan halves

1 tbsp butter

1-2 tsps of ground pink Himalayan salt

Preheat the air fryer to 180°C.

Using a pan over medium heat or the microwave, melt butter and stir in the salt.

Toss the pecan halves into the butter and stir until fully coated.

Place in the basket of the air fryer and cook for 5 minutes, tossing once or twice during cooking.

Remove and allow to cool to room temperature before transferring to a storage container.

MAKES 2 CUPS

Spiced Almonds

1 tbsp garlic powder

1 tbsp soy sauce

1½ tsps paprika

¼ tsp pepper

Pinch of chilli powder

1 tsp honey

2 cups (250g) raw almonds

1 tbsp egg white, whisked

Place all the ingredients except the almonds and egg white in a large bowl and stir well. Add the almonds and egg white and stir to thoroughly and evenly coat them.

Place in the basket of the air fryer and cook for 6 minutes at 180°C. Taste for readiness: the almonds should be hard but chewy inside. Continue to cook for a further 2-3 minutes until desired consistency is reached.

Remove and allow to cool to room temperature before transferring to a storage container.

MAKES 2 CUPS

Note: Will keep in a storage container for up to a week.

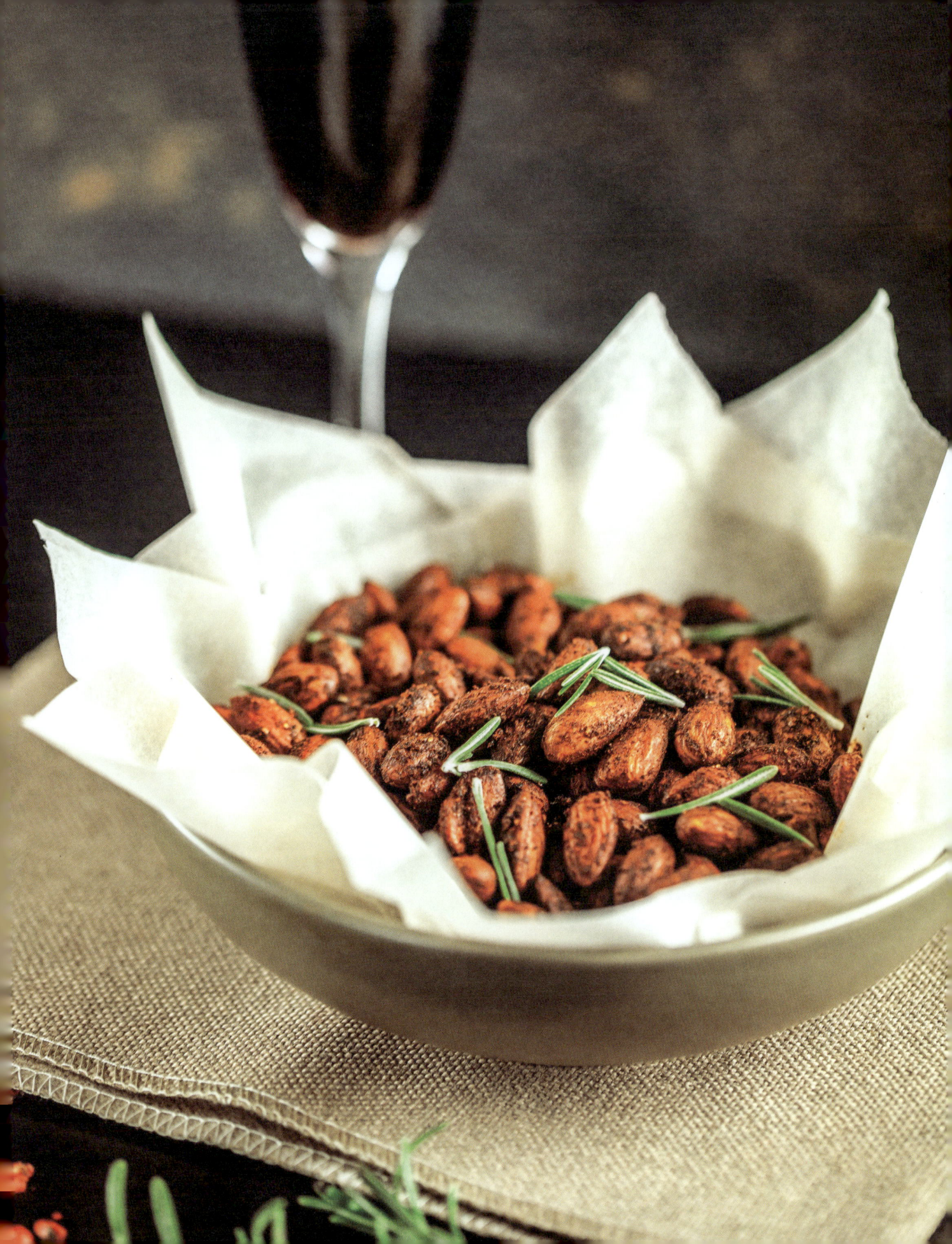

Wasabi Peas

40g wasabi paste

1 tbsp mirin

1 tbsp rice vinegar

1 tbsp salt

2 cups (350g) freeze-dried peas

Baking tray, sprayed with oil

Whisk together the wasabi, mirin, rice vinegar and salt in a mixing bowl.

Place the peas in the bowl and toss well to coat with the mixture.

Arrange the peas on the prepared tray, ensuring they are spaced apart.

Place in the air fryer basket. Cook for 15 minutes at 180°C, removing the basket and shaking once or twice during cooking.

SERVES 4

Spicy Roasted Peanuts

2 tbsps olive oil

3 tsps all-purpose seasoning

2 cups (250g) unsalted peanuts, shelled

Salt, to taste

Preheat the air fryer to 160°C.

Combine the olive oil and all-purpose seasoning in a large bowl and stir to combine. Add the peanuts and stir until well coated.

Transfer the peanuts to the air fryer basket. Cook for 10 minutes. Remove the basket, toss and return to the air fryer to cook for a further 10 minutes.

Again remove the basket from the air fryer and salt peanuts to taste. Toss peanuts again and cook for a further 5 minutes.

SERVES 4

Roasted Almonds and Cashews

1 cup (125g) almonds

1 cup (125g) cashew nuts

1 tsp melted ghee (or butter)

1 tsp salt

½ tsp pepper

Preheat the air fryer to 180°C.

Place the almonds and cashews in a large mixing bowl. Add the ghee, salt and pepper and mix well until the nuts are fully coated.

Transfer the nuts to the air fryer basket and cook for 7 minutes, removing and shaking the basket halfway through cooking.

SERVES 4

Masala Roasted Chickpeas

1 x 400g can chickpeas

1 tbsp olive oil

Pinch of salt

½ tsp garlic powder

¼ tsp onion powder

½ tsp paprika

¼ tsp cayenne

Preheat the air fryer to 190°C.

Drain and rinse the chickpeas. Transfer to a large mixing bowl. Add the olive oil, salt and spices and toss well to coat.

Place the chickpeas in the air fryer basket. Cook for 15 minutes, removing the basket and shaking once or twice during cooking.

SERVES 2

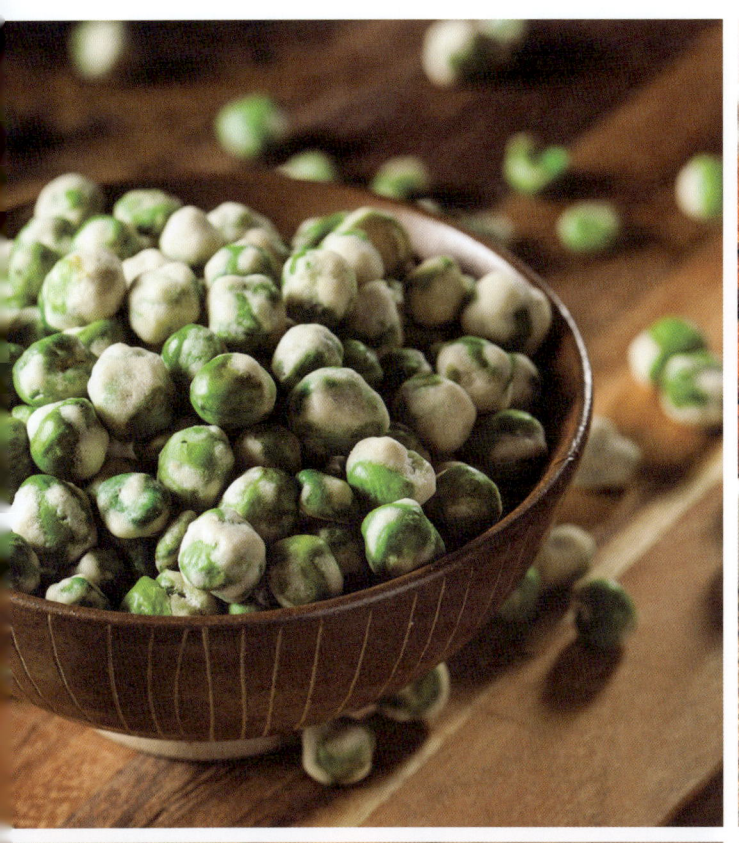
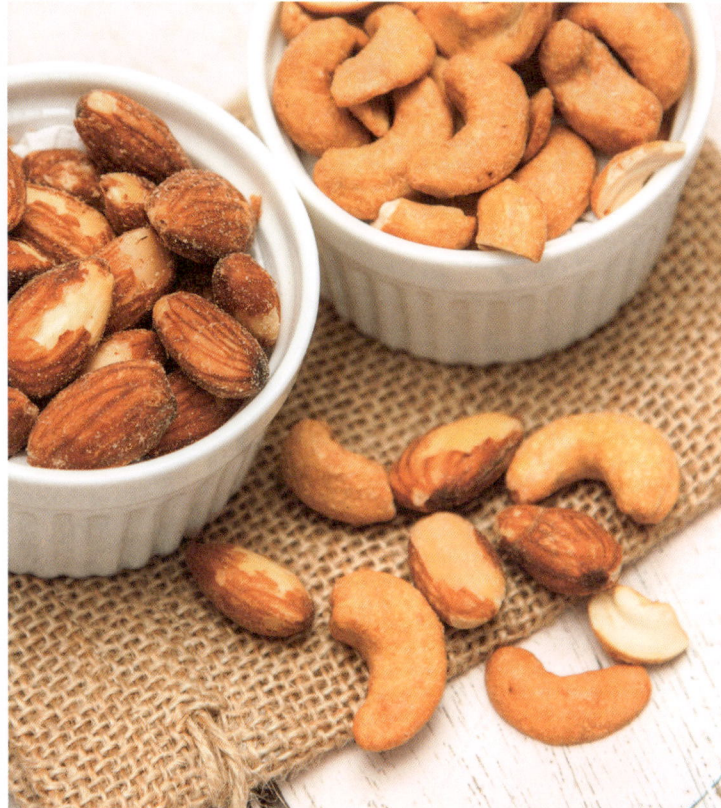
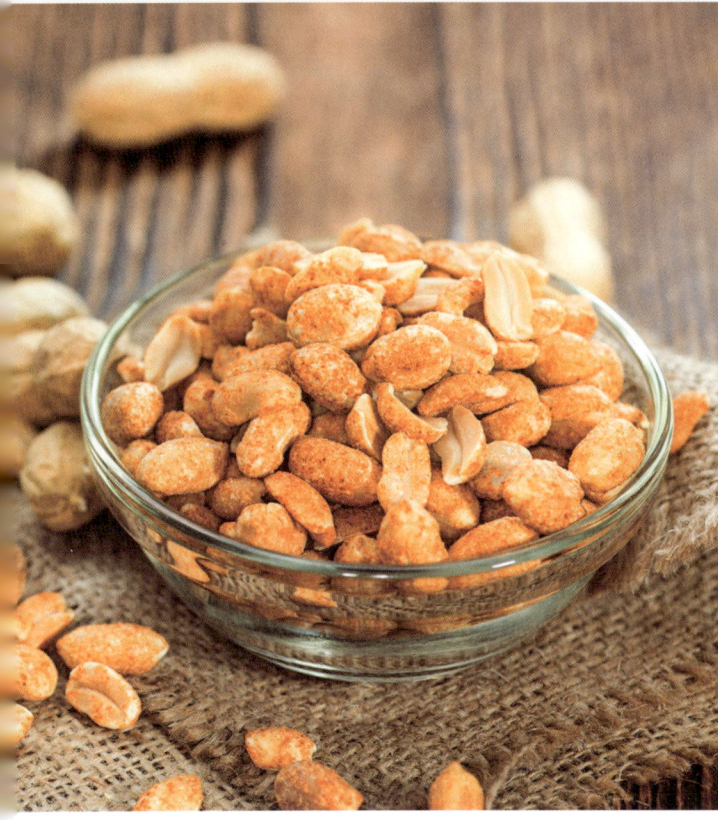
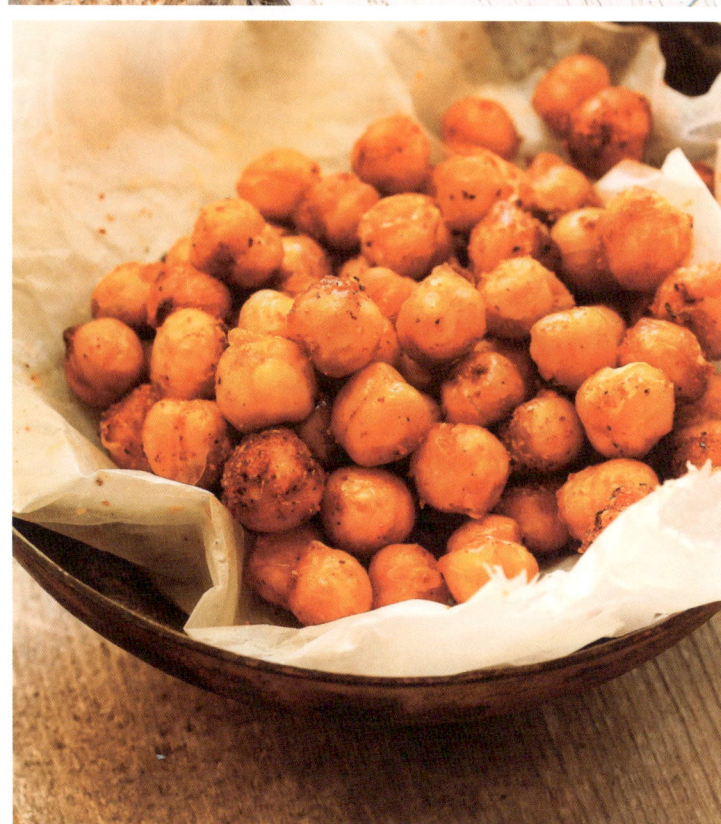

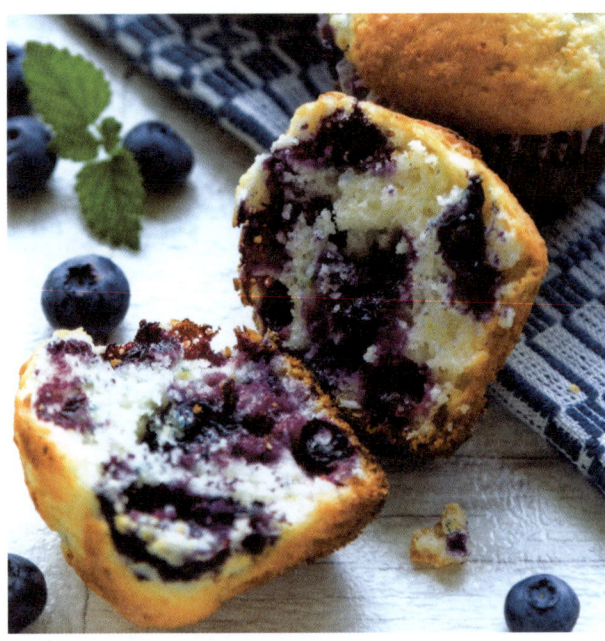

Blueberry Muffins

1 cup (125g) plain flour

1 tsp baking powder

2 tbsps sugar

1 egg, beaten

2 tsps vanilla extract

⅓ cup (80ml) milk

3 tbsps melted butter

1 cup (100g) blueberries (fresh or frozen)

Muffin tray (or silicone muffin cups)

Preheat the air fryer to 160°C.

Combine all the ingredients except the blueberries in a large mixing bowl and stir well to form a smooth batter. Gently fold in the blueberries.

Spray the muffin cups. Spoon the batter into each cup up to about two-thirds full.

Place in the air fryer and cook for 15 minutes, checking and moving the cups around halfway through cooking.

When cooked, a toothpick inserted in the centre should come out clean.

Cool on a wire rack.

MAKES 6

Pumpkin Scones

2 tbsps butter

½ cup (110g) sugar

¼ tsp salt

1 egg

1 cup (225g) mashed cooked pumpkin

2 cups (250g) self-raising flour

1 tbsp milk

Preheat the air fryer to 200°C.

Beat the butter and sugar until pale and creamy. Add salt and combine.

Add the egg and beat again, then add the mashed pumpkin and stir to fully combine.

Slowly add the sifted flour and stir with a wooden spoon to bring the dough together.

Roll the dough out onto a floured surface, form into a ball, flatten, and then cut into scones. Brush the tops with milk using a pastry brush.

Spray the basket of the air fryer.

Place the scones inside the basket and bake for 4 minutes. Reduce the temperature to 160°C and continue cooking for a further 7 minutes or until golden brown.

When cooked, a toothpick inserted in the centre should come out clean.

MAKES 6

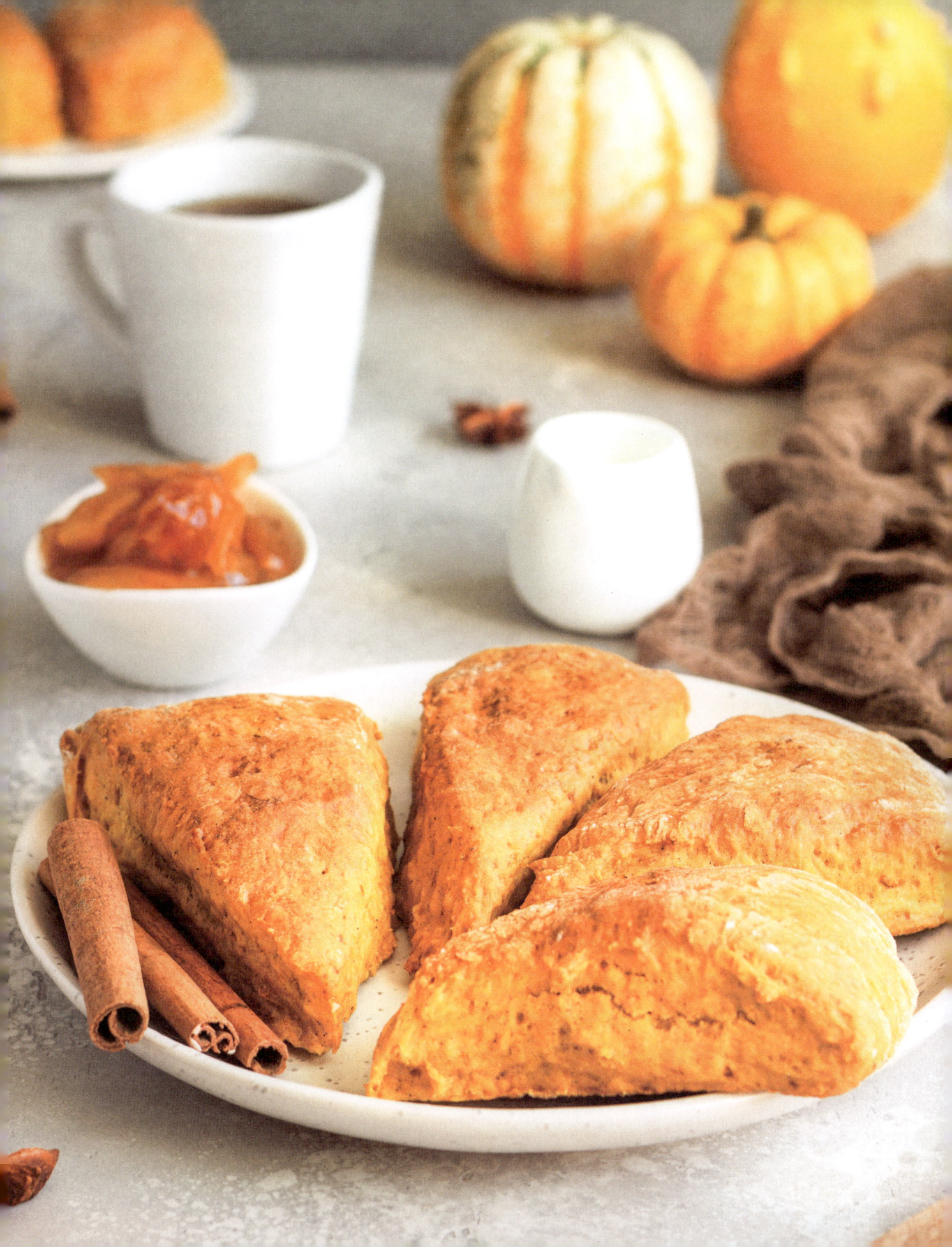

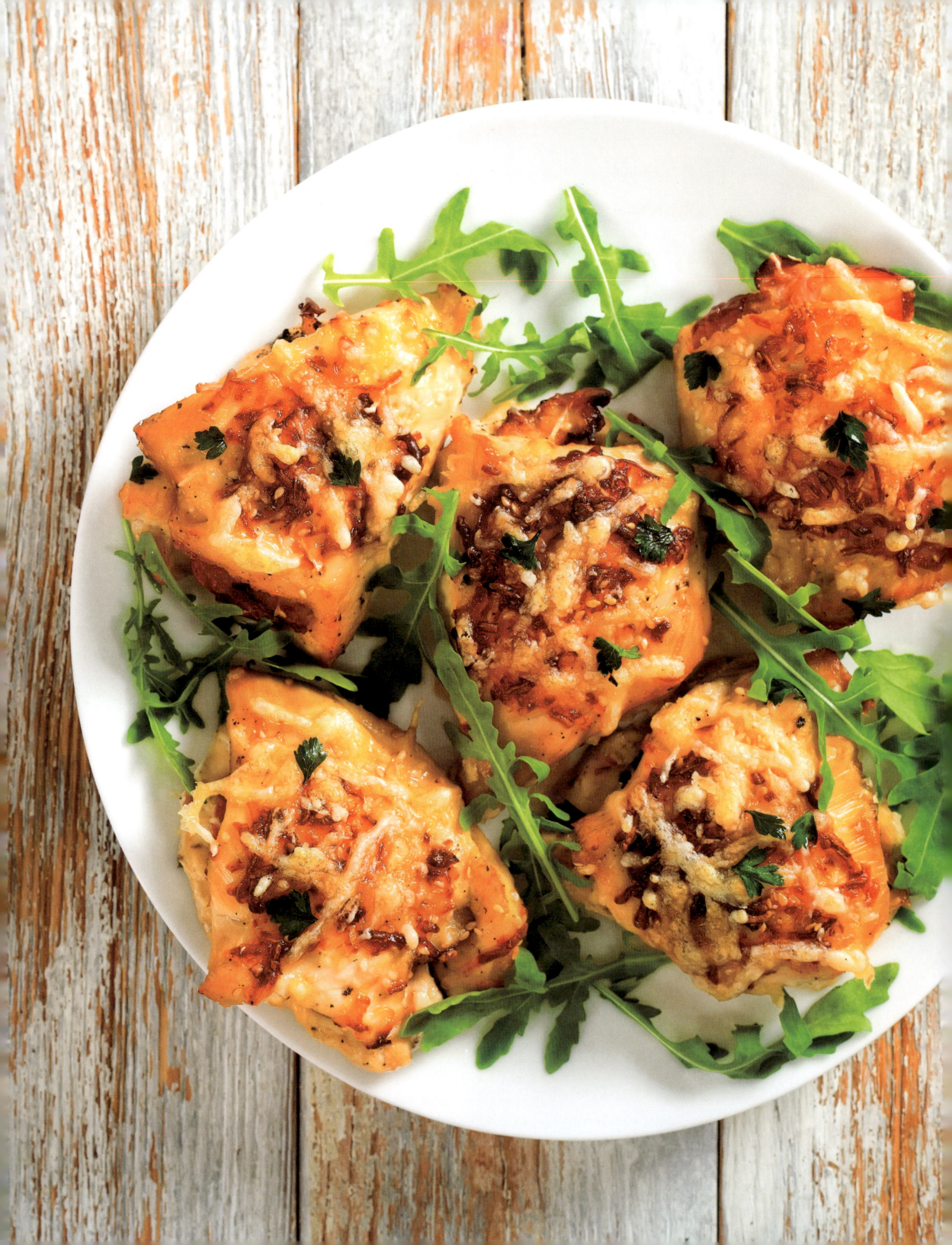

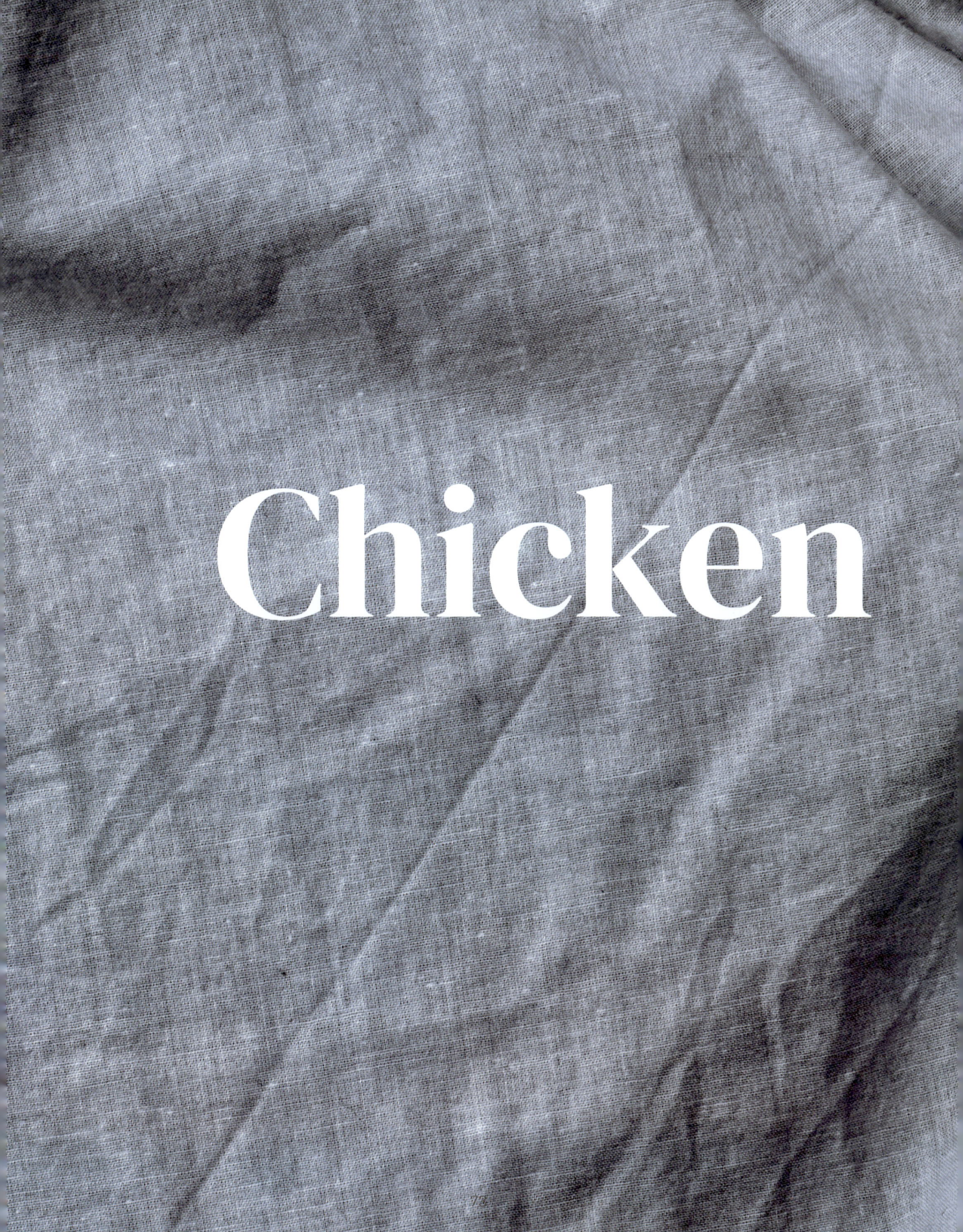

Chicken

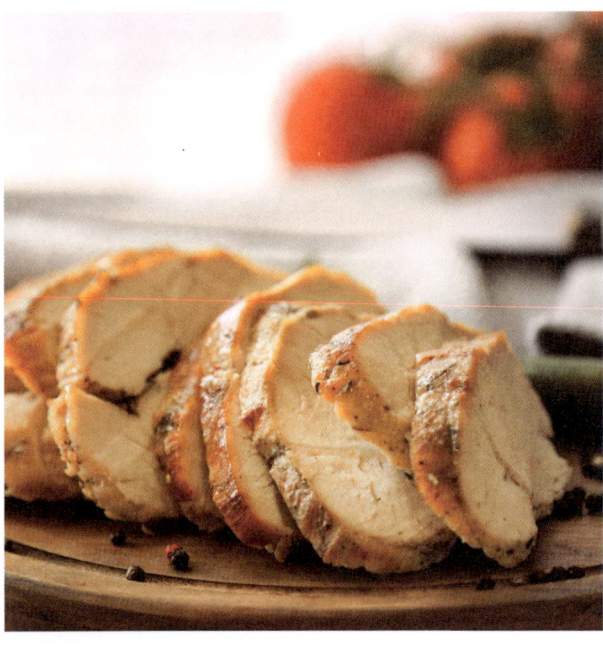

Simple Chicken Breast

2 chicken breasts

2 tsps mixed herbs

1 tbsp salt

Preheat the air fryer to 180°C.

Spray olive oil on the chicken breasts then sprinkle with herbs and salt and rub into the chicken breast.

Transfer to the air fryer basket and cook for 15 minutes, turning halfway.

SERVES 2

Popcorn Chicken

3 cups (90g) cornflakes, crushed

1 tsp Kentucky-style chicken seasoning

½ tsp salt

Pinch of pepper

½ cup (50g) plain flour

1 egg, beaten

500g chicken mince

Blitz the cornflakes into fine crumbs using a food processor. If you don't have one, place in a bag and crush with a rolling pin. Add the Kentucky seasoning, salt and pepper and stir to combine. Place on a flat plate and set aside.

Place the flour in a shallow bowl. Place the egg in a second shallow bowl.

Roll the chicken mince into small balls. Dredge the balls in the flour, shaking off excess. Dip in the beaten egg, and then roll in the cornflake crumbs until well coated.

Place the crumbed chicken balls in the air fryer basket, leaving a little space between them.

Cook at 180°C for 10 minutes or until chicken is cooked through and crispy on the outside.

SERVES 6

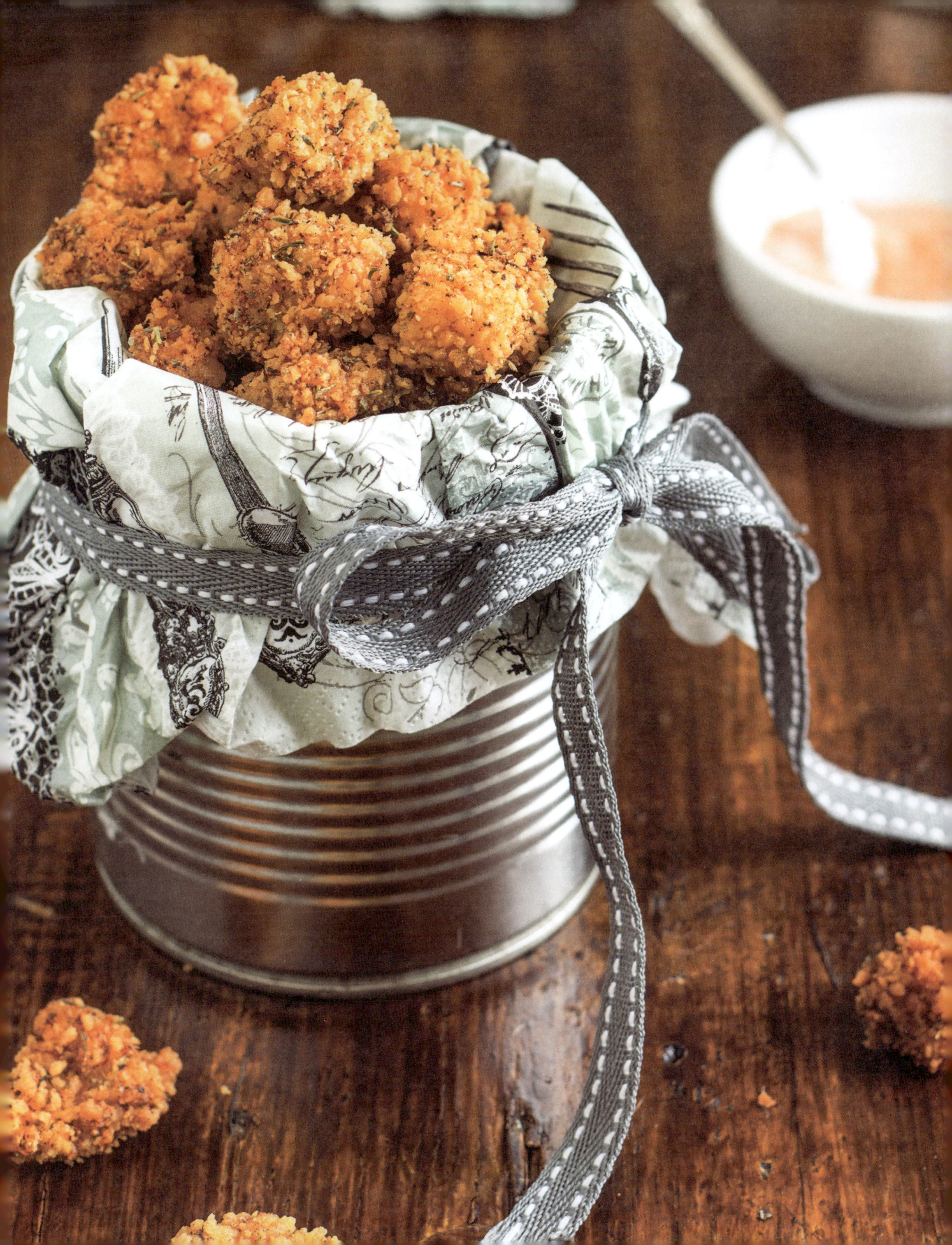

Roast Chicken

2kg whole chicken

1 tbsp all-purpose seasoning or homemade chicken rub (see below)

Knob of butter, softened

Preheat the air fryer to 170°C.

Pat the chicken dry with paper towel.

Mix the seasoning with the butter in a small bowl. Rub the mixture over the chicken and into the skin.

Spritz the air fryer basket with cooking spray.

Place chicken into the basket with the legs facing down.

Roast chicken for 30 minutes.

Remove the basket and flip chicken carefully using tongs.

Return to the air fryer and cook for a further 20 minutes.

SERVES 6

Roast Chicken Salad

2 cooked chicken breasts (see recipe for Simple Chicken Breast on page 74)

2 tsps mixed herbs

1 tbsp salt

1 apple, finely sliced

60g baby spinach

½ cup (60g) walnuts, finely chopped

½ cup (80g) dried cranberries

Slice the cooked chicken breasts with a sharp knife.

Assemble the salad by placing the baby spinach leaves in two serving bowls. Arrange the chicken and apple slices on top of the spinach, and then sprinkle with walnuts and cranberries.

SERVES 2

Chicken Dry Rub

¾ cup (290g) salt

4 tbsps paprika

4 tbsps onion powder

4 tbsps garlic powder

4 tbsps Italian seasoning

4 tbsps brown sugar

2 tbsps dried thyme

2 tbsps dry mustard

2 tbsps cayenne pepper

1 tsp chilli flakes (optional)

Place all the ingredients in a sealed jar or container. Shake well to combine. Store in an airtight container.

MAKES 2½ CUPS

Garlic Butterflied Chicken

1 butterflied chicken

1 tbsp minced garlic

½ tsp salt

¼ tsp pepper

1 punnet cherry tomatoes

1 lemon, cut into pieces

Preheat the air fryer to 180°C.

Sprinkle the chicken generously with minced garlic and salt and pepper and massage into both sides.

Spritz the air fryer basket with cooking spray.

Cook for 25 minutes. Remove from the basket and turn the chicken over. Add the tomatoes and lemon slices and return to the air fryer to cook for a further 25 minutes.

SERVES 6

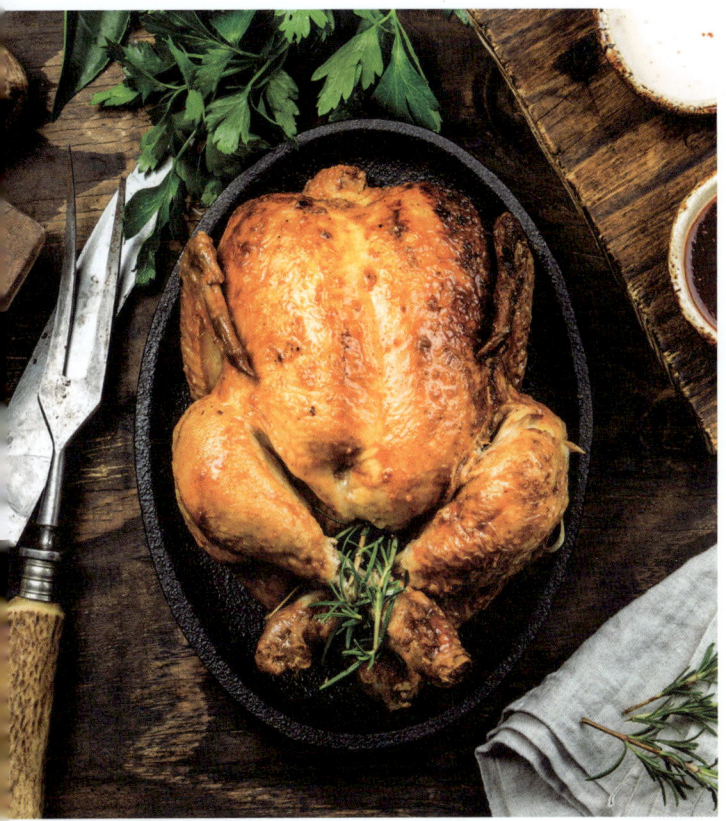
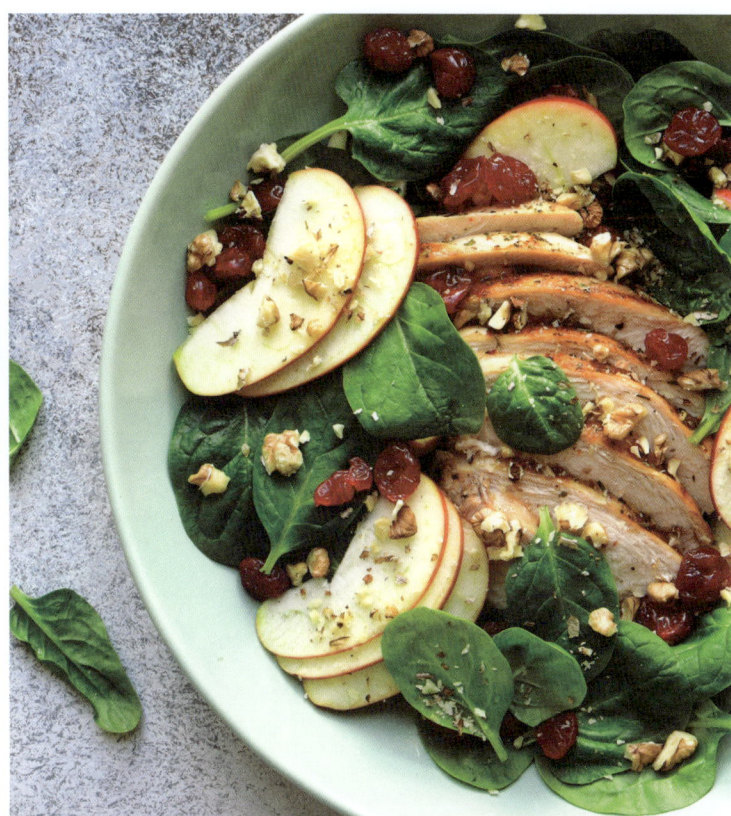
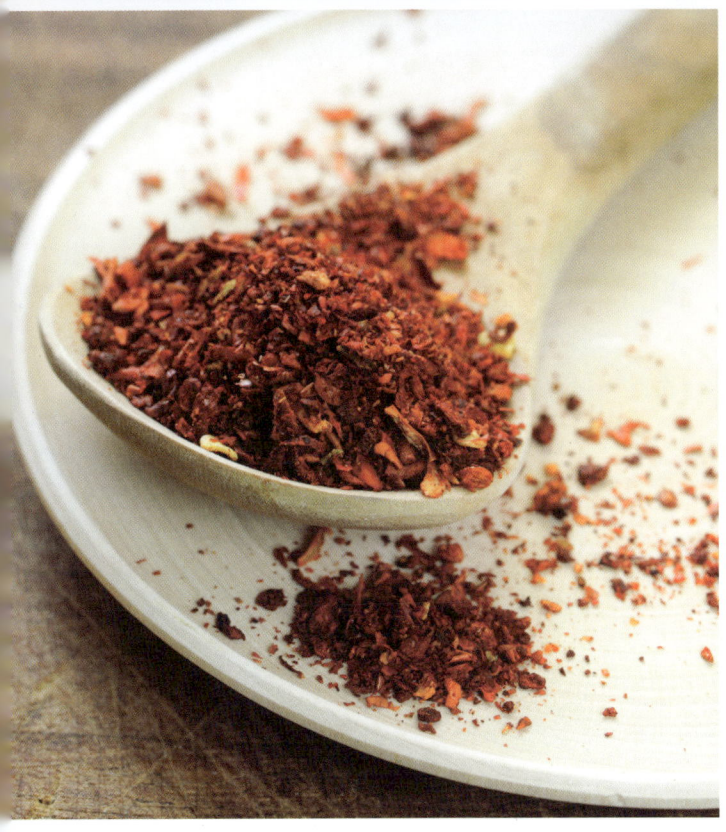
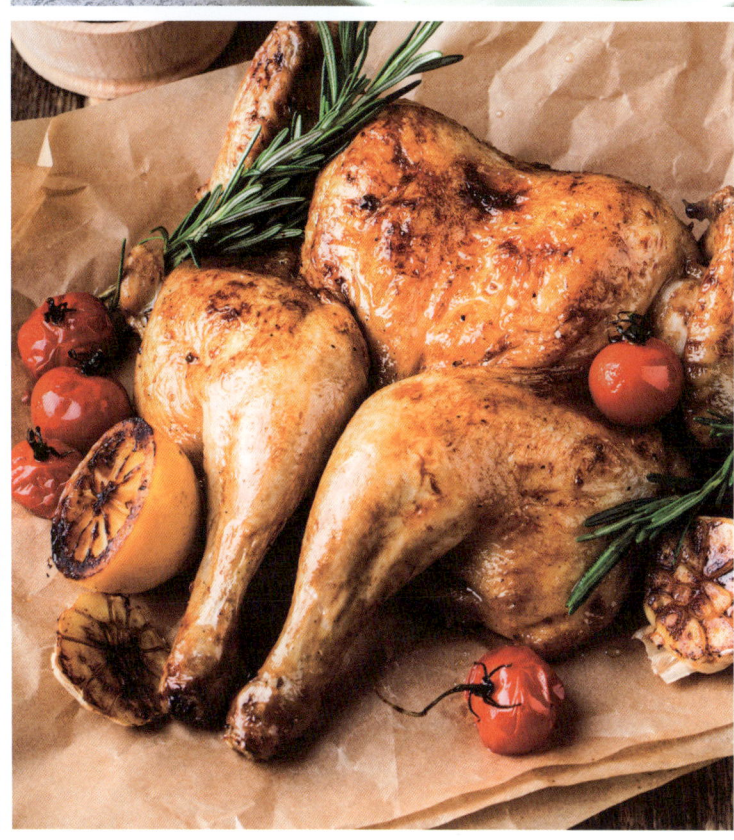

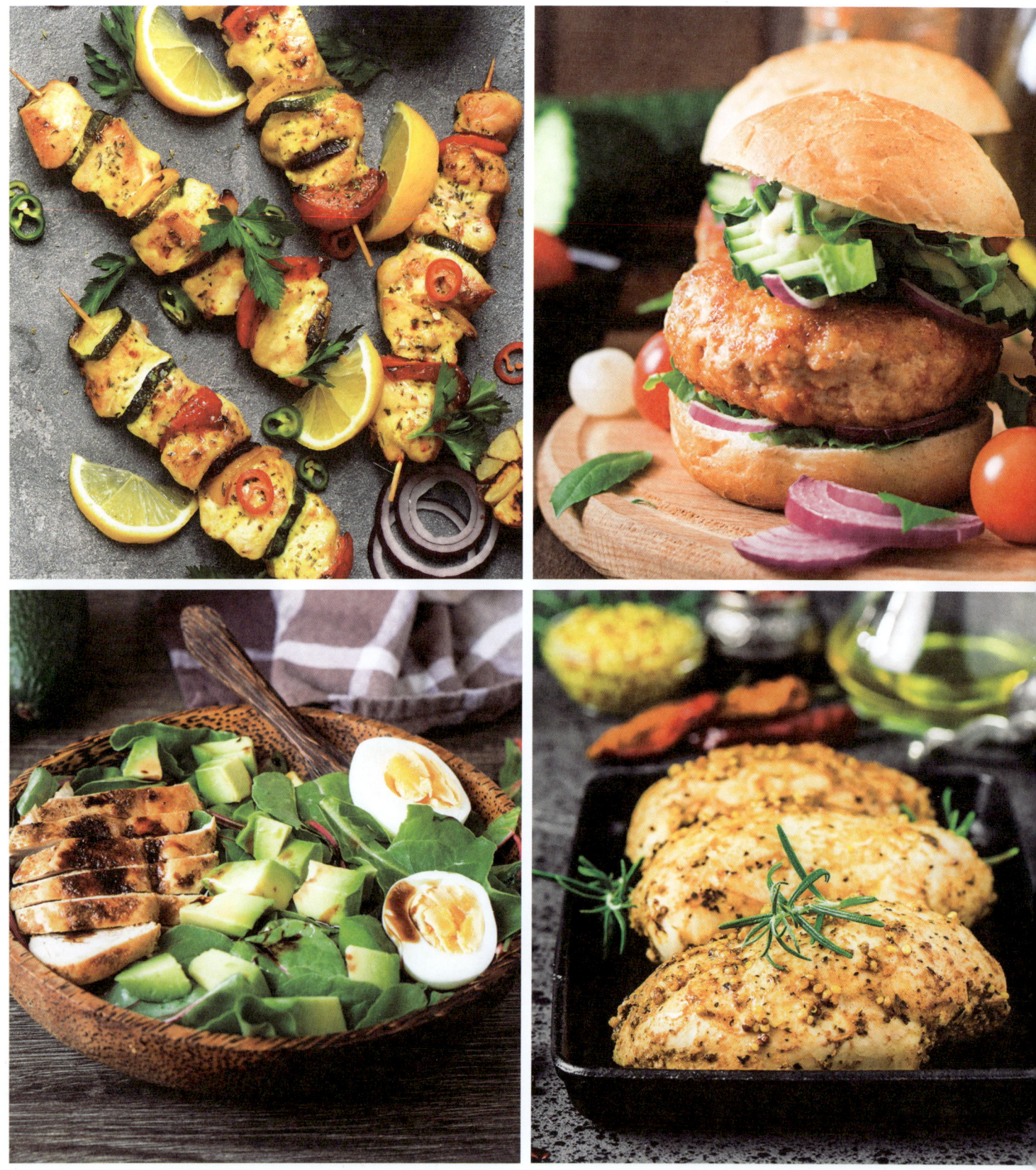

Honey Chicken Kebabs

2 chicken breasts, diced

Pinch of salt and pepper

⅓ cup (115g) honey

⅓ cup (80ml) soy sauce

1 small zucchini, sliced into rounds

1 red capsicum, deseeded and cut into chunks

Skewer tray

Spray the chicken breasts with oil and season with salt and pepper.

Put the honey and soy sauce in a small bowl and whisk to combine.

Thread the chicken, zucchini and capsicum onto the skewers.

Coat kebabs with the sauce and transfer to the fridge for a minimum of 1 hour.

Preheat the air fryer to 170°C.

Place the kebabs on the skewer tray and place in the air fryer. Cook for 15 minutes.

SERVES 2

Easy Chicken Salad

¼ cup (60ml) olive oil

1 tbsp balsamic vinegar

1 tbsp wholegrain mustard

2 cooked chicken breasts (see recipe for Simple Chicken Breast on page 74)

1 avocado, peeled and chopped

2 eggs, hard-boiled and halved

200g mixed salad leaves

Place the olive oil, balsamic vinegar and mustard in a sealed jar and shake vigorously to combine. Set aside.

Slice the chicken breasts.

Place the mixed greens in two serving bowls and top with avocado, chicken and eggs. Drizzle a generous amount of dressing over the top and serve.

SERVES 2

Chicken Burger

500g chicken mince

1 tsp olive oil

1 tsp Worcestershire sauce

1 tsp salt

¼ tsp pepper

4 hamburger buns, to serve

Salad vegetables, to serve

Combine all the ingredients apart from the buns and salad in a large bowl and mix well.

Using damp hands, gently shape into 4 burger patties.

Preheat the air fryer to 180°C.

Spritz the air fryer basket with cooking spray and gently slide two burgers into the basket.

Cook for 5 minutes. Increase the temperature to 200°C and flip the burger over in the basket. Return to cook for a further 4 minutes.

Repeat with the remaining two burgers.

Serve in buns with salad.

SERVES 4

Honey Mustard Chicken Breasts

2 tbsps wholegrain mustard

1 tbsp honey

2 tsps fresh rosemary, finely chopped

½ tsp salt

¼ tsp pepper

2 chicken breasts

Preheat the air fryer to 180°C.

Mix the mustard, honey, rosemary, salt and pepper together in a small bowl.

Rub the mustard mixture all over chicken breasts.

Spritz the air fryer basket with cooking spray.

Place the chicken breasts in the air fryer basket. Cook for 15 minutes, turning halfway.

SERVES 2

BBQ Marinade

1 cup (250ml) BBQ sauce

¼ cup (60ml) white vinegar

¼ cup (40g) brown sugar

2 tbsps paprika

1 tbsp olive oil

1 tbsp chilli powder

2 tsps garlic powder

½ tsp cayenne powder (optional)

Combine all ingredients in medium bowl and stir until sugar is dissolved.

MAKES 1¼ CUPS

BBQ Chicken Thighs

4 chicken thighs

BBQ marinade (see opposite)

Rub the chicken thighs with BBQ marinade. Place in a sealed container and transfer to the fridge. Leave to marinate overnight.

Preheat the air fryer to 180°C.

Place the chicken thighs in the air fryer basket and slide into the air fryer.

Cook for 25 minutes, turning halfway through cooking.

SERVES 2

Turmeric-Paprika Chicken

2 chicken breasts

1 tbsp olive oil

½ tsp paprika

¼ tsp turmeric

¼ tsp chilli powder

¼ tsp pepper

¼ tsp garlic powder

¼ tsp onion powder

½ tsp salt

Cut each chicken breast in half. Drizzle with olive oil, and rub to coat thoroughly.

In a shallow dish, combine paprika, turmeric, chilli powder, pepper, garlic powder, onion powder and salt.

Dredge each chicken piece in spice mix and transfer to the air fryer basket.

Cook in the air fryer at 200°C for 15 minutes, flipping halfway.

SERVES 2

Sweet and Sour Chicken

½ cup (60g) cornflour

1 tsp salt

1 tsp five-spice powder

1 egg, beaten

1 red chilli, deseeded and sliced (optional)

1 tsp sesame oil

500g chicken breast, cut into pieces

Sweet and sour sauce, to serve

Mix the cornflour, salt and five-spice in a shallow bowl.

Mix the egg, chilli and sesame oil in a second shallow bowl.

Preheat the air fryer to 190°C and spritz the basket with cooking spray.

Dip each chicken piece in the cornflour mixture, then into the egg mixture, then back into the cornflour mixture. Place in the air fryer basket. Spray the pieces with cooking spray. Cook for 10 minutes, turning and spraying again halfway through cooking.

Toss with the sweet and sour sauce to serve.

SERVES 4

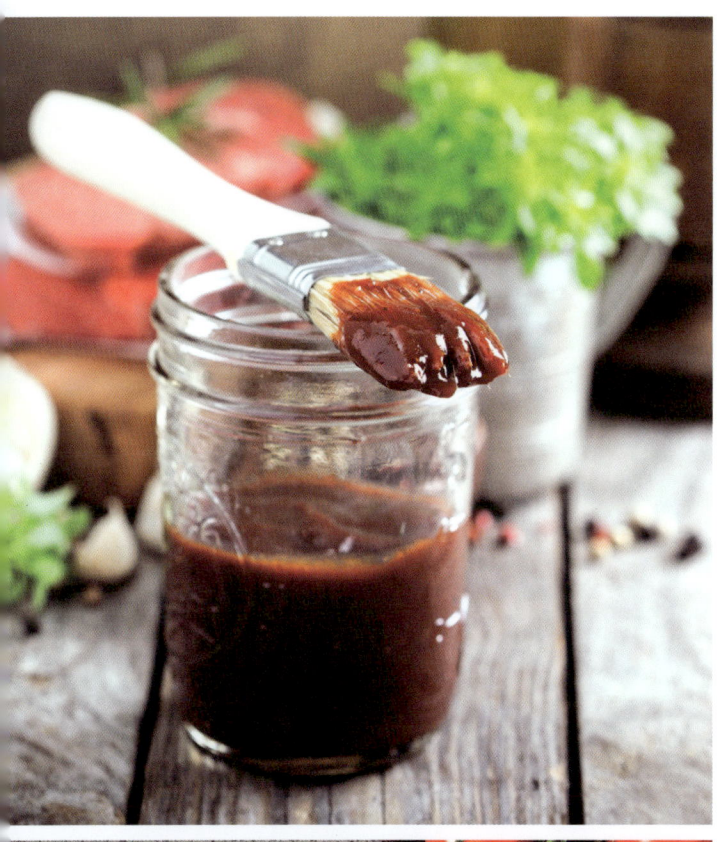
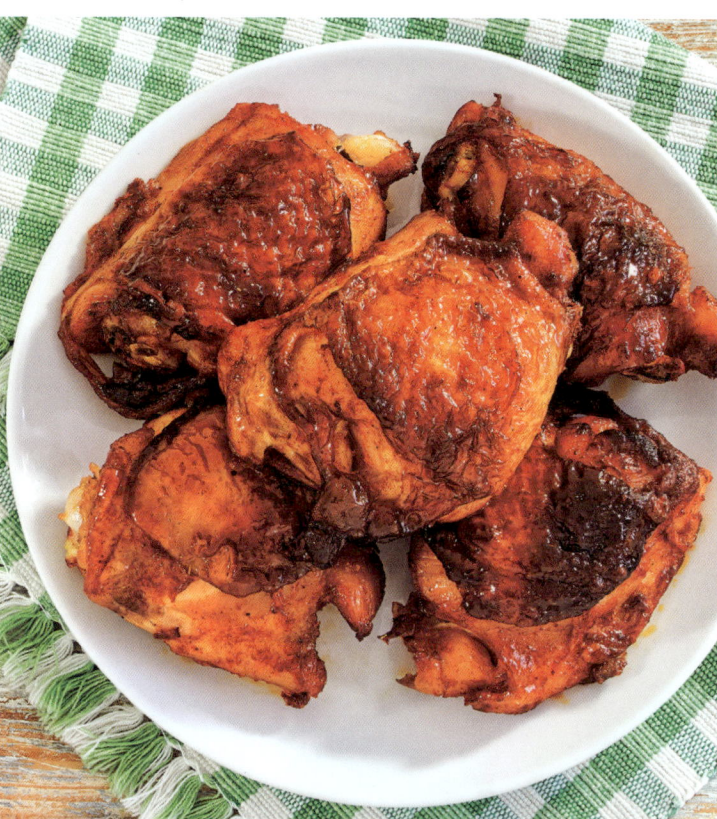
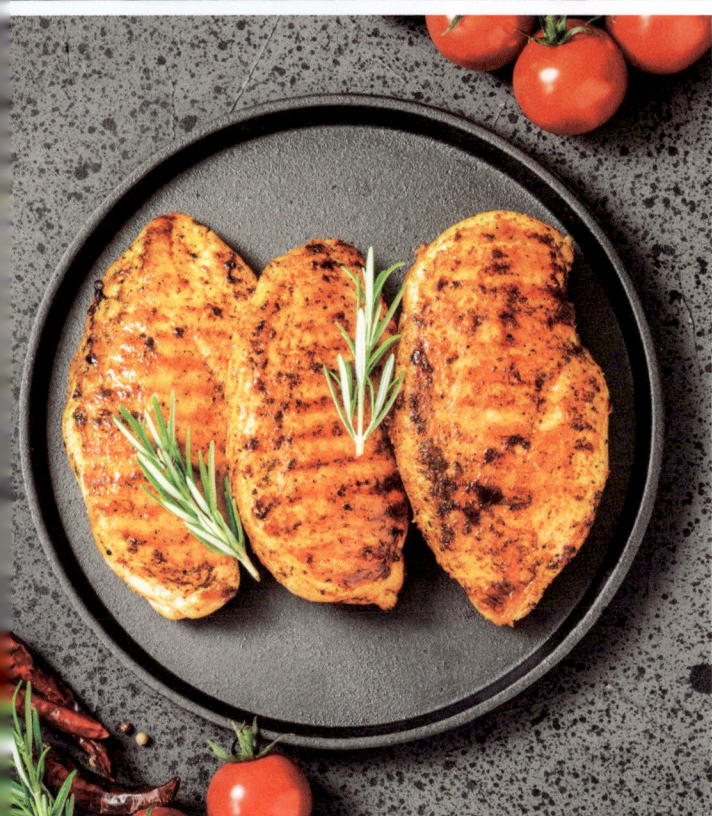
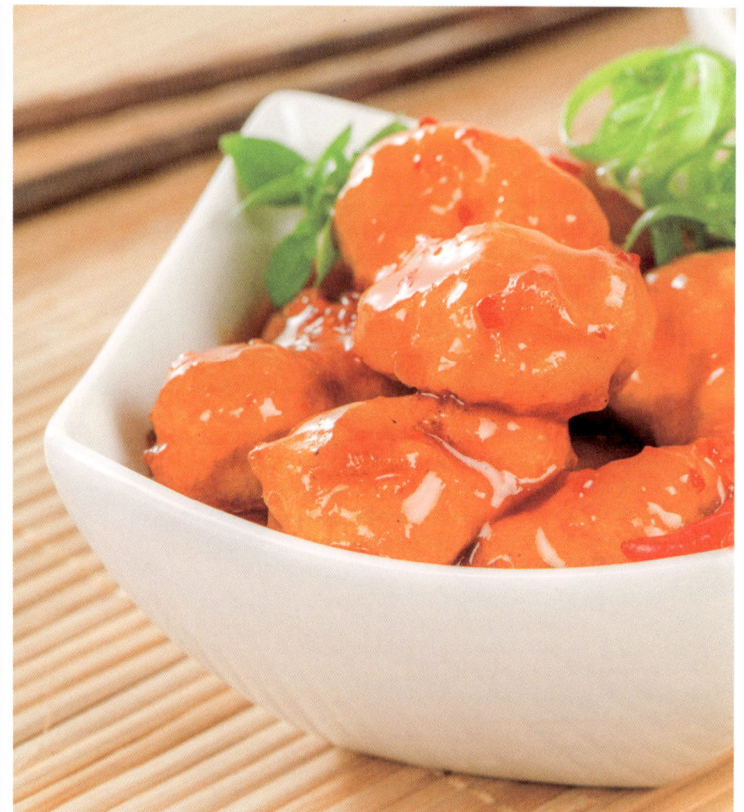

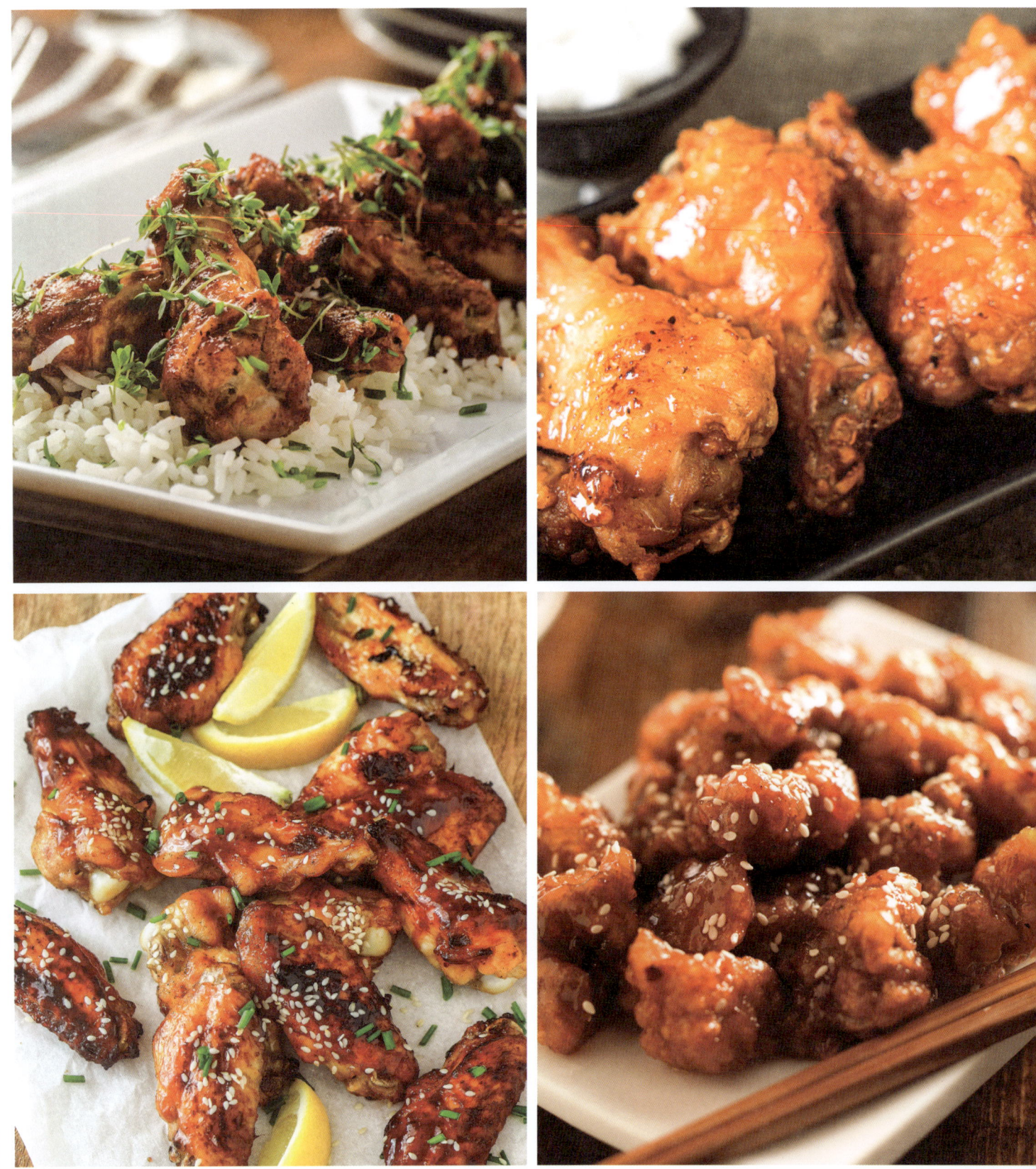

Spicy Barbecue Drumsticks

6 chicken drumsticks

2 cloves garlic, crushed

1 tbsp mustard

2 tbsps olive oil

3 tsps brown sugar

1 tsp chilli powder

Combine all the ingredients except for the chicken in a small bowl and whisk to combine. Completely coat the drumsticks in the marinade. Place in a container with a lid. Cover and transfer to the refrigerator for 30 minutes.

Preheat the air fryer to 200°C.

Shake off any excess marinade then transfer the drumsticks (top to tail) into the air fryer basket and cook for 10 minutes until browned. Turn down the temperature to 150°C and cook for a further 10 minutes.

SERVES 2

Korean-Style Drumsticks

4 chicken drumsticks

1 cup (250ml) Korean BBQ sauce

Place the chicken and sauce in a large bowl and combine well to ensure the chicken is fully coated.

Transfer to the fridge to marinate for 1 hour, or longer if convenient.

Place the chicken drumsticks (top to tail) in the air fryer basket and cook for 14 minutes at 180°C , turning once during cooking.

SERVES 2

Chinese Chicken Wings

6 chicken wings

1 tbsp soy sauce

1 tsp mixed spice

1 tbsp Chinese five-spice powder

Pinch of salt and pepper

Combine all the ingredients except for the chicken wings in a small bowl and whisk to combine.

Add the chicken wings and rub the seasoning over the chicken. Massage into the chicken until thoroughly coated.

Place a piece of foil into the bottom of the air fryer. Place the chicken on it and pour over any remaining seasoning.

Cook for 15 minutes at 180°C. Remove the chicken and flip it over using tongs then return to the air fryer. Increase the temperature to 200°C and cook for a further 15 minutes.

SERVES 2

Orange Sesame Chicken

6 boneless chicken thighs (or 3 large breasts), cubed and tossed in cornflour

¼ cup (60ml) soy sauce

2 tbsps brown sugar

2 tbsps orange juice

4 tbsps hoisin sauce

1 clove garlic, minced

1 tbsp cold water

1 tbsp cornflour

2 tsps sesame seeds

Place the chicken in the air fryer basket and cook for 20 minutes at 200°C, turning halfway.

Meanwhile, make the sauce. Place soy sauce, sugar, orange juice, hoisin sauce and garlic in a small saucepan over medium heat. Stir until sugar has dissolved, then whisk in the cold water and cornflour. Stir in the sesame seeds and remove from the heat. Set aside.

When chicken is cooked, remove from the air fryer and coat with the sauce.

SERVES 6

Honey Chicken Wings

6 chicken wings

3 tsps honey

1 tsp sesame oil

2 tsps soy sauce

1 tsp dark soy sauce

Pinch of pepper

1 tbsp sesame seeds

Whisk all the ingredients except the chicken wings in a large bowl. Add the chicken wings and stir to fully coat them.

Cover and transfer to the refrigerator to marinate for 2 hours.

Place the wings in the air fryer basket and cook for 20 minutes at 180°C, turning halfway.

Sprinkle with sesame seeds to serve.

SERVES 2

Nando's Honey Garlic Drumettes

1kg chicken drumettes

1 bottle (250g) Nando's Peri-Peri Marinade (choose the heat you prefer)

1 tbsp olive oil

2 tbsps honey

1 tsp garlic powder

Pinch of salt and pepper

Coat the drumettes in the peri-peri marinade and transfer to the refrigerator to marinate for at least 1 hour.

Preheat the air fryer to 180°C.

Remove drumettes from the fridge. Drizzle with the olive oil and honey and season with garlic powder, salt and pepper. Stir until all pieces are coated.

Place drumettes in a single layer in the air fryer basket and cook for 20 minutes, shaking halfway.

SERVES 6

BBQ-Glazed Chicken Meatballs

450g chicken mince

½ cup (60g) breadcrumbs

1 egg

½ cup (125ml) Buffalo sauce, divided

1 tsp garlic powder

½ tsp onion powder

½ tsp salt

Combine the chicken, breadcrumbs, egg, half of the Buffalo sauce, the garlic powder, onion powder and salt in a large bowl and stir to fully combine.

Spritz the air fryer basket with cooking spray.

Using clean hands, roll meat into 12 golf-ball-size meatballs.

Place the meatballs into the air fryer basket. (You may need to cook in batches or use a double layer accessory). Cook on 200°C for 12 minutes.

Toss meatballs with the remaining Buffalo sauce before serving.

SERVES 4

Easy BBQ Wings

1kg chicken wings

½ cup (125ml) BBQ sauce

Preheat the air fryer to 190°C.

Toss the wings in sauce to fully coat. Cover and transfer to the fridge to marinate for 30 minutes.

Liberally spray wings with oil.

Place wings in a single layer in the air fryer basket and cook for 20 minutes, shaking halfway.

SERVES 6

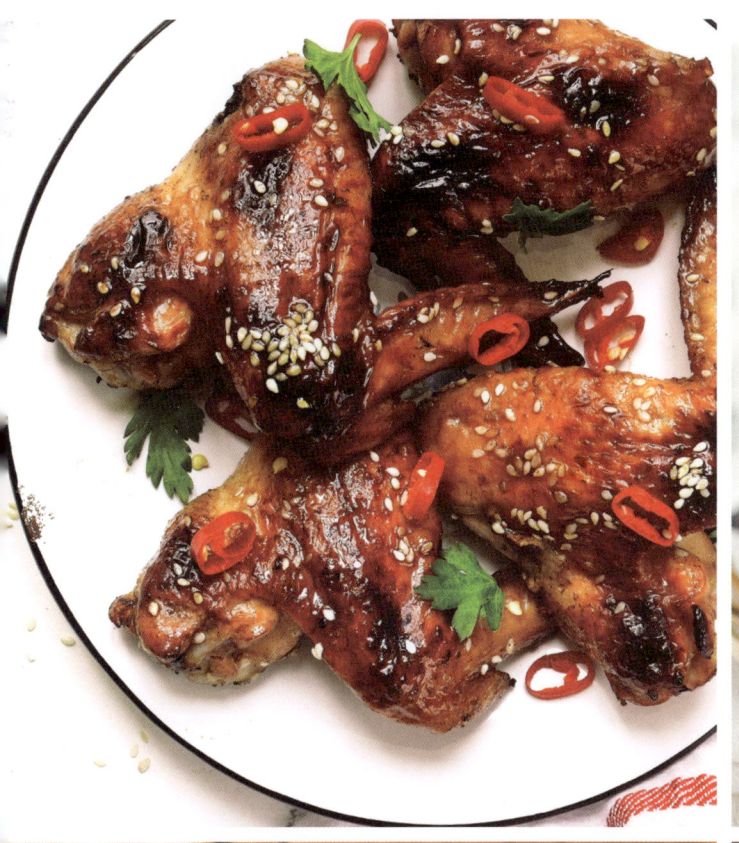
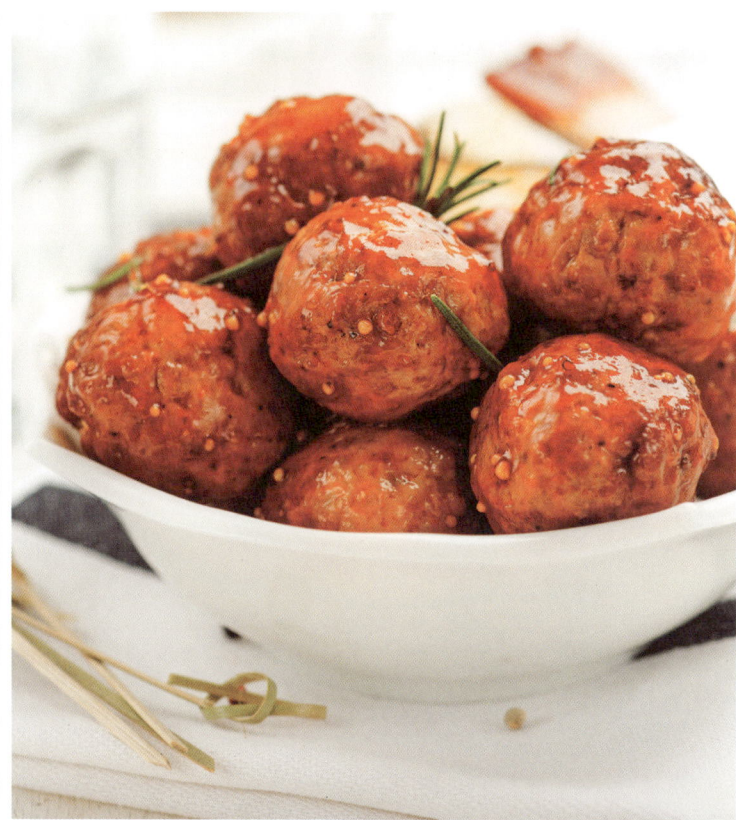
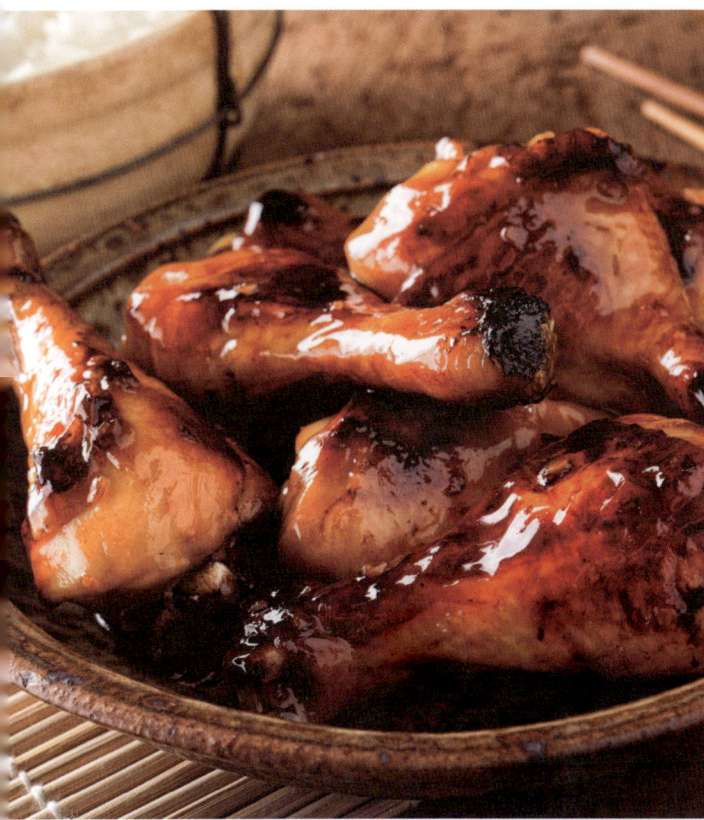
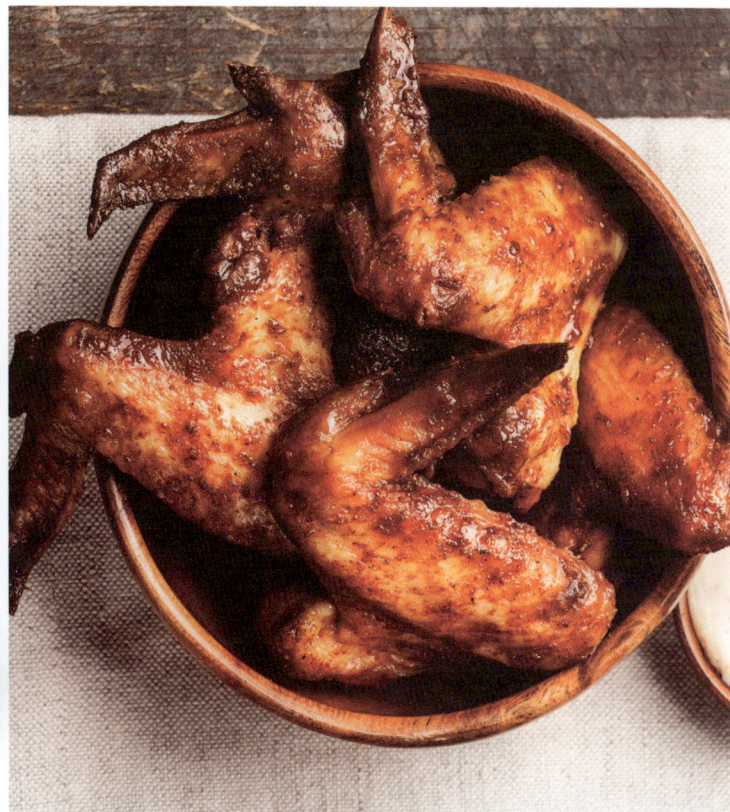

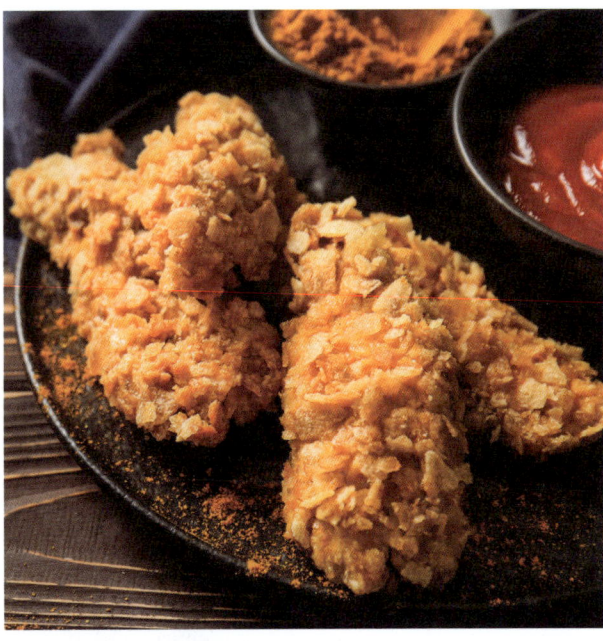

Crispy Chicken

1 egg, beaten

½ cup (60g) plain flour

1 cup (125g) panko breadcrumbs or rice crumbs

2 chicken breasts, cut into thick strips

Preheat the air fryer to 200°C.

Place the egg, flour and panko in three separate shallow bowls.

Dredge the chicken strips through the flour mixture, then into the egg, then through the panko, pressing in firmly to ensure they are covered. Spray the chicken lightly with cooking spray.

Place the chicken into the air fryer basket. Be careful not to overcrowd the basket. Cook in batches or use a double layer accessory if needed. Cook for 20 minutes, turning halfway.

SERVES 6

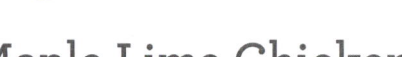

Maple Lime Chicken

6 skin-on chicken thighs

½ tsp salt

3 tbsps olive oil

1 tbsp sesame oil

5 tbsps soy sauce

1 tbsp Worcestershire sauce

1 lime, juiced (or 2 tbsps lime juice)

3 tbsps maple syrup

1 tsp garlic powder

1 tbsp onion powder

Wire rack

Place all the ingredients except for the chicken into a large mixing bowl and whisk to combine. Add the chicken and coat well using your fingers to rub the mixture into the skin.

Place chicken pieces on the wire rack with the skin-side facing up, leaving space around them so they don't touch. You may need to cook in batches.

Fry at 200°C for 10 minutes. Remove the basket and turn the chicken. Replace in the air fryer and cook for a further 10 minutes.

SERVES 6

Note: Substitute honey for maple syrup if preferred.

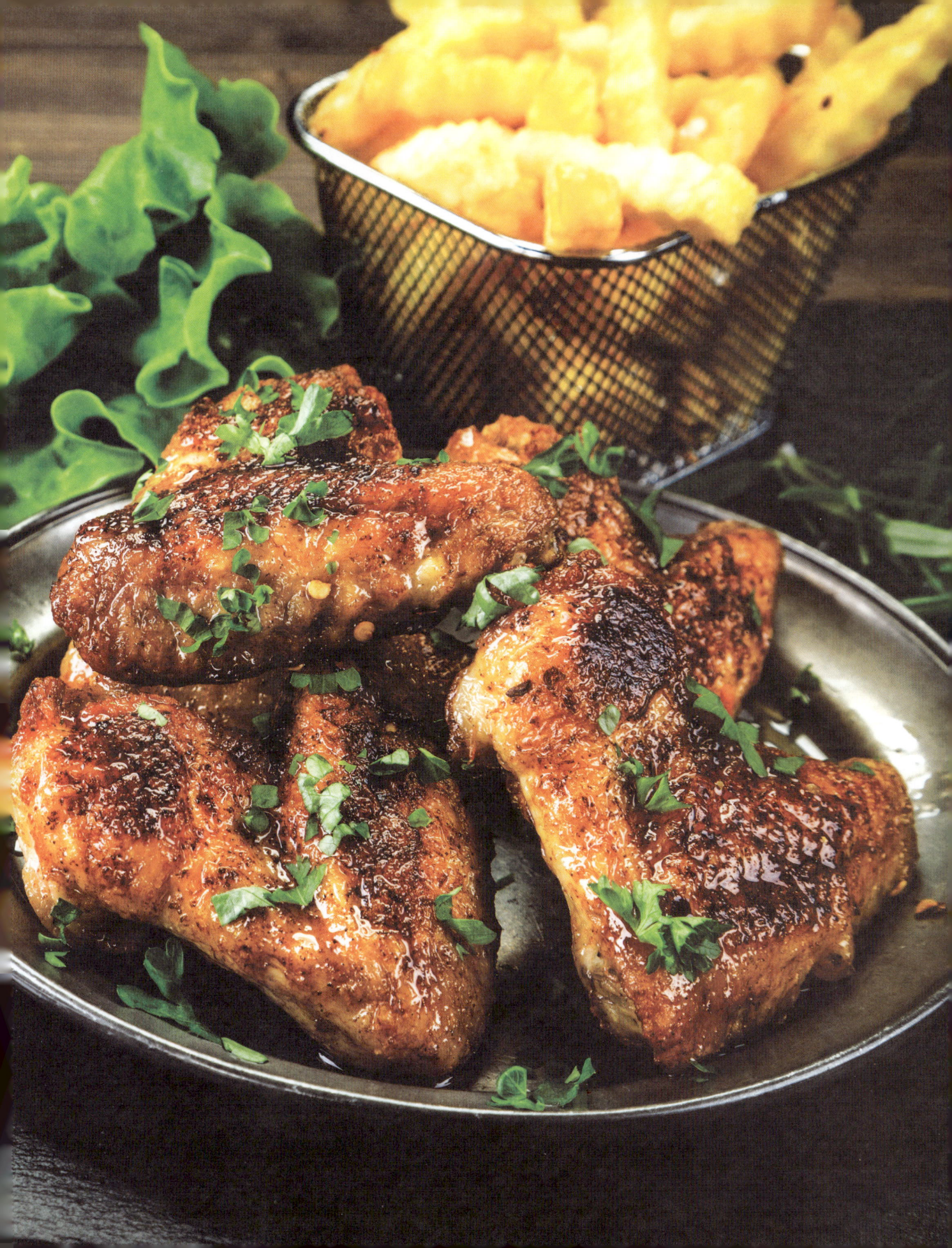

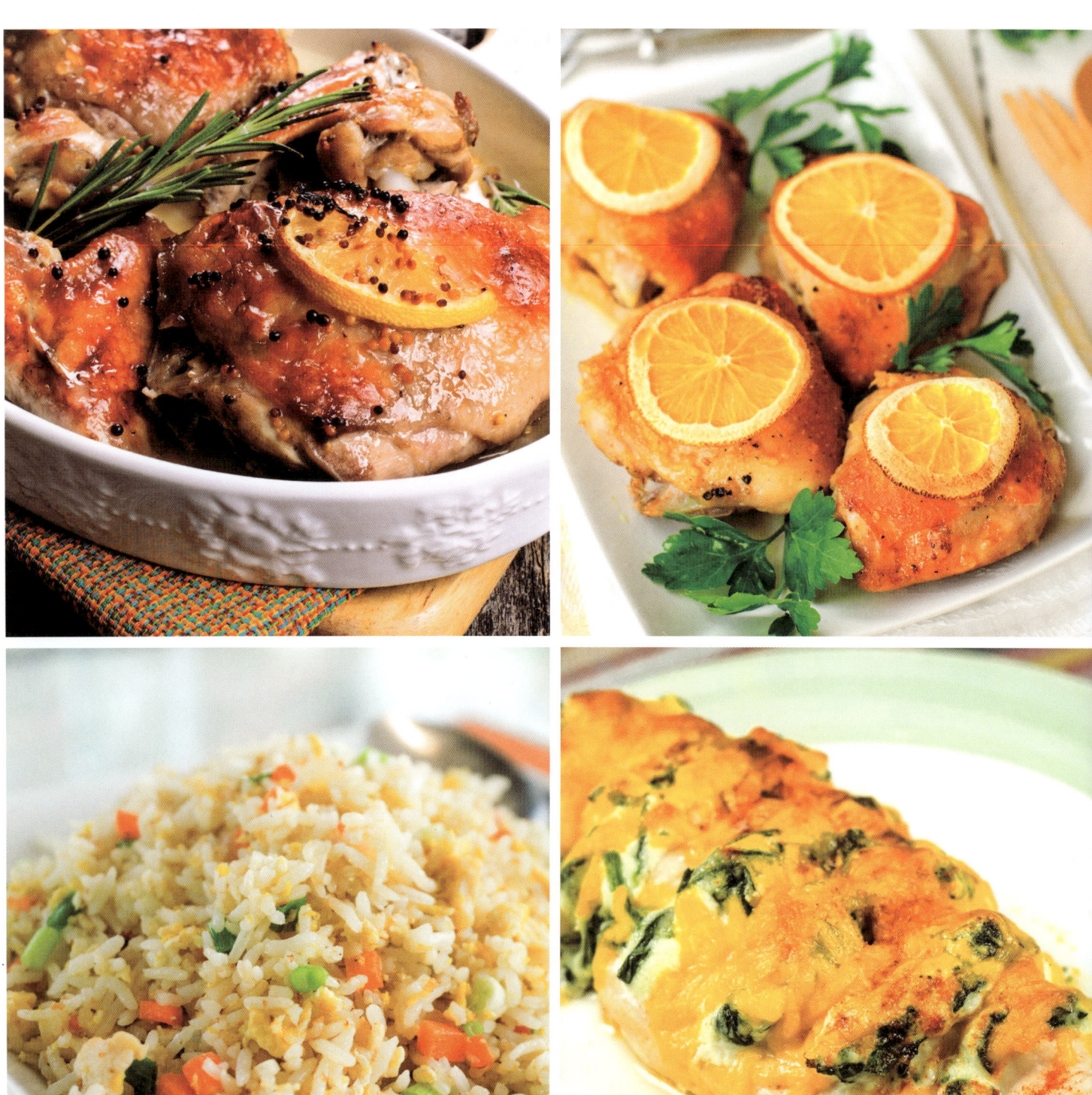

Honey Mustard Chicken

4 skin-on chicken thighs

1 packet (165g) honey mustard finishing sauce

Line the air fryer basket with foil and lay the chicken pieces skin-side up in a single layer.

Spoon the honey mustard sauce over the chicken. Cover the top with foil to bake the chicken.

Bake for 12 minutes at 200°C, then take out of the air fryer. Discard the foil and reduce temperature to 185°C. Return to cook for a further 10 minutes.

SERVES 2

Duck Breast with Orange Sauce

4 duck breasts

¾ cup (185ml) orange juice (+ 2 tbsps, if needed)

¾ cup (185ml) chicken stock

1 cup (325g) marmalade

1 tbsp cornflour (if needed)

Place the duck breasts in the air fryer basket.

Cook at 180°C for 20 minutes, turning halfway.

Meanwhile, make the sauce. Combine the orange juice, chicken stock and marmalade in a small saucepan over a high heat. Bring to a boil, then lower the heat and simmer for 15 minutes. If the mixture is too thin, then combine the cornflour with 2 tablespoons orange juice in a small bowl and stir to make a slurry. Add the slurry to the sauce and briefly return to a boil. Keep warm until ready to serve.

Drizzle the duck breasts with orange sauce to serve.

SERVES 2-4

Chicken Fried Rice

3 cups (495g) cold cooked white rice

6 tbsps soy sauce

1 tbsp vegetable oil

1 cup (170g) chopped mixed veg (frozen is fine)

1 cup (125g) cooked and sliced chicken

1 large onion, diced

1 egg

Cake tin

Preheat the fryer to 180°C.

Place the rice into a large mixing bowl. Add the soy sauce and vegetable oil and stir to combine.

Add the remaining ingredients except the egg and combine well.

Empty the mixture into the cake tin.

Place the pan into the air fryer and cook for 20 minutes. Stir a few times. Break the egg on top in the last 5 minutes and stir to combine.

SERVES 2

Hasselback Chicken

75g spinach, lightly wilted and chopped

⅓ cup (75g) ricotta

2 chicken breasts

Pinch of salt and pepper

¼ cup (20g) Cheddar cheese, grated

1 tsp paprika

Place the cooked spinach and the ricotta in a mixing bowl and combine well.

Spritz the air fryer basket with cooking spray.

Using a sharp knife, cut deep slits in the chicken breasts about 1cm apart. Place the chicken into the air fryer basket.

Spoon the spinach and ricotta mixture into the slits, pressing in well. Season the chicken with salt and pepper. Sprinkle the cheese generously over the top and dust with paprika.

Slide the basket into the air fryer and cook for 20-25 minutes at 200°C until the cheese has melted and the chicken is cooked.

SERVES 2

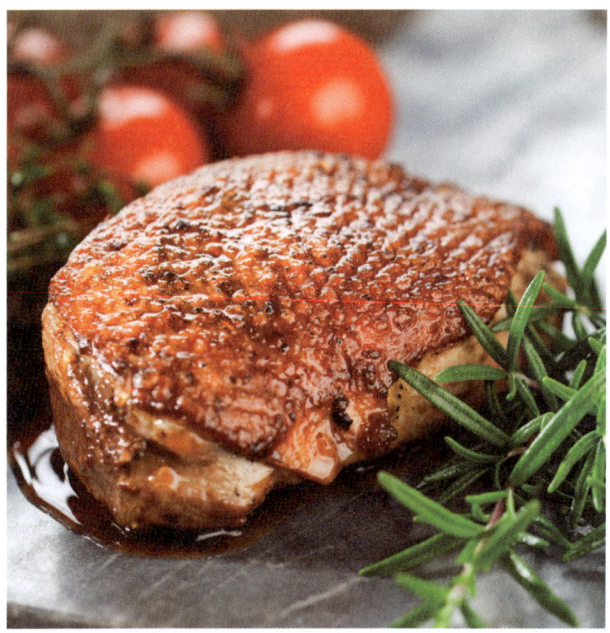

Maple Duck Breast

2 duck breasts, skin on

¼ cup (80g) maple syrup

½ tsp cayenne pepper

1 tbsp brown sugar

Pinch of salt and pepper

Using kitchen scissors or a sharp knife, trim off any extra skin around the duck breasts. The skin should just cover the meat and not overhang.

Place the duck breasts in the air fryer basket with the skin-side facing down. Cook at 180°C for 12 minutes.

Meanwhile, make the sauce. Combine the maple syrup, cayenne and brown sugar in a small saucepan over a high heat. Bring to a boil, then simmer for a few minutes. Remove from the heat and set aside.

Remove the breasts from air fryer, turn them over and baste with maple glaze. Return to cook for a further 5 minutes, until golden brown.

Remove from the air fryer and allow to rest for 5 minutes before serving.

SERVES 2

Gluten-Free Chicken Nuggets

2 eggs

¾ cup (75g) almond flour

¼ cup (40g) ground flaxseed

1 tbsp black sesame seeds

1 tsp garlic powder

1 tsp salt

⅛ tsp pepper

2 large chicken breast, cut into slices

Spritz the air fryer basket with cooking spray.

Whisk the eggs in a mixing bowl.

Place the flour, flaxseed, sesame seeds, garlic powder, salt and pepper in a second bowl and stir to combine.

Dip a slice of chicken into the egg mixture and shake off any excess. Then press into the flour mixture ensuring the chicken is well coated on all sides. Place on a plate. Repeat until all chicken is coated.

Preheat the air fryer to 200°C.

Transfer the chicken slices into the air fryer basket. (Be careful not to overcrowd the basket. Cook in batches or use a double layer accessory if needed.)

Cook for 20 minutes, turning once during cooking.

SERVES 2

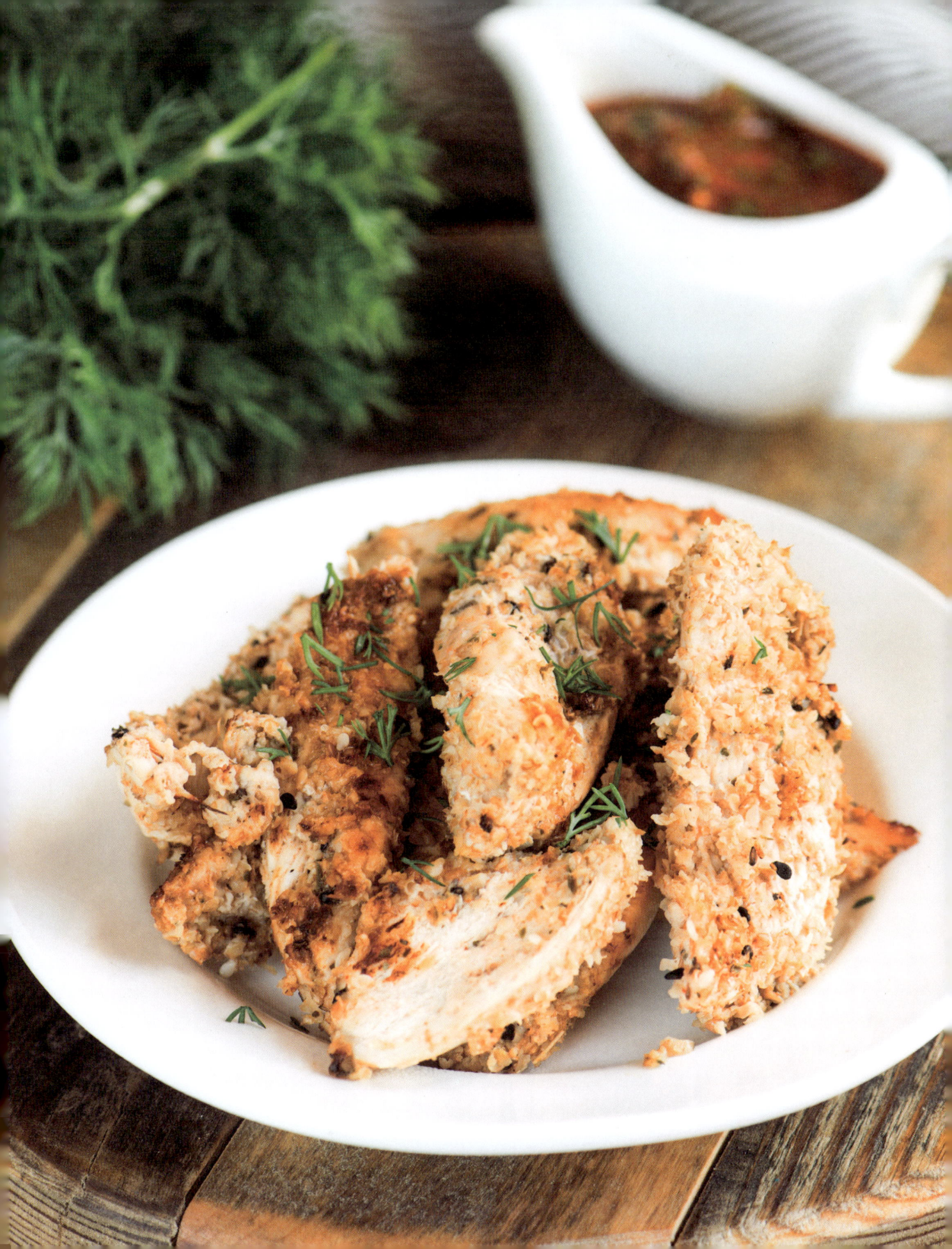

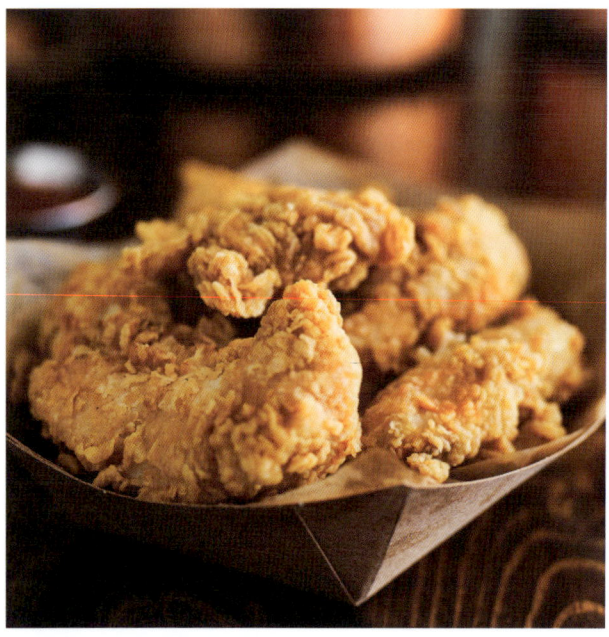

'KFC' Chicken

6 chicken pieces

2 cups (250g) breadcrumbs

¼ cup (30g) 'KFC' spice mix (see next page)

1 egg

½ cup (50g) plain flour

Pat dry the chicken pieces.

Place the breadcrumbs and spice mix in a shallow bowl.

Beat the egg in a second bowl.

Place the flour in a third shallow bowl.

Dip the chicken pieces in the egg, shaking off any excess, then dredge through the flour again shaking off excess. Roll in the breadcrumb mixture until well coated.

Cook for 20 minutes at 180°C, turning halfway through cooking.

SERVES 2-3

Traditional Southern Fried Chicken

1kg chicken pieces

¼ cup (60ml) buttermilk

¾ cup (90g) plain flour

1 packet (75g) coating mix for southern fried chicken

Salt and pepper, to taste

Place the chicken in a large bowl. Drizzle over the buttermilk and toss to coat. Cover and transfer to the fridge for 1 hour minimum (longer is better).

When you are ready to cook the chicken, begin by combining the flour, chicken coating mix, salt and pepper in a large, shallow bowl. Stir and mix well.

Dredge the chicken in seasoning mix, ensuring that both sides are fully coated.

Spritz the air fryer basket with cooking spray.

Preheat the air fryer to 200°C.

Place the chicken in the air fryer, being careful not to overcrowd the basket. Cook in batches if necessary.

Cook for a total of 20 minutes on 190°C, flipping the chicken every 5 minutes.

SERVES 4

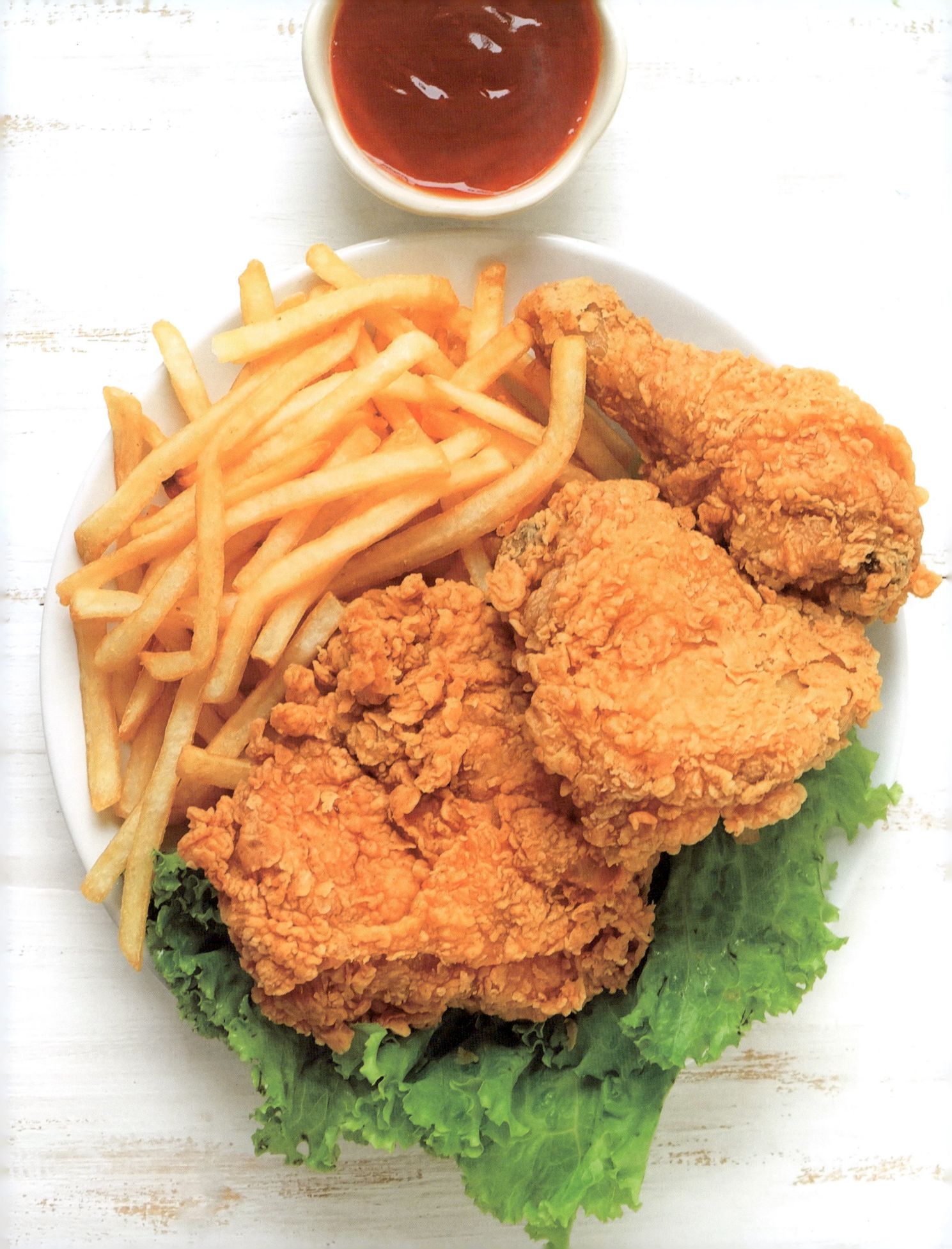

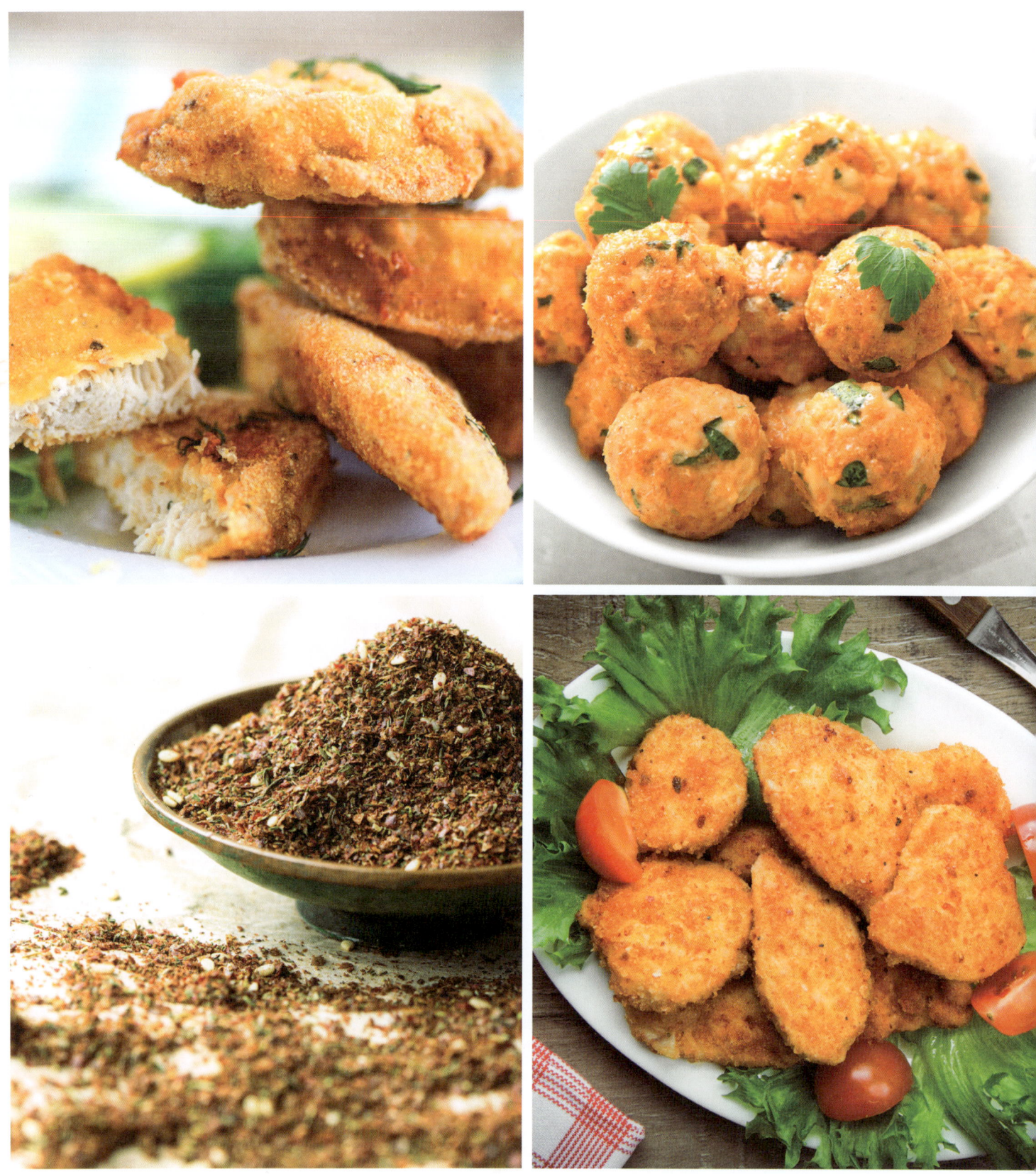

Parmesan Chicken

2 eggs

½ cup (50g) Parmesan cheese, grated

1 tsp garlic salt

1 tsp mixed herbs

½ cup (60g) breadcrumbs

500g chicken tenderloins

Preheat the air fryer to 180°C.

Beat the eggs in a small bowl.

Combine the Parmesan cheese, garlic salt, herbs and breadcrumbs in a shallow baking dish.

Dredge the chicken pieces in the egg and shake off any excess. Then dredge through the cheese and breadcrumb mixture, pressing in with your fingers.

Spritz the air fryer basket with cooking spray.

Place the chicken breasts in the air fryer – ensuring they don't overlap.

Cook for 14 minutes, shaking halfway.

SERVES 4

Chicken and Parsley Meatballs

675g chicken mince

1 egg, beaten

¾ cup (90g) Cheddar cheese, grated

½ cup (20g) fresh parsley, finely chopped

Salt and pepper, to taste

Preheat the air fryer to 200°C.

Combine all the ingredients together in a bowl.

Using your hands, roll into golf-ball-sized meatballs.

Place half the meatballs a single layer in the air fryer basket.

Cook for 8 minutes until lightly browned, shaking the basket halfway through cooking.

Repeat with the remaining meatballs.

SERVES 4

'KFC' Spice Mix

6 tsps paprika

4 tsps dried oregano

4 tsps dried tarragon

3 tsps dried parsley

3 tsps dried chives

2 tsps dried thyme

1 tsp garlic powder

1 tsp onion powder

2 tsps cayenne pepper

1 tbsp chicken seasoning

Pinch of salt and pepper

Place all the ingredients in a mixing bowl and stir well to combine. Place in a sealed jar and store in a cool place until needed.

When using as an ingredient, combine with plain flour in a ratio of 1:4. For example, 1 tablespoon of spice mix with 4 tablespoons of flour.

Perfect for chicken nuggets.

MAKES ½ CUP

Spicy Chicken Nuggets

1 chicken breast

1 egg, beaten

2 tbsps curry powder

½ cup (60g) breadcrumbs

2 tbsps vegetable oil

Preheat the air fryer to 180°C.

Cut chicken into pieces.

Place the egg in a small bowl.

Combine the curry powder, breadcrumbs and oil together in a second bowl.

Dredge the chicken breasts in the egg mixture and shake off any excess. Then dredge through the breadcrumb mixture, pressing in with your fingers.

Arrange chicken in the air fryer basket in an even layer. Cook for 12 minutes, turning once.

SERVES 1-2

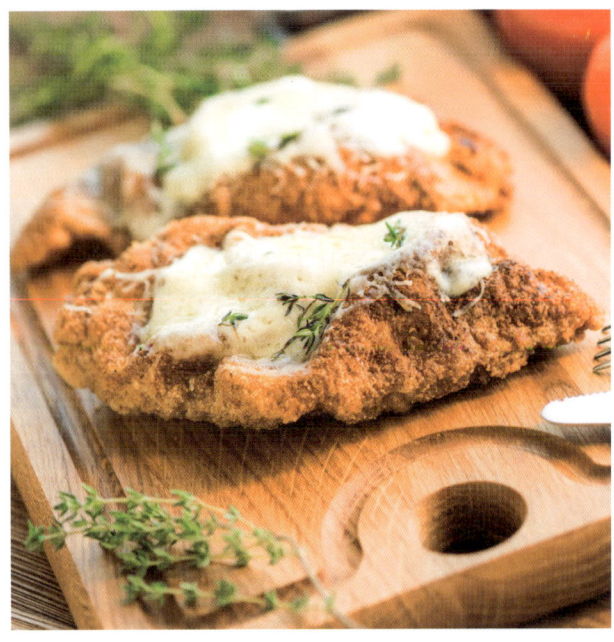

Homemade Chicken Schnitzel

½ cup (50g) Parmesan cheese, grated

1 tsp garlic salt

1 tsp mixed herbs

½ cup (60g) breadcrumbs

2 boneless chicken breasts, pounded to 3mm thickness

2 eggs, beaten

4 slices Swiss cheese

Preheat the air fryer to 180°C.

Combine the Parmesan cheese, garlic salt, herbs and breadcrumbs in a shallow baking dish. Place the egg in a second shallow dish.

Dredge the chicken breasts in the beaten egg and shake off any excess. Then dredge through the cheese and breadcrumb mixture, pressing in with your fingers.

Spritz the air fryer basket with cooking spray.

Place the chicken breasts in the air fryer in an even layer.

Cook for 6 minutes, then remove from the air fryer. Turn over the chicken pieces and place two slices of cheese on top of each. Return to cook for a further 6 minutes.

SERVES 2

Parmesan Chicken Nuggets

1 chicken breast

½ tsp salt

Pinch of pepper

115g butter

½ cup (60g) breadcrumbs

2 tbsps Parmesan cheese, grated

1 tbsp chicken seasoning

Preheat the air fryer to 200°C.

Trim any excess fat from the chicken breast, then cut into thick slices. Cut each slice into 3 or 4 nuggets. Season with salt and pepper.

Melt the butter in a small saucepan over medium heat (or in the microwave). Place melted butter in a small, shallow bowl. Combine the breadcrumbs, Parmesan and chicken seasoning and place in a second shallow bowl.

Dredge each piece of chicken in butter, then breadcrumbs.

Place in a single layer in the air fryer basket. (You may need to do multiple batches.)

Cook for 12 minutes, removing and shaking the basket halfway through.

SERVES 2

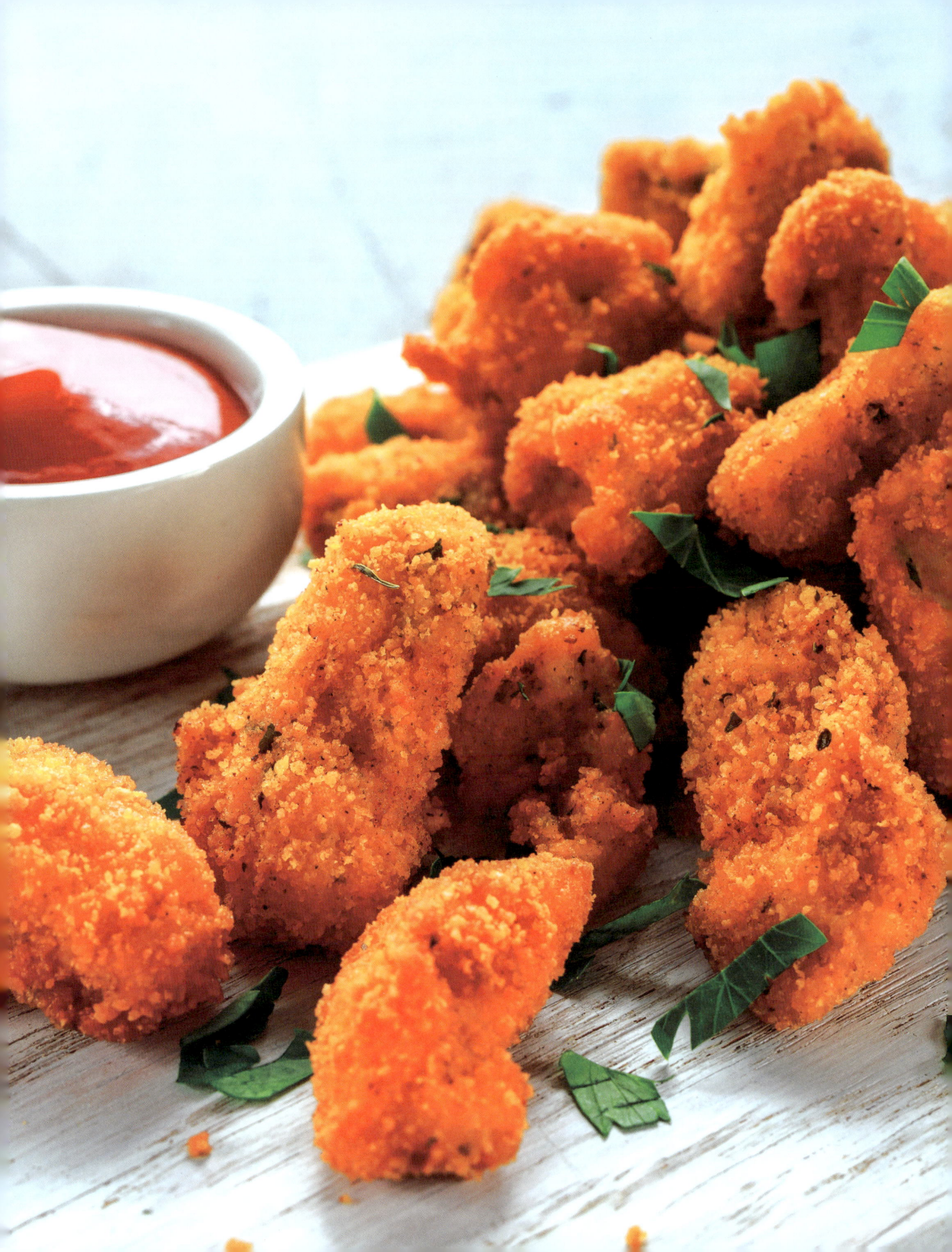

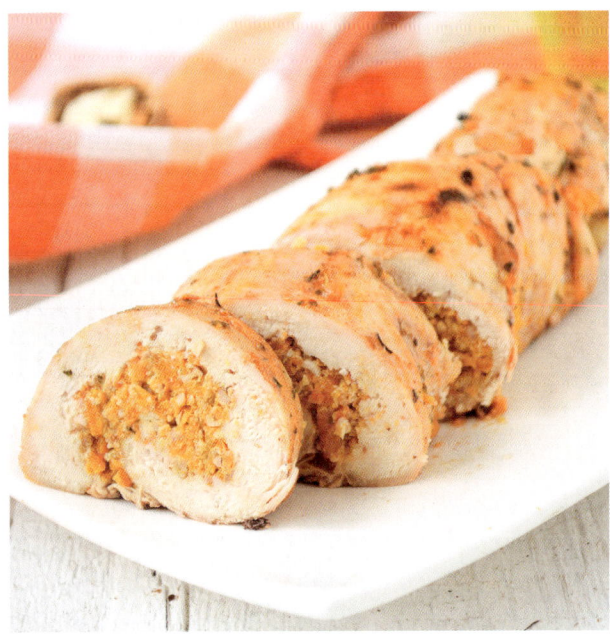

Apricot Stuffed Chicken

2 chicken breasts

Pinch of salt and pepper

1 cup (125g) breadcrumbs

¼ cup (50g) dried apricots, roughly chopped

2 tbsps pine nuts, toasted

½ lemon, zested

30g butter

½ small onion, finely diced

1 egg, beaten

Insert a sharp knife into the thick end of each chicken breast and cut across it lengthwise to create a deep pocket. Be careful not to cut through the breast. Open out the butterflied breast and season with salt and pepper.

Place the breadcrumbs, apricots, pine nuts and lemon zest in a mixing bowl and stir to combine.

Melt the butter in a small frying pan and cook the onion until soft. Transfer to the breadcrumb mixture and stir.

Spread the mixture over each opened chicken breast.

Starting with the long edge, roll the chicken up to the other side. Use one or two toothpicks to hold the roll together.

Preheat the air fryer to 180°C.

Place the stuffed chicken roll ups in the air fryer basket and spray with oil. Cook for 20 minutes, turning halfway.

SERVES 2

Bacon and Tomato Stuffed Chicken

1 tbsp olive oil

4 rashers bacon

1 small onion, finely chopped

1 clove garlic, minced

1 tomato, chopped

4 chicken breasts

Pinch of salt and pepper

2 eggs

½ cup (60g) plain flour

¼ tsp garlic powder

¼ tsp paprika

½ cup (120g) sun-dried tomato pesto

½ cup (50g) Colby cheese, grated

Heat the olive oil in a large frying pan. Cook the bacon on both sides for 1-2 minutes. Remove from the pan and set aside. Add the chopped onion to the pan and cook for 2-3 minutes on medium heat. Add the minced garlic and tomato and cook for 1 minute. Set aside to cool.

Insert a sharp knife into the thick end of each chicken breast and cut across it lengthwise to create a deep pocket. Be careful not to cut through the breast. Open the pocket and stuff with the onion mixture. Place a slice of bacon in each and season with salt and pepper.

Whisk the eggs in a shallow bowl.

In a second shallow bowl place the flour, garlic powder and paprika and mix together.

Dip each stuffed chicken breast into the flour mixture, then into the eggs, and then back into the flour mixture.

Preheat the air fryer to 200°C.

Place the chicken into the air-fryer basket. Lightly spritz with oil.

Cook for about 20 minutes, turning halfway through cooking.

Reduce temperature to 190°C. Spoon tomato pesto on top of each chicken breast and sprinkle with cheese. Cook for a further 10 minutes.

SERVES 4

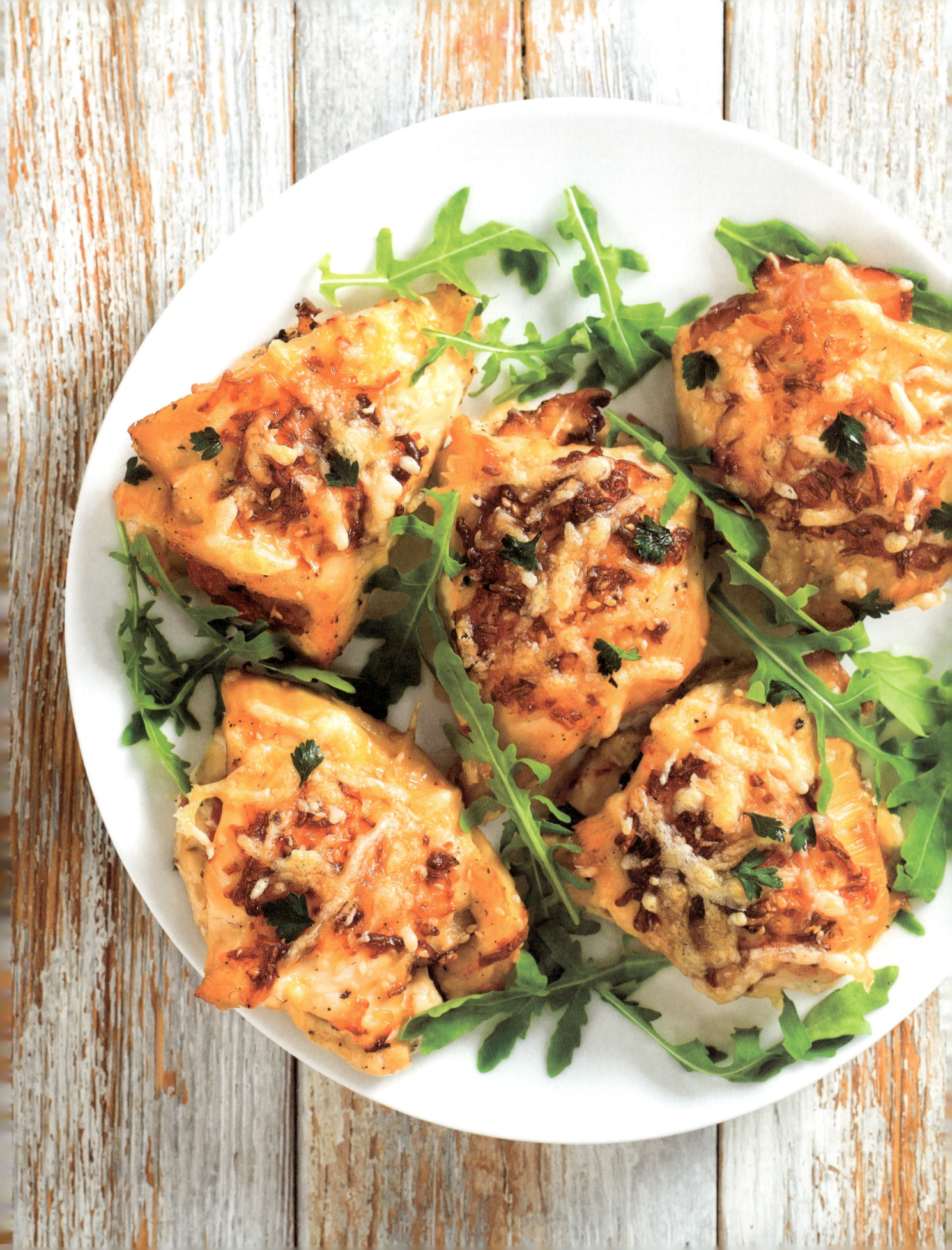

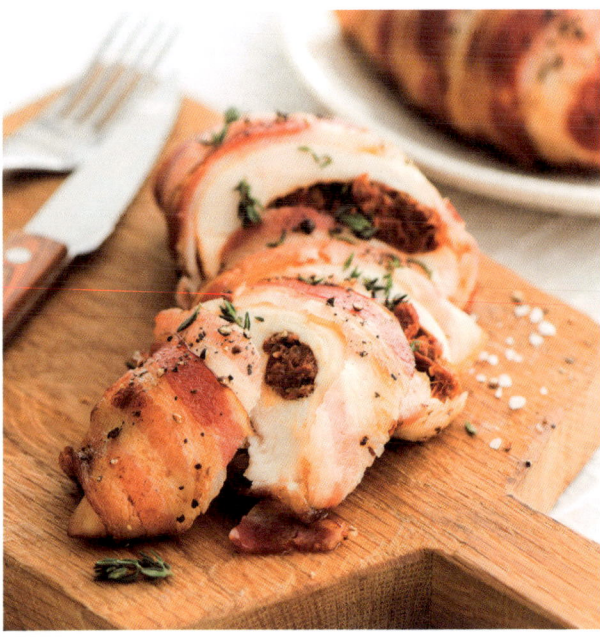

Sun-Dried Tomato Stuffed Chicken Roll Up

2 chicken breasts

Salt and pepper, to season

2 tbsps tahini

6-8 rashers bacon

1 cup (240g) sun-dried tomato pesto

Place a piece of plastic wrap over the chicken breast and gently pound it with a meat mallet to create an even thickness. Flatten to approximately ¼-inch thickness. Season with salt and pepper. Spread the tahini chicken on the chicken, then spoon on the sun-dried tomato pesto.

Starting with the long edge of the chicken breast, roll the chicken up to the other side then wrap strips of bacon around the chicken roll. Use one or two toothpicks to hold the roll together.

Preheat the air fryer to 180°C.

Place the stuffed chicken roll ups in the air fryer basket and cook for 20 minutes, turning halfway.

SERVES 2

Parmesan-Crusted Chicken Cordon Bleu

2 chicken breasts

½ tsp salt

¼ tsp pepper

1 tbsp Dijon mustard

4 slices Swiss cheese

4 slices thick-cut ham

1 tsp dried oregano

¼ cup (30g) plain flour

1 egg, beaten

¾ cup (90g) breadcrumbs

⅓ cup (30g) Parmesan cheese, grated

Place a piece of plastic wrap over the chicken breast and gently pound it with a meat mallet to create an even thickness. Flatten to approximately ¼-inch thickness. Season with salt and pepper.

Spread the Dijon mustard on the chicken. Layer one slice of cheese on top of the mustard, then top with two slices of ham and another slice of cheese. Sprinkle with oregano.

Starting with the long edge of the chicken breast, roll the chicken up to the other side. Use one or two toothpicks to hold the roll together.

Preheat the air fryer to 180°C.

Place the flour in a shallow dish. Place the beaten egg in a second shallow dish. Combine the breadcrumbs and Parmesan cheese together in a third shallow dish.

Dredge the stuffed and rolled chicken breasts in the flour and then the beaten egg, shaking off any excess. Roll in the breadcrumbs-cheese mixture, pressing in with fingers to ensure they are well covered. Spray with olive oil and transfer to the air fryer basket.

Cook for 20 minutes, turning the chicken roll over halfway through the cooking time.

SERVES 2

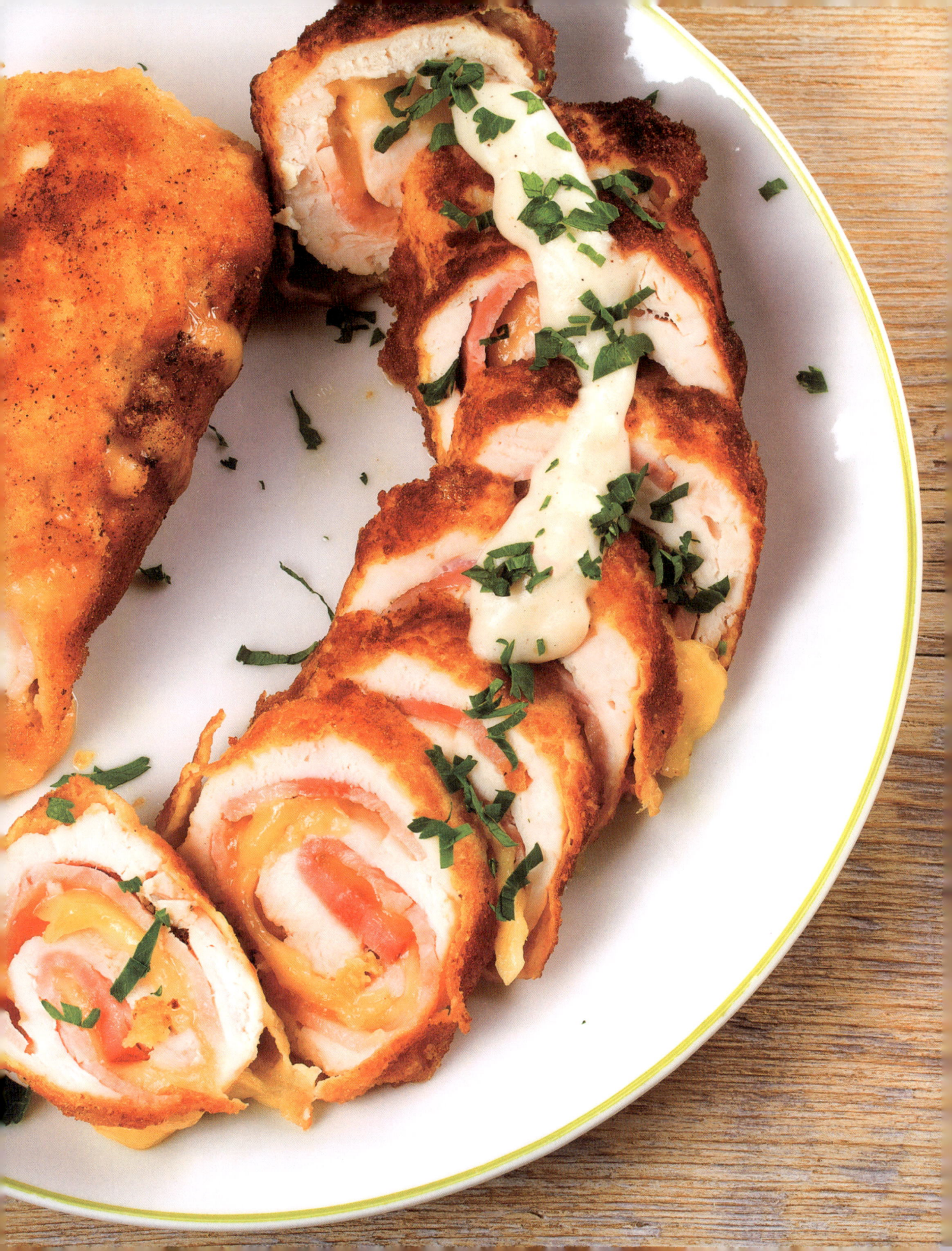

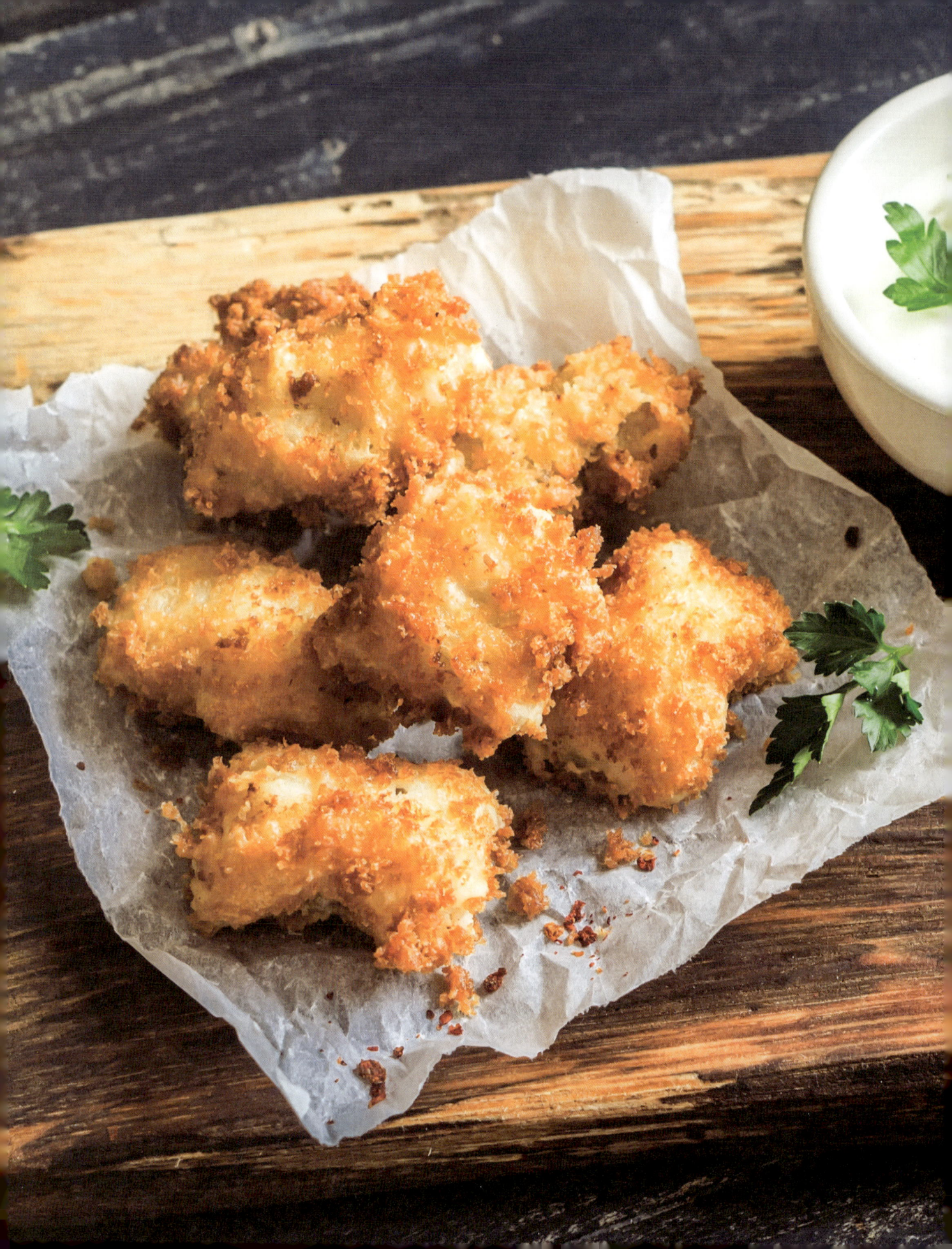

Seafood

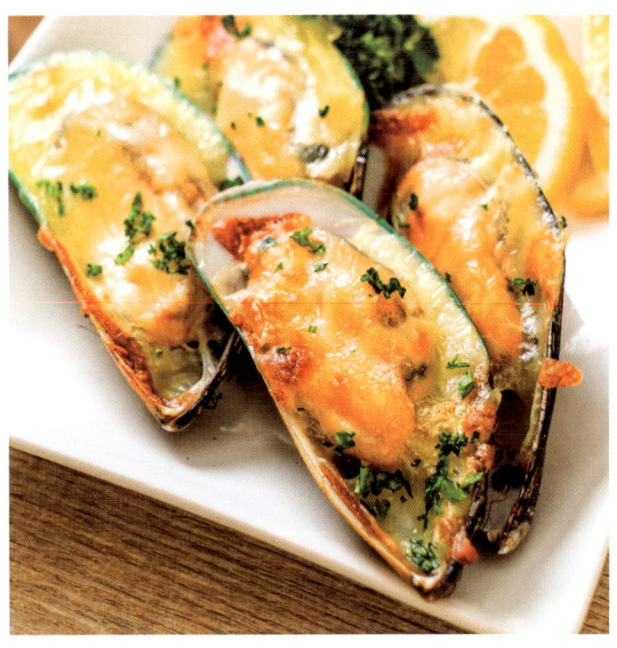

Cheesy Mussels

60g unsalted butter, melted

1 tbsp panko breadcrumbs

1 clove garlic, minced

½ tsp salt

¼ tsp pepper

2 tbsps parsley, finely chopped

10 mussels on the half shell

¼ cup (25g) Parmesan cheese, finely grated

Combine the butter, panko, garlic, salt, pepper and parsley in a small bowl and whisk together.

Pour the mixture evenly on top of the open mussels.

Place the mussels in the air-fryer cook for 7 minutes at 180°C. Remove from the air fryer and sprinkle the cheese on top. Return to the air fryer for 3 minutes.

SERVES 2

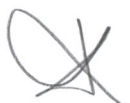

Oysters Kilpatrick

2 rashers thick-cut bacon

2 tbsps butter, melted

4 tbsps balsamic vinegar

2 tbsps Worcestershire sauce

1 dash of Tabasco sauce

16 oysters (shucked)

Lemon wedges, to serve

Grill or fry the bacon in a frying pan. Slice into small strips.

Preheat the air fryer to 180°C.

Combine the butter, vinegar, Worcestershire sauce and Tabasco sauce in a small bowl.

Pour a tablespoon of the sauce over each oyster, then sprinkle on a few strips of bacon. Finish by pouring any remaining sauce over the top.

Cook for 10 minutes.

SERVES 4

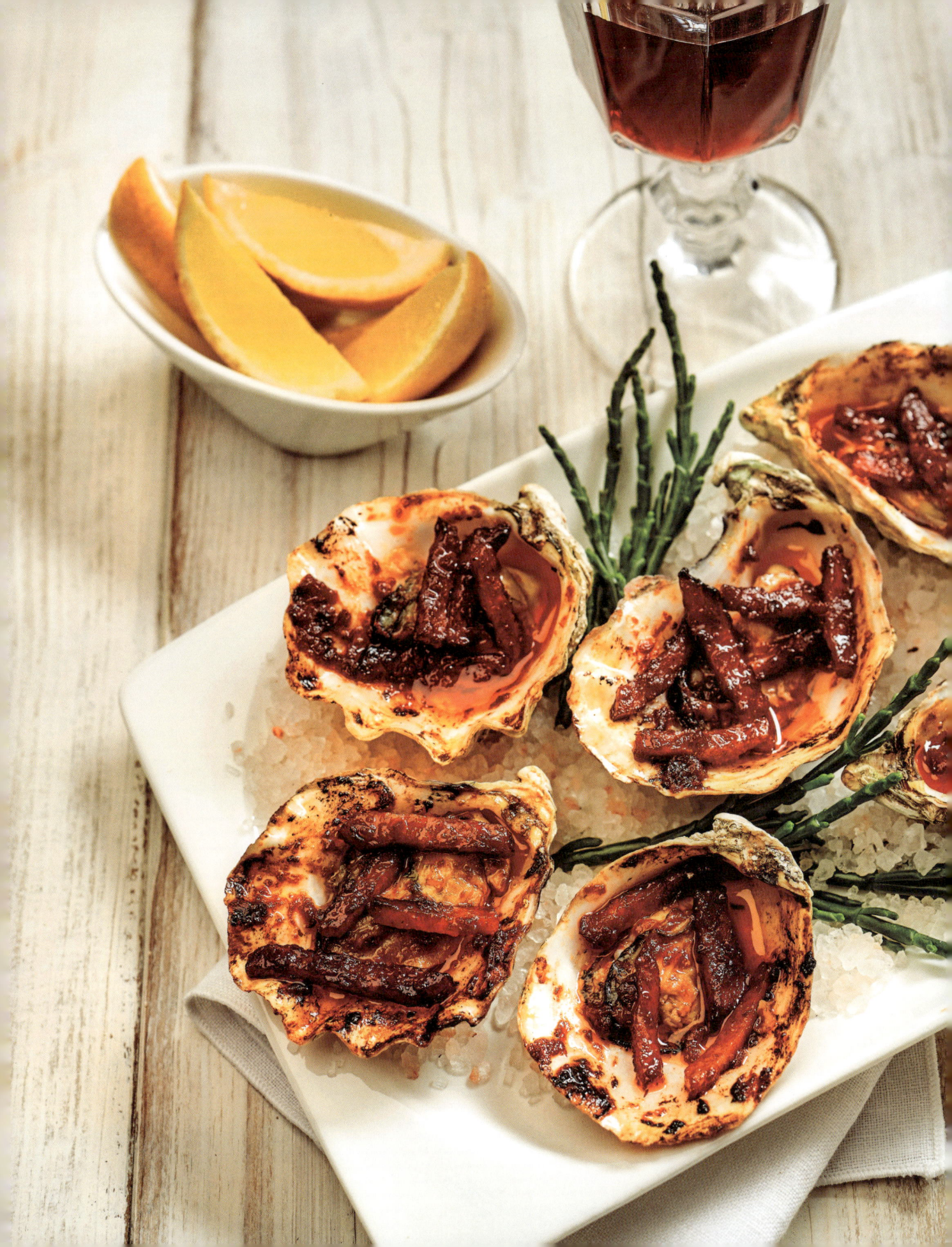

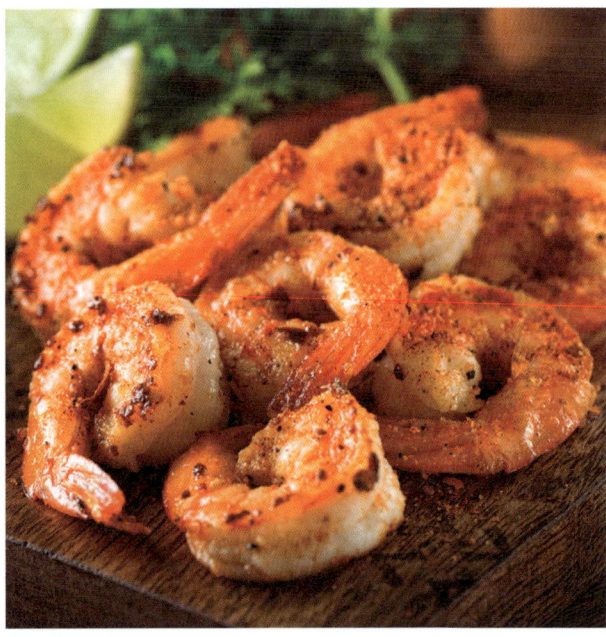

Salt and Pepper Prawns

1 tsp black peppercorns

1 tsp Sichuan peppercorns

½ tsp salt

½ tsp sugar

300g raw prawn meat (frozen)

1 tbsp rice flour

2 tsps oil

Toast and grind the peppercorns using a spice grinder (or pestle and mortar). Allow to cool slightly.

Add the salt and sugar to the grinder and pulse until a coarse powder forms.

Place the prawns in a large bowl. Add the spice mix, rice flour and oil and toss until prawns are fully coated.

Preheat the air fryer to 190°C.

Place the prawns in the air fryer basket in a single layer. (Be careful not to overcrowd the basket. Cook in batches or use a double layer accessory if needed.)

Spray with oil.

Cook for 4-6 minutes, shaking the basket once or twice during cooking.

SERVES 2

Note: You can use fresh prawns in this recipe if you prefer.

Garlic Butter Prawns

125g butter, just melted

5 cloves garlic, minced

1 tsp fresh parsley + more to garnish

½ lemon, juiced

1kg king prawns, tails intact

Salt and pepper, to season

Combine the butter, garlic, parsley and lemon juice in a large bowl. Set aside.

Peel, devein and rinse the prawns, and then pat dry using paper towels to remove any moisture.

Cut the outside edge and open the prawns up. Press down gently.

Place the prawns in the mixing bowl with the butter mixture and toss to ensure that they are evenly coated. Generously season the prawns with salt and pepper.

Preheat the air fryer to 200°C.

Arrange the prawns in the basket in an even layer, making sure they are not crowded.

Cook for 6-8 minutes, until bright pink and cooked through.

Serve with lemon slices.

SERVES 3

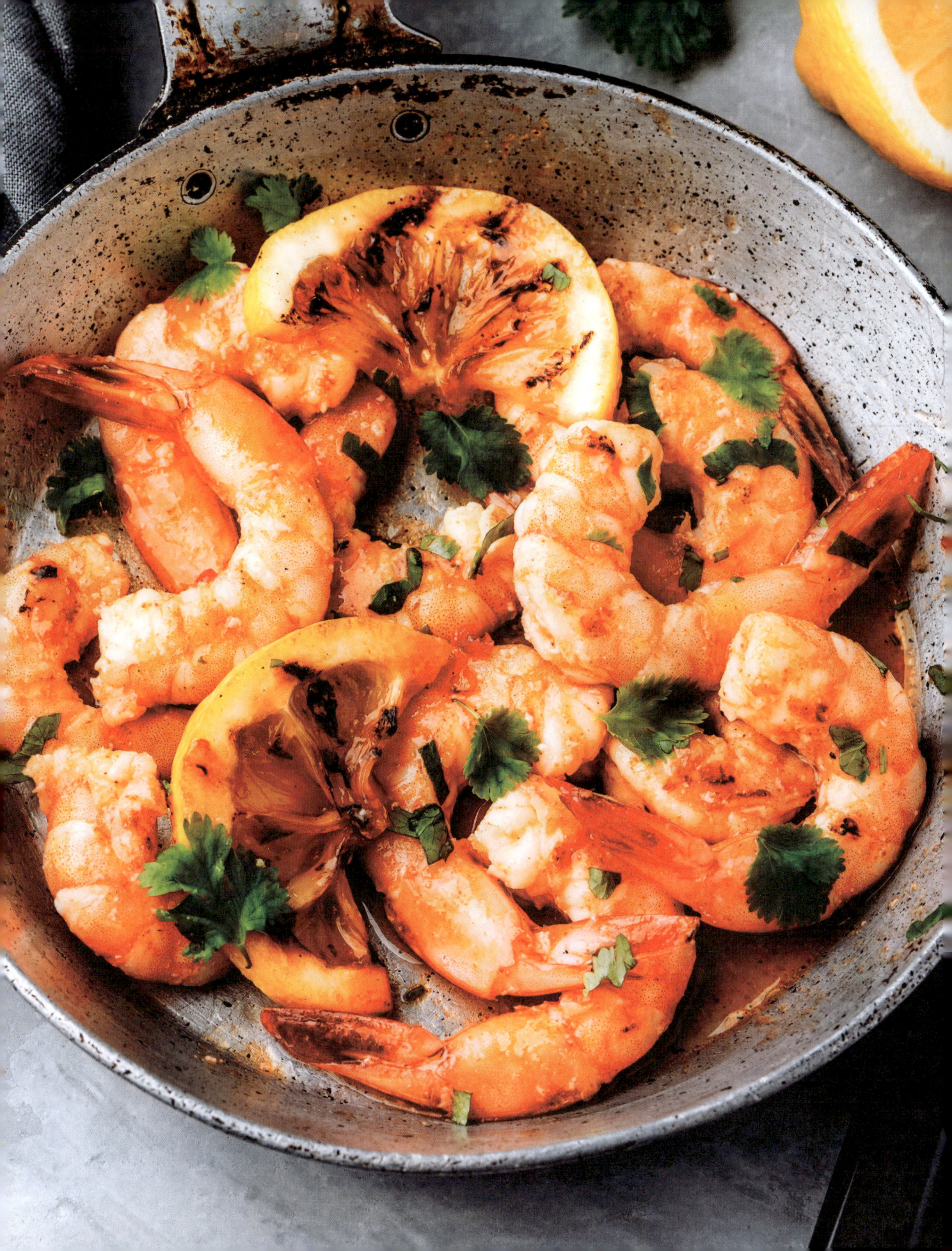

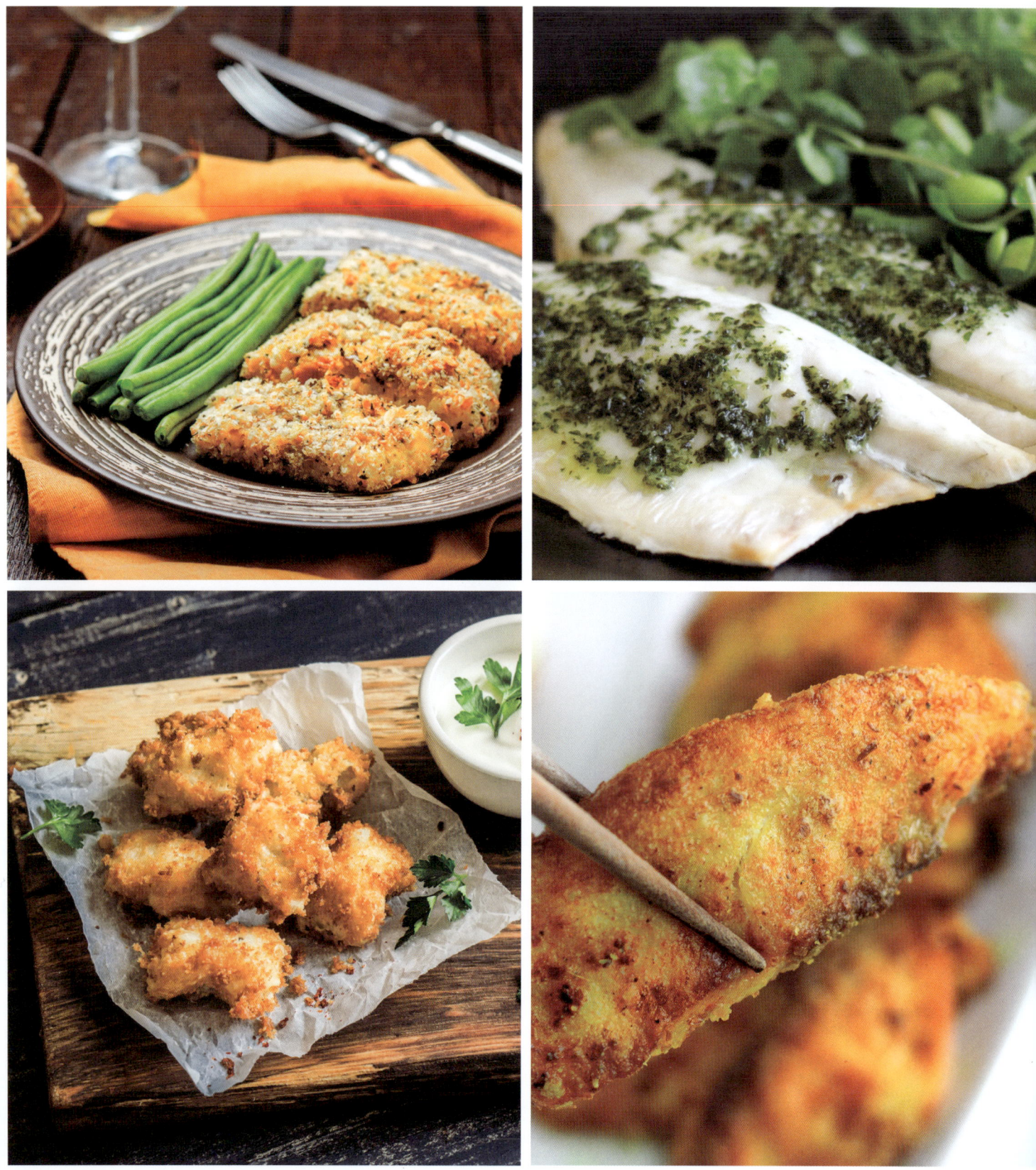

Crumbed Fish

4 tbsps vegetable oil

¾ cup (100g) breadcrumbs

1 tbsp mixed herbs

Pinch of salt and pepper

1 egg, beaten

4 white fish fillets (such as snapper)

Preheat the air fryer to 180°C.

Mix the oil, breadcrumbs, mixed herbs, salt and pepper together until the mixture is crumbly. Transfer to a shallow bowl or plate.

Place the egg in a shallow bowl.

Dredge the fish fillets into the egg, shaking off any excess. Dredge the fish fillets into the crumb mixture. pressing in to ensure even and full coverage.

Spritz the air fryer basket with cooking spray, then lay the fillets in the air fryer basket and cook for 12 minutes.

SERVES 4

Fish with Pesto Sauce

3 white fish fillets (such as snapper)

1 tsp salt

Pinch of pepper

1 bunch fresh basil, leaves picked

3 cloves garlic

¼ cup (35g) pine nuts

1 tbsp Parmesan cheese, grated

1 cup (250ml) extra virgin olive oil

1 tbsp lemon juice

Preheat the air fryer to 180°C.

Lightly spritz fish with oil and season with salt and pepper. Place in the air fryer basket and cook for 8 minutes.

Place the basil leaves, garlic, pine nuts, Parmesan cheese, olive oil and lemon juice in a food processor. Process until a coarse sauce consistency is reached.

Serve fish drizzled with the pesto sauce.

SERVES 3

Fish Nuggets

1 cup (30g) cornflake crumbs

1 tbsp vegetable oil

2 white fish fillets (such as snapper)

Salt and pepper, to season

½ cup (60g) flour

1 egg, beaten

Pulse cornflakes and vegetable oil in a food processor until a rough crumb forms. Place in a shallow bowl. Place the flour in a second shallow bowl. Place the egg in a third.

Preheat the air fryer to 180°C.

Cut the fish into nuggets (approximately 12). Season with salt and pepper then dredge in the flour, shaking off any excess. Dip into the egg and then into the crumbs, pressing in to ensure even and full coverage.

Place half the nuggets in the basket (or use a double layer accessory) and cook for 15 minutes. Repeat with the remaining half.

SERVES 2

Turmeric Fish

4 small white fish fillets (such as flathead)

1 tbsp olive oil

½ tsp salt

1 tsp turmeric powder

Pat fish dry using a paper towel.

Rub olive oil into the fillets. Next rub the salt and turmeric into the flesh. Cover and transfer to the fridge to marinate for 30 minutes.

Preheat the air fryer to 180°C.

Place the fish in an even layer in the air fryer basket. Cook for 5 minutes. Increase the temperature of the air fryer to 200°C and cook for a further 7 minutes.

SERVES 4

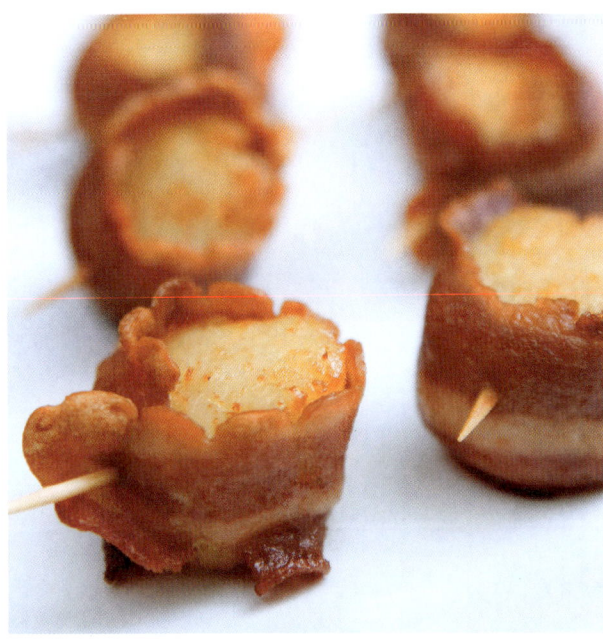

Bacon-Wrapped Scallops

8 rashers bacon

10 scallops

1 tbsp lemon juice

1 tsp balsamic vinegar

Cut the bacon rashers in half lengthwise, trimming off any extra fat.

Wrap the bacon around each scallop and pierce the scallop with a toothpick from one side through to the other side, keeping the bacon in place.

Preheat the air fryer to 200°C.

Place five scallops in the basket, leaving space between them.

Cook for 12 minutes, turning halfway during cooking.

Remove from the air fryer and cover with foil to keep warm. Repeat with the remaining five scallops.

Drizzle with balsamic and lemon juice to serve.

SERVES 2

Fish Tacos

2 white fish fillets (such as snapper)

⅓ cup (35g) spice mix for soft tacos

4 tortillas

¼ cup (70g) salsa

1 cup (100g) red cabbage, sliced

1 avocado, sliced

1 tbsp fresh parsley, chopped

1 cup (200g) avocado dip

1 lemon, juiced

Prepare the fish by cleaning and cutting into four small fillets.

Place the seasoning mix in a large plastic bag and then add the fish. Seal the bag and gently rub the seasoning mix into the flesh of the fish.

Preheat the air fryer to 180°C.

Cook the fish for 10 minutes.

To serve place each fish piece inside a tortilla, then top with salsa, red cabbage, avocado, fresh parsley and avocado dip. Squeeze over the fresh lemon juice to serve.

SERVES 2 (MAKES 4)

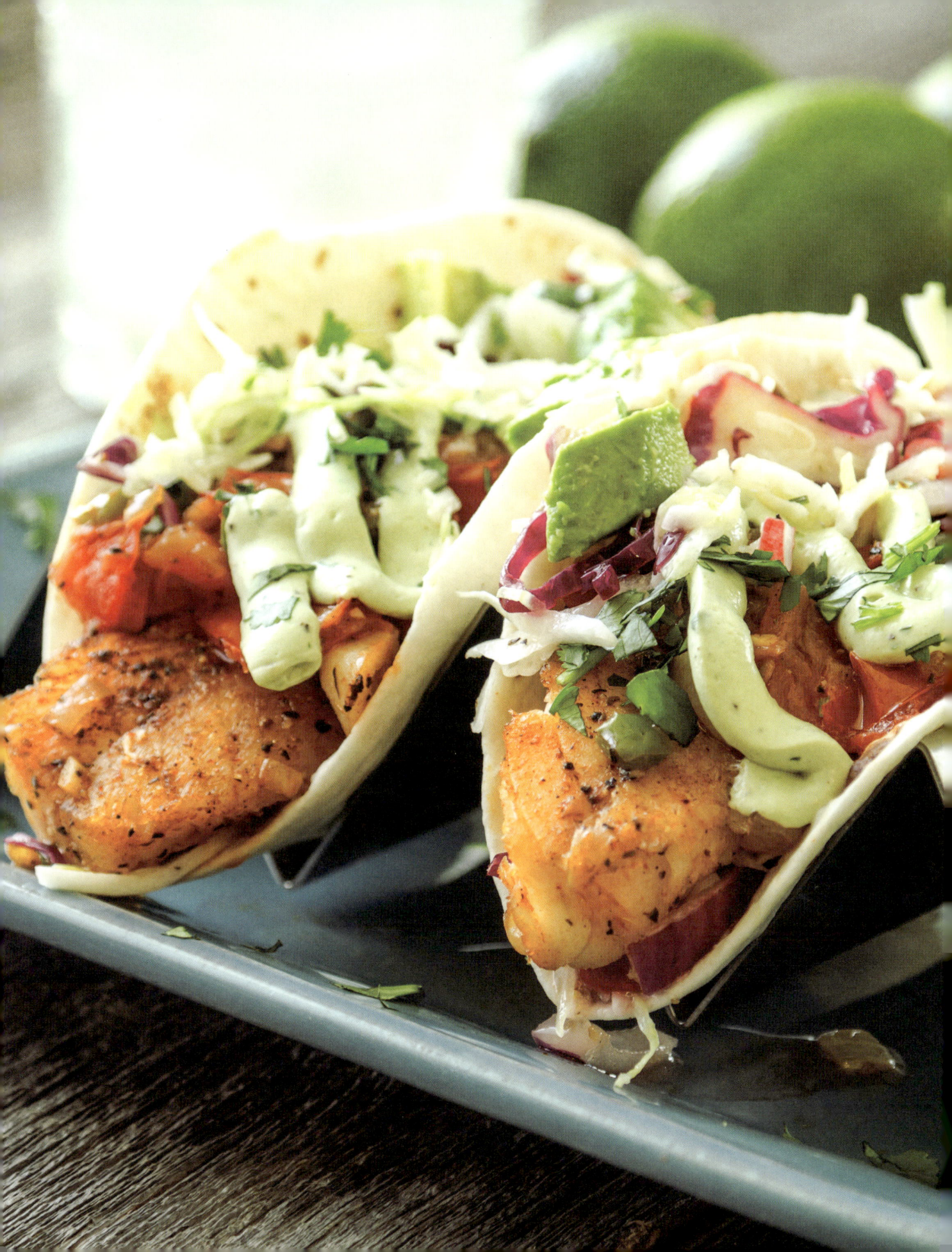

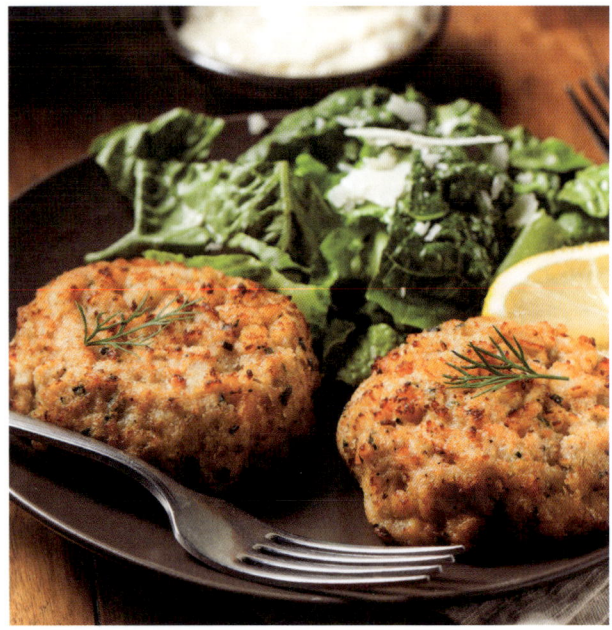

Crab Cakes

1 cup (125g) breadcrumbs + ½ cup (60g) breadcrumbs

1 onion, diced

1 egg

2 tbsps fresh dill (or 1 tbsp dried)

2 tbsps mayonnaise

1 tsp Worcestershire sauce

1 tbsp all-purpose seasoning

½ tsp Dijon mustard

¼ tsp salt

140g fresh crab meat

Combine 1 cup breadcrumbs, onion, egg, dill, mayonnaise, Worcestershire sauce, seasoning, Dijon mustard and salt in a large mixing bowl. Add the crab meat and gently stir to combine.

Place the remaining breadcrumbs on a plate.

Shape the crab mixture into patties and press each patty into the breadcrumbs, coating both sides.

Cover and place in the refrigerator for 1 hour.

Preheat air fryer to 180°C.

Spray crab patties on both sides and place in the basket of the air fryer.

Cook for 15 minutes until crisp on the outside and cooked through.

SERVES 2

Thai Fish Cakes

1 white fish fillet (such as snapper)

Milk, for poaching (approximately 2 cups)

125g frozen chopped spinach, drained

1½ cups (390g) mashed potatoes

2 tbsps red curry paste

½ cup (60g) breadcrumbs

Sweet chilli sauce, to serve

Place the fish in a large pan and cover with milk. Bring milk just to the boil and then reduce the heat to low and cover the pan. Cook for 7 minutes until fish is cooked. Drain and set aside. Retain the poaching liquid if desired for use in other recipes.

When cooled slightly, place the fish in a large mixing bowl. Add the drained spinach, mashed potato and red curry paste and stir to fully combine.

Place breadcrumbs on a shallow bowl.

Shape the into patties and press each patty into the breadcrumbs, coating both sides.

Cover and place in the refrigerator for 2 hours.

Preheat air fryer to 180°C.

Cook for 15 minutes until crisp on the outside and cooked through.

Serve with sweet chilli sauce.

SERVES 2

Note: Make a poaching liquid of half milk and half water if you prefer.

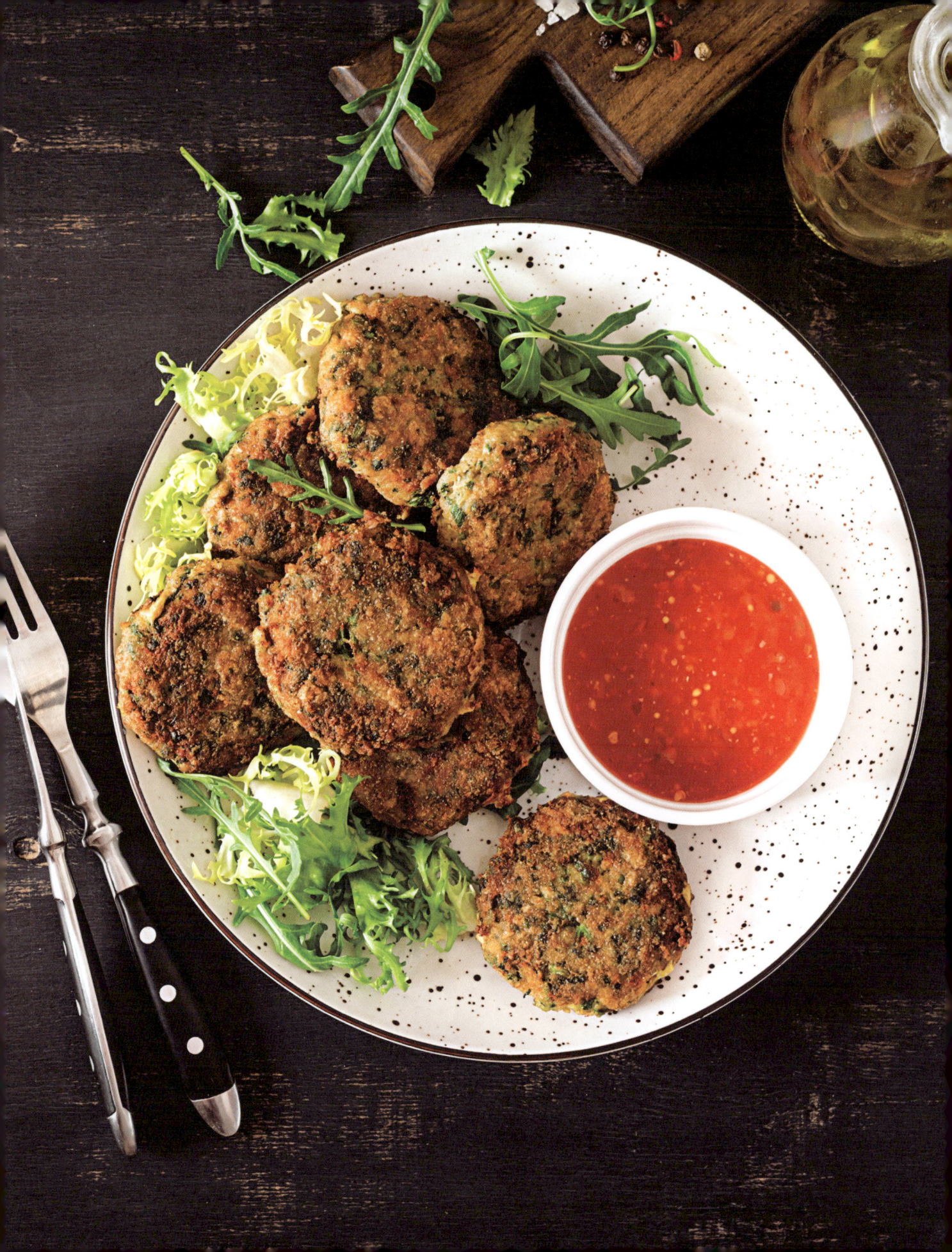

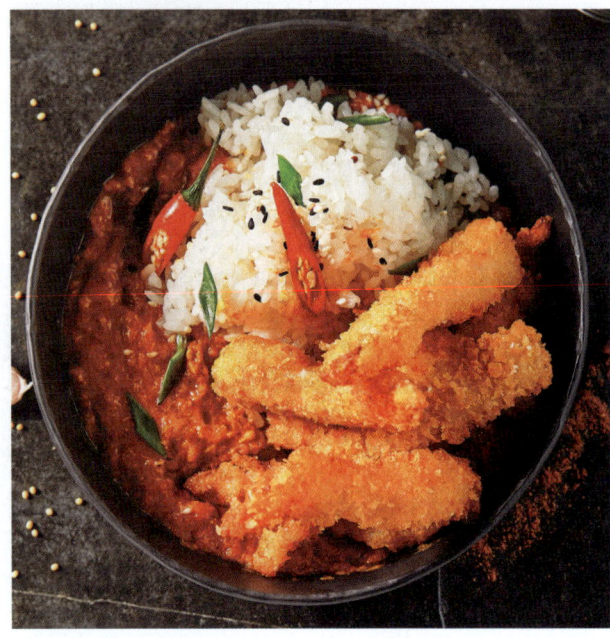

Coconut Prawns

½ cup (60g) plain flour

2 eggs

1 cup (90g) desiccated coconut

⅓ cup (40g) panko breadcrumbs

450g green king prawns, peeled and deveined

Place the flour in a shallow bowl.

Beat the eggs in a shallow bowl.

Combine the coconut and breadcrumbs in a third bowl.

Dip the prawns first into the flour, then into the eggs, shaking off any excess. Next press into the panko mixture, being sure to fully coat each prawn.

Preheat the air fryer to 200°C.

Spritz the air fryer basket with cooking spray.

Spray the prawns generously with olive oil spray.

Cook for 6 minutes, turning halfway through cooking.

SERVES 2

Crispy Chilli Fish

2 white fish fillets (such as snapper)

1 tbsp olive oil

1 cup (125g) breadcrumbs

½ tsp paprika

¼ tsp chilli powder

¼ tsp pepper

¼ tsp garlic powder

¼ tsp onion powder

½ tsp salt

Preheat the air fryer to 200°C.

Drizzle the fish fillets with olive oil and rub in to fully coat the fish.

Place the breadcrumbs, paprika, chilli powder, pepper, garlic powder, onion powder and salt in a shallow bowl and stir to combine.

Place egg in a small bowl and whisk.

Dip each fillet in the egg, shaking off the excess, and then press into the breadcrumb mixture so that the fish is fully coated.

Transfer to the air fryer and cook for 14 minutes, turning halfway.

SERVES 2

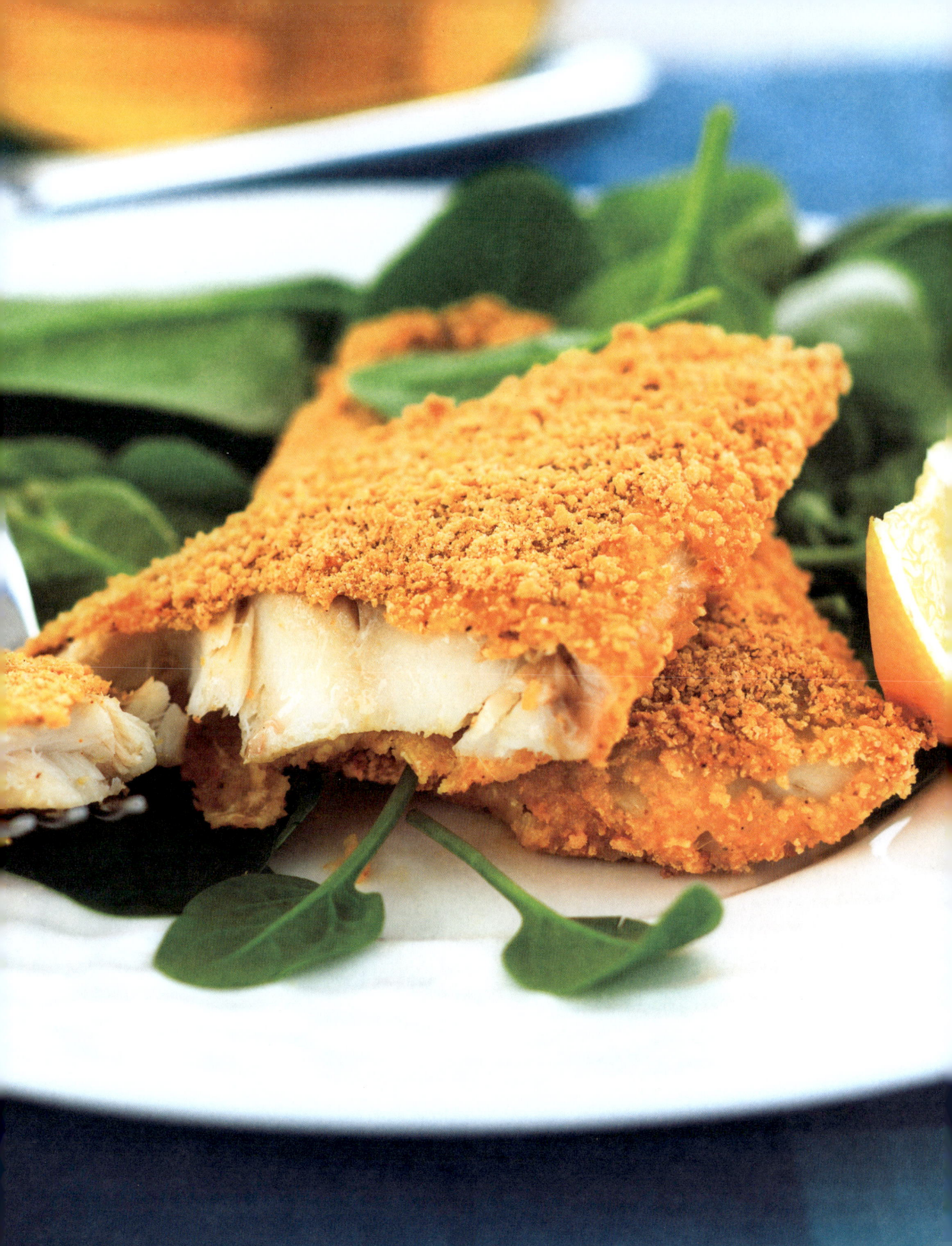

Baked Lemon Salmon

2 medium salmon fillets, bones removed

1 tsp dried dill

½ tsp salt

Pinch of pepper

1 tsp lemon rind, finely grated

Preheat the air fryer to 180°C.

Spray the salmon with oil and gently rub into the flesh. Sprinkle with dill, salt, pepper and lemon rind.

Place salmon in the air fryer basket. Cook for 8 minutes.

Check the salmon with a fork to make sure it's cooked to your preference. Cook for an additional minute or longer as needed.

SERVES 2

Herbed Salmon Patties

1 x 415g can salmon

1 egg

2 spring onions, finely sliced

½ cup (60g) breadcrumbs

1 tbsp mixed herbs

Empty the canned salmon into a sieve. Drain off any fluid and check for small bones.

Place the salmon in a large mixing bowl. Add the egg, spring onion, breadcrumbs and mixed herbs. Stir well to combine.

Preheat air fryer to 200°C.

Shape the mixture into patties.

Place patties in the air fryer. (Cook in batches if necessary.)

Cook for 10 minutes, flipping halfway through cooking.

SERVES 2

Ahi Tuna Steaks

2 yellowfin tuna steaks

2 tbsps soy sauce

1 tbsp toasted sesame oil

1 tbsp runny honey

½ tsp salt

¼ tsp pepper

Rinse the tuna steaks.

Place the other ingredients in a small bowl and whisk together until honey has dissolved. Pour into a large ziplock bag.

Add the tuna steaks to the bag and gently rub the sauce into the flesh. Marinate in the fridge for 1 hour or proceed to the next step.

Transfer to the air fryer basket.

Cook at 170°C for 7 minutes (for rare) or 8 minutes (for medium) then remove and allow to rest for a few minutes before serving.

SERVES 2

Cajun Salmon

1 salmon fillet

1 tbsp Cajun seasoning (or enough to fully coat)

½ tsp salt

1 tsp brown sugar

Preheat the air fryer to 180°C.

Pat fish dry using paper towel.

Lightly spray the fish with olive oil. Sprinkle over the seasoning, salt and sugar.

Place skin-side down in the air fryer basket or grill pan accessory. Cook for 8 minutes.

Check the salmon with a fork to make sure it's cooked to your preference. Cook for an additional minute or longer as needed.

SERVES 1

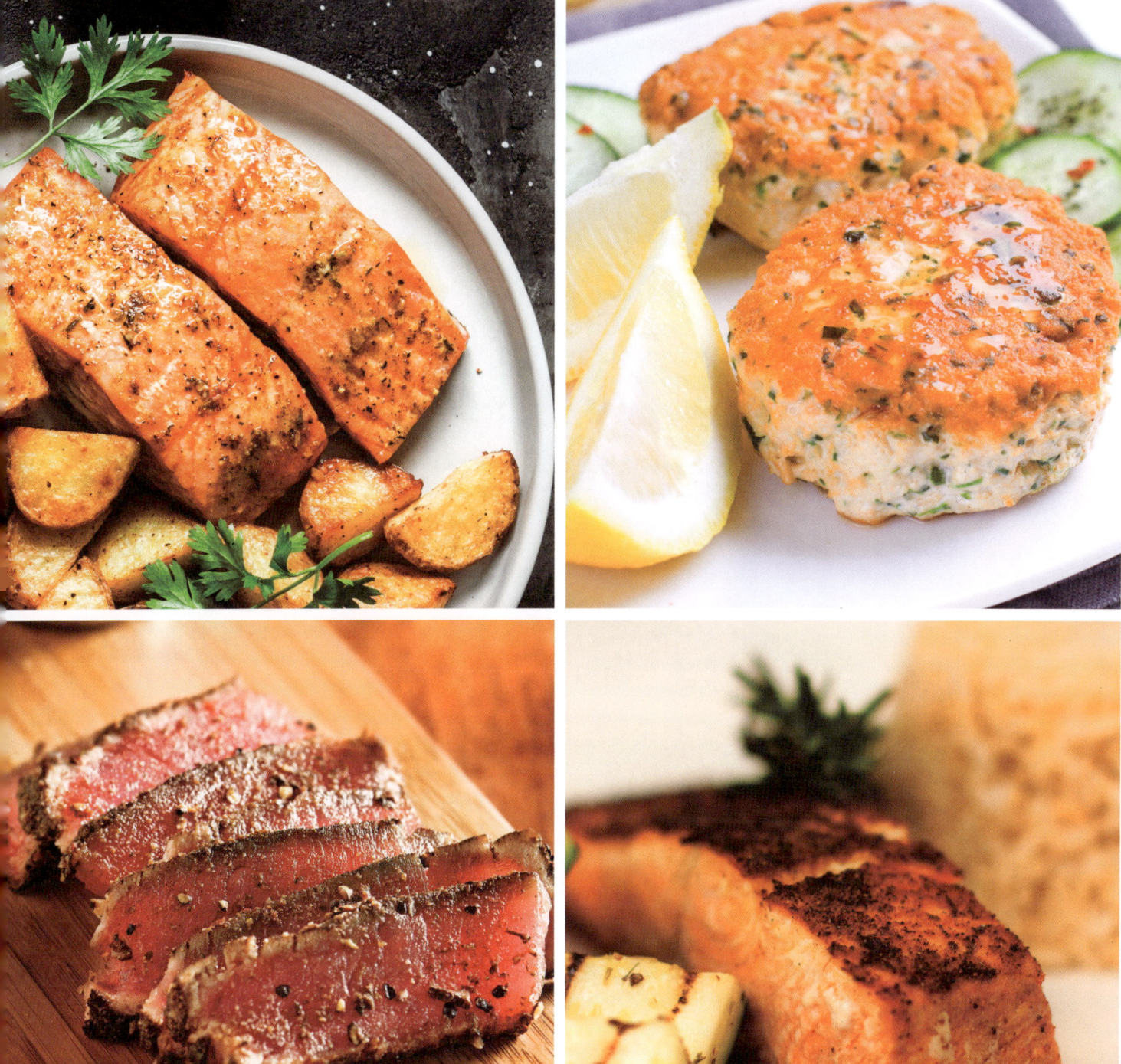

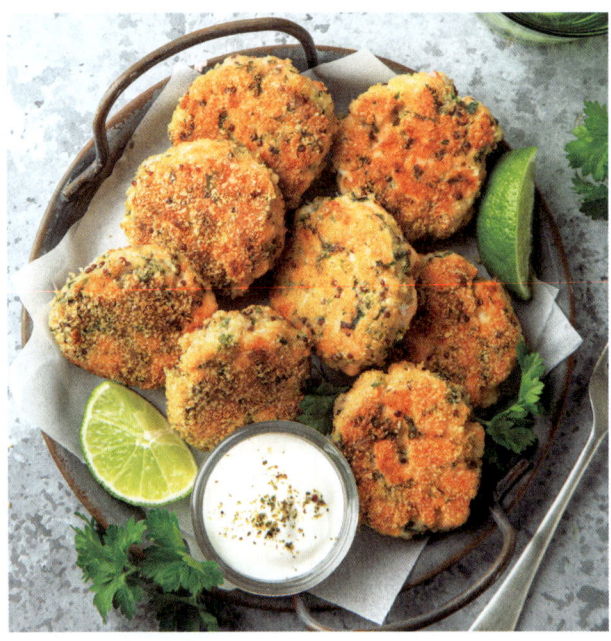

Salmon Quinoa Patties

6 medium florets broccoli

2 cups (370g) cooked quinoa

1 salmon fillet

¼ red onion, finely chopped

2 tbsps parsley, chopped

½ tsp salt

¼ tsp pepper

1 egg

1 cup (125g) panko breadcrumbs

¼ cup (25g) Parmesan cheese, grated

Boil the broccoli until well done (about 5 minutes). Drain, transfer to a large mixing bowl and set aside. When cool, mash with a potato masher.

Preheat the air fryer to 180°C. Cook the salmon in the air fryer for 7 minutes. Flake with a fork and set aside.

Place the quinoa in the bowl with the broccoli. Add the salmon, onion, parsley, salt, pepper and egg and stir well to fully combine.

Mix the panko and cheese together on a plate.

With dry hands, shape the salmon mixture into 6-8 patties. Roll the patties in the breadcrumb mixture, spray with some oil and cook for 12 minutes until golden, turning halfway through cooking.

SERVES 2-3

Homemade Calamari Rings

300g calamari tubes

1⅔ cups (400ml) buttermilk

⅓ cup (50g) cornflour

Salt and pepper, to season

½ cup (60g) panko breadcrumbs

1 egg

Baking mat (optional)

Clean and debone the calamari tubes (or get your fishmonger to do this).

Place the calamari tubes in a large bowl and cover with the buttermilk. Place in the fridge to soak overnight.

Place cornflour in a shallow bowl. Season with salt and pepper. Place breadcrumbs in second shallow bowl. Whisk egg in a third shallow bowl.

Lightly toss calamari rings in cornflour. Dip in the egg, shaking off any excess, then roll in breadcrumbs.

Preheat the air fryer to 180°C.

Spray calamari rings with oil, ensuring each one is lightly coated.

Spritz the air fryer basket with cooking spray.

Place in the air fryer basket or onto a baking mat and cook for 8 minutes, removing and gently shaking the basket halfway through cooking.

SERVES 2

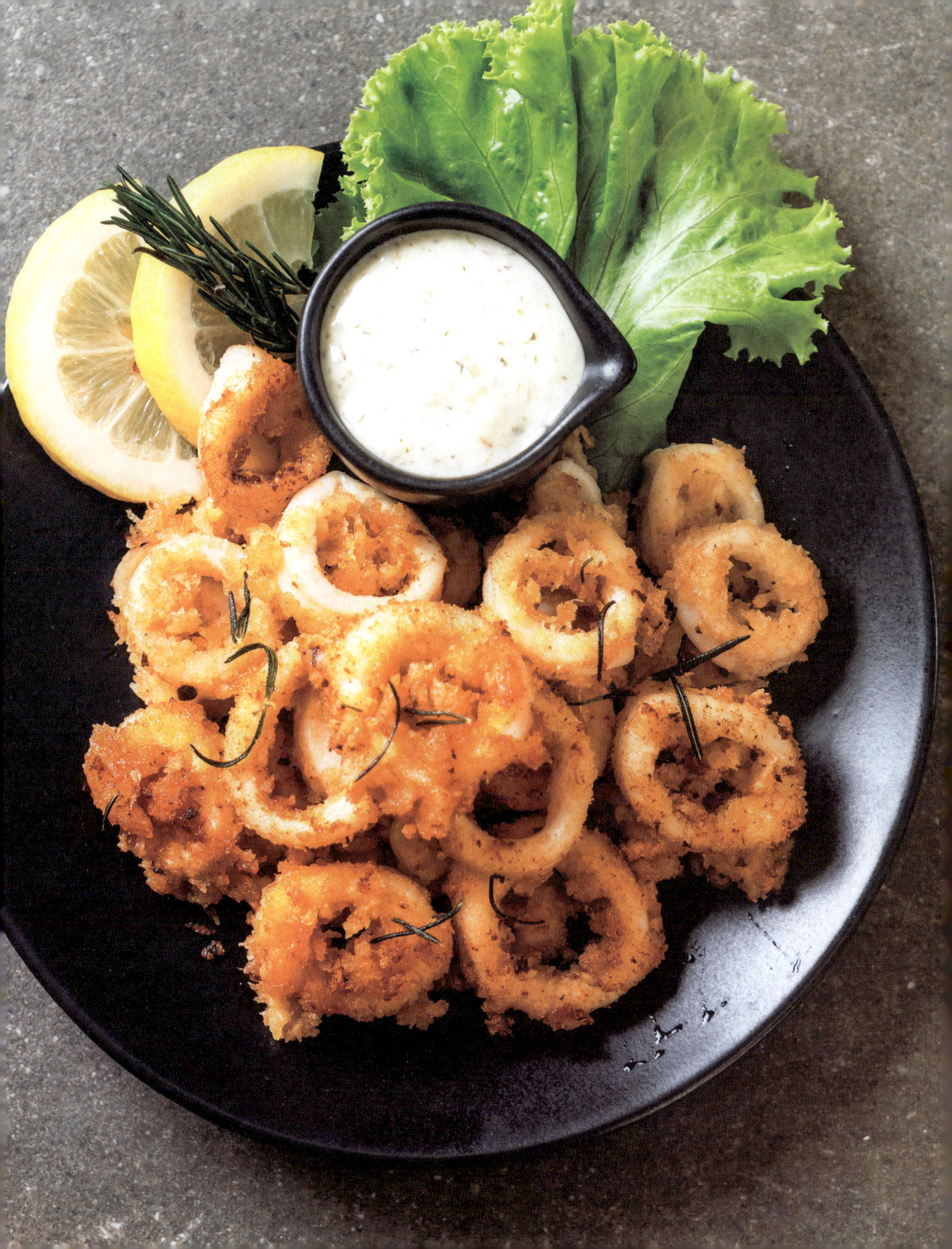

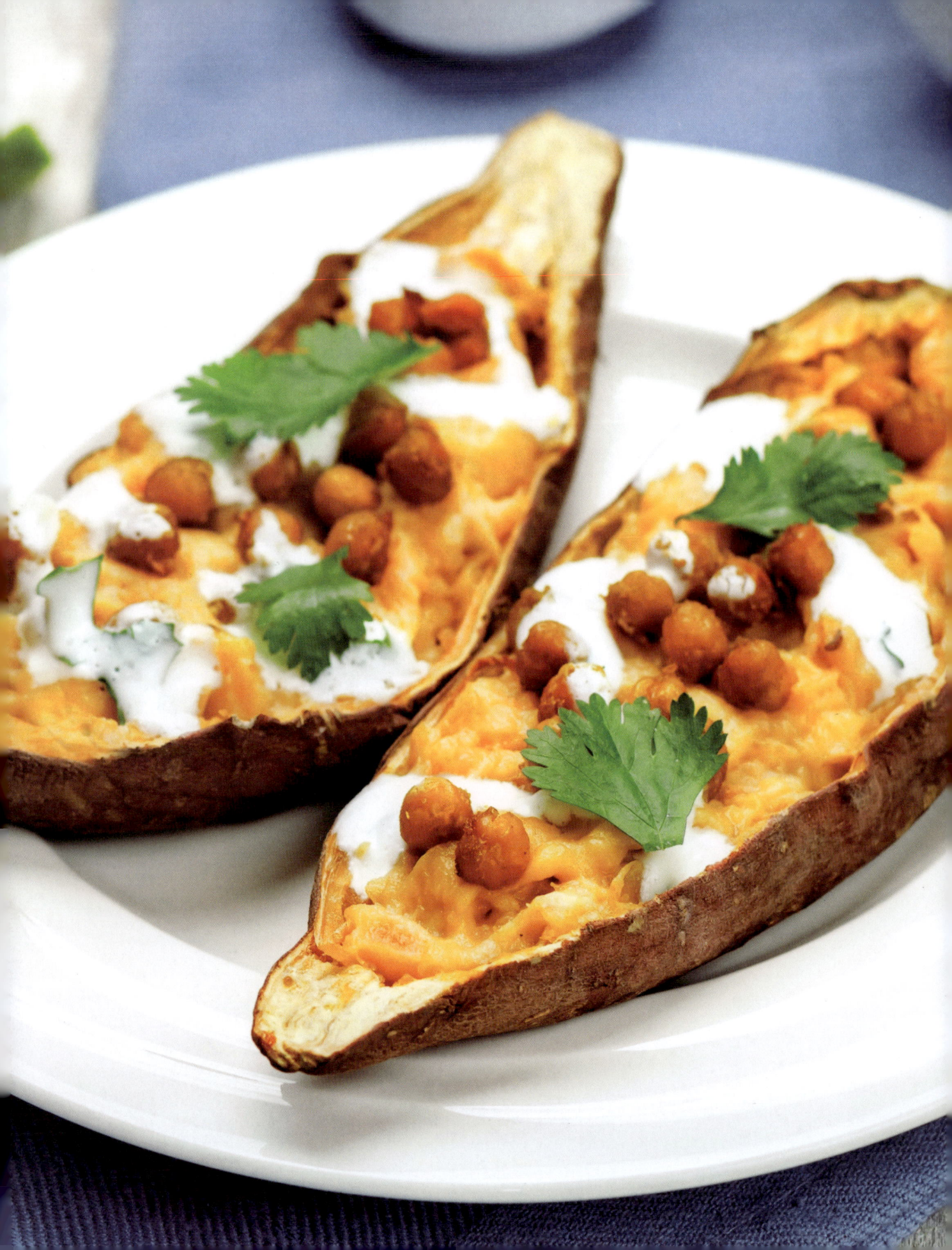

Vegetables

Baked Potatoes

4 potatoes

2 tbsps olive oil

Pinch of salt and pepper

Sour cream, to serve

Clean the potatoes and pat dry. Rub with olive oil and season with salt and pepper.

Place in the air fryer and cook at 200°C for 45 minutes.

Serve with sour cream.

SERVES 4

Homemade Fries

4 medium potatoes

4 tbsps olive oil

Salt and pepper, to season

Preheat the air fryer to 180°C.

Peel the potatoes and cut into fries of the desired thickness. Place in a bowl and add the olive oil. Toss to coat the potatoes in oil.

Place in the air fryer basket and slide into the air fryer. Cook for 20 minutes, shaking after the first 2 minutes and twice more during cooking.

Cook for an additional 5 minutes, if required, to further crisp the fries.

Season with salt and pepper to serve.

SERVES 4

Cajun Wedges

4 potatoes

1 tbsp olive oil

½ tsp salt

½ tsp pepper

1 tbsp Cajun seasoning

Scrub the potatoes and pat dry with a paper towel. Cut into wedges and place in a large bowl. Drizzle with olive oil and toss to coat.

Preheat the air fryer to 190°C.

Place potatoes in the air fryer basket and slide into the air fryer. (Be careful not to overcrowd the basket. Cook in batches or use a double layer accessory if needed.)

Cook for 25 minutes, shaking after the first 2 minutes and twice more during cooking.

When cooked, transfer to a bowl. Sprinkle with salt and pepper and Cajun spice and toss to combine until potato wedges are evenly coated.

SERVES 4

Rosemary Roast Potatoes

12 baby new potatoes

1 tbsp olive oil

1 small stem rosemary, leaves picked (or 1 tsp dried)

½ tsp salt

½ tsp pepper

Scrub potatoes well and cut in half.

Place in a bowl with the olive oil and rosemary, and toss until well coated.

Preheat the air fryer to 180°C.

Place the potatoes in the air fryer basket, being careful not to overcrowd the basket. (Cook in batches or use a double layer accessory if needed.)

Cook for 18 minutes, shaking a few times during cooking.

When cooked, transfer to a bowl. Sprinkle with salt and pepper and toss to combine.

SERVES 4

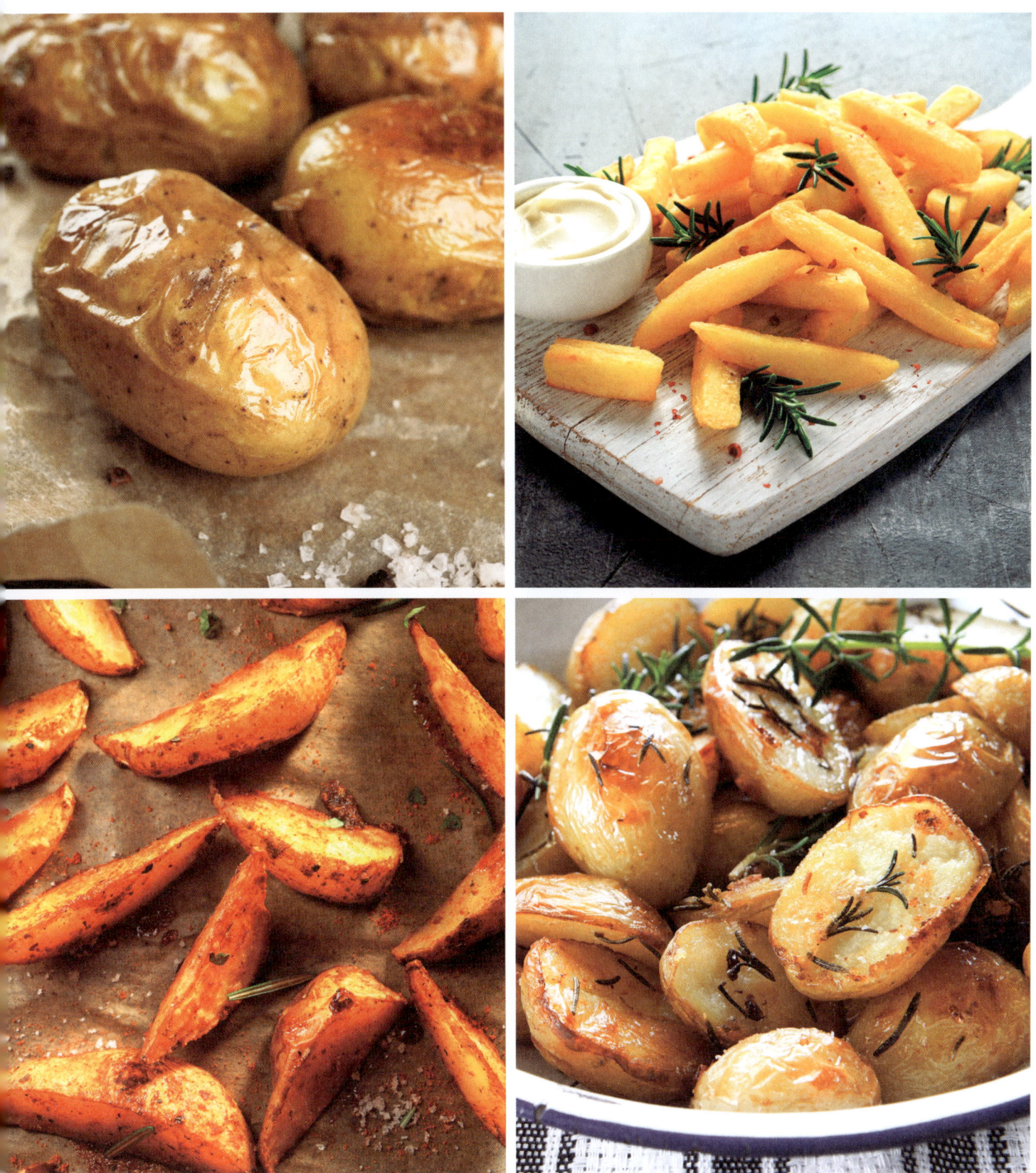

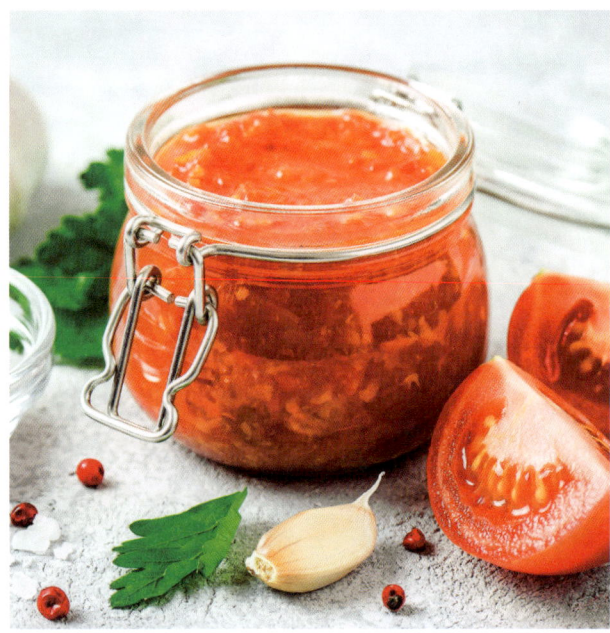

Homemade Tomato Sauce

10 ripe tomatoes

2 tbsps olive oil

2 tbsps butter

1 onion, chopped

3 cloves garlic, minced

¼ tsp mixed herbs

3 tbsps tomato paste

Water, as needed

Bring a pot of salted water to the boil over a medium-high heat. Have ready a large bowl of iced water. Plunge whole tomatoes into the boiling water for 1 minute. Remove with a slotted spoon and transfer to the ice bath. Set aside until cool enough to handle, then remove skin and discard. Chop tomatoes or puree in a blender.

Place oil and butter in a large pot over medium heat. Add onion and garlic and cook, stirring, for 5 minutes, until onion is soft. Add pureed tomatoes and mixed herbs.

Bring sauce to a boil, then reduce heat to low. Cover and simmer for 1 hour. Stir in tomato paste and simmer for a further 30 minutes. Check occasionally and add water to thin, if needed.

SERVES 4

Note: This sauce is the perfect accompaniment to fries, nuggets and many of the other recipes in this book.

Golden Wedges

4 medium potatoes (such as Russet Burbank or Sebago)

1 tbsp olive oil

Salt, to season

Scrub the potatoes and pat dry with a paper towel. Cut into wedges and place in a large bowl.

Toss in the olive oil and sprinkle with salt.

Preheat the air fryer to 200°C.

Place in the air fryer basket and slide into the air fryer. (Be careful not to overcrowd the basket. Cook in batches or use a double layer accessory if needed.)

Cook for 20 minutes, turning over once or twice during cooking.

SERVES 2

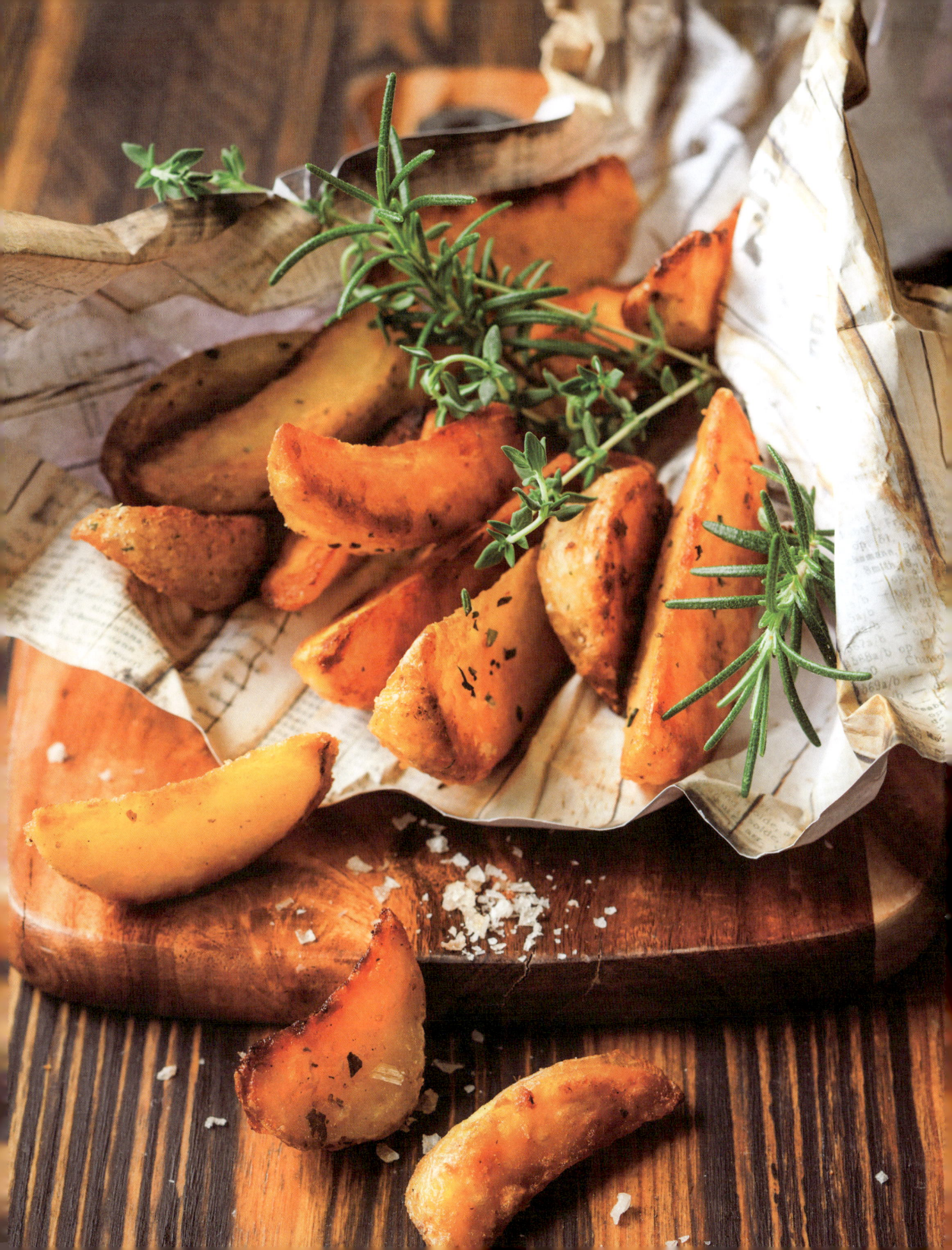

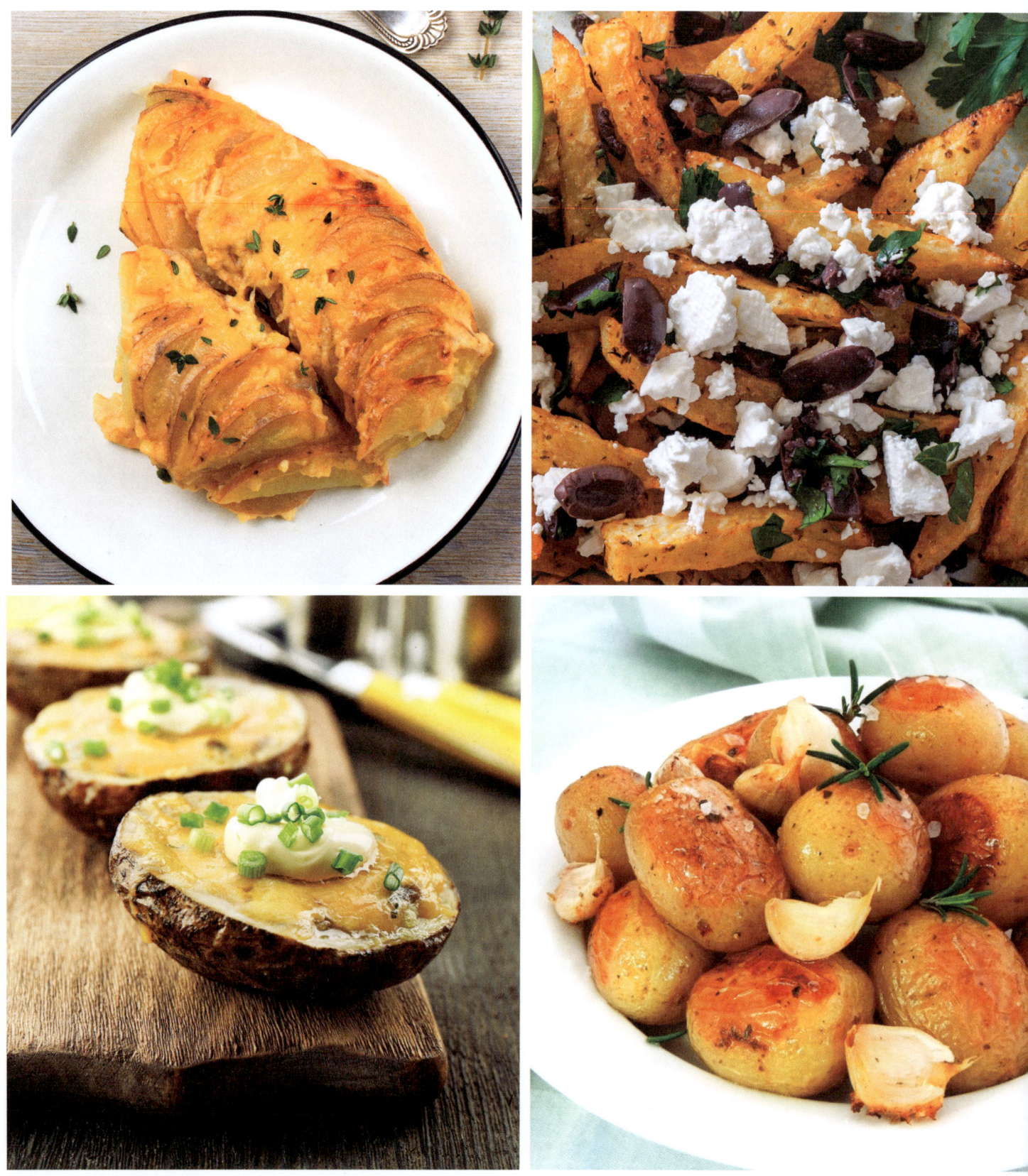

Potatoes Au Gratin

6 potatoes, peeled

½ cup (125ml) milk

½ cup (125ml) cream

Salt and pepper, to taste

½ cup (60g) Cheddar cheese, grated

Baking dish

Preheat the air fryer to 200°C.

Slice the potatoes thinly. In a mixing bowl, stir together the milk and cream and season to taste with salt and pepper.

Transfer the potato slices to the baking dish and pour the cream mixture over the top of the potatoes.

Place the baking dish in the air fryer.

Cook for 25 minutes. Remove basket and sprinkle the cheese evenly over the potatoes.

Cook for a further 10 minutes until golden brown and cheese has melted.

SERVES 4

Greek Fries

2 potatoes, peeled

2 tbsps olive oil

½ tsp salt

¼ tsp pepper

2 tbsps dried oregano

10 Kalamata olives, pitted and chopped

50g feta cheese, crumbled

Preheat air fryer to 180°C.

Cut the potatoes into chips of even size. Place in a bowl of cold water and soak for 30 minutes.

Drain and pat dry. Place in a large mixing bowl and add the olive oil, salt, pepper and oregano. Toss well to coat the potatoes evenly.

Cook the potatoes in the air fryer for 25 minutes, shaking the basket a couple of times during cooking.

Serve with the feta cheese, Kalamata olives and chopped parsley over the top.

SERVES 4

Cheesy Baked Potatoes

2 potatoes

2 tsps butter

½ cup (60g) Cheddar cheese, grated

Salt and pepper, to taste

2 tbsps sour cream

1 spring onion, sliced

Poke holes into the top of each potato with a fork.

Lightly spray with cooking spray.

Place the potatoes in the air fryer. Cook for 40 minutes at 190°C.

Remove the potatoes from the air fryer and set aside until cool enough to handle.

Slice each of the potatoes in half lengthwise. Top with the butter, cheese and salt and pepper and return to the air fryer to cook for a further 5 minutes until cheese has melted.

Serve with a dollop of sour cream and sprinkled with spring onion.

SERVES 2

Garlic Baby Potatoes

500g baby potatoes

1 tbsp olive oil

¼ tsp salt

½ tsp garlic powder

8 cloves garlic

Preheat the air fryer to 175°C.

Combine the potatoes, oil, salt, garlic powder and garlic cloves in a mixing bowl and toss to coat.

Place potatoes and garlic into the air fryer basket and slide into the air fryer.

Cook for 20 minutes, shaking the basket a couple of times during cooking.

SERVES 4

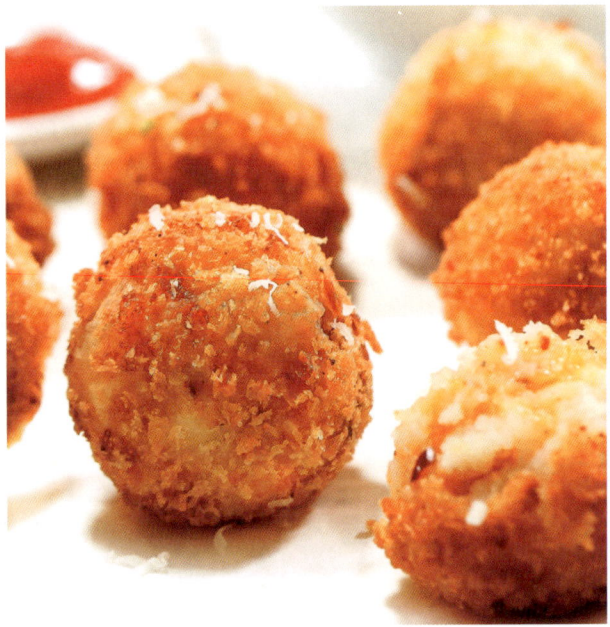

Mashed Potato Croquettes

3 medium potatoes, peeled and cut into chunks

30g butter

1 egg yolk

½ cup (50g) Parmesan cheese, grated

2 tbsps flour

Salt and pepper, to season

½ cup (50g) breadcrumbs

2 tbsps olive oil

Place the potatoes in a large saucepan of cold salted water and bring to the boil. Cook for 15 minutes, until soft. Drain and mash with butter until creamy. Set aside until cool enough to handle.

Add the egg yolk, cheese and flour to the bowl with the mashed potato. Season with salt and pepper and mix to fully combine.

Preheat the air fryer to 200°C.

Combine the breadcrumbs and olive oil and place on a shallow bowl or plate.

Form the croquettes into balls and roll in the breadcrumb mixture. Press in to ensure fully coated.

Transfer to the basket of the air fryer in an even layer. (Be careful not to overcrowd the basket. Cook in batches or use a double layer accessory if needed.)

Cook for 5 minutes per batch, shaking halfway through.

SERVES 4

Mashed Potato Cakes

2 cups (520g) mashed potatoes

1 cup (125g) Cheddar cheese, grated

1 tsp salt

½ tsp pepper

2 eggs, beaten

1 cup (125g) plain flour

2 cups (250g) breadcrumbs

Baking pan

Place mashed potato, cheese and salt and pepper in a mixing bowl and stir to combine.

Line the baking pan with greaseproof paper. Spread the mixture evenly on top.

Transfer to the freezer for 30 minutes.

Using a cookie cutter, create circles from the mixture until all the mixture is used up.

Put flour in a shallow bowl. Place eggs in a second bowl and the breadcrumbs in a third bowl.

Dredge the potato cakes into the flour and then the eggs, shaking off any excess. Next press into the breadcrumbs, ensuring the potato cakes are fully and evenly covered.

Preheat the air fryer to 190°C.

Place the potato cakes in the air fryer basket in a single layer. (Be careful not to overcrowd the basket. Cook in batches or use a double layer accessory if needed.)

Cook for 7 minutes.

SERVES 4

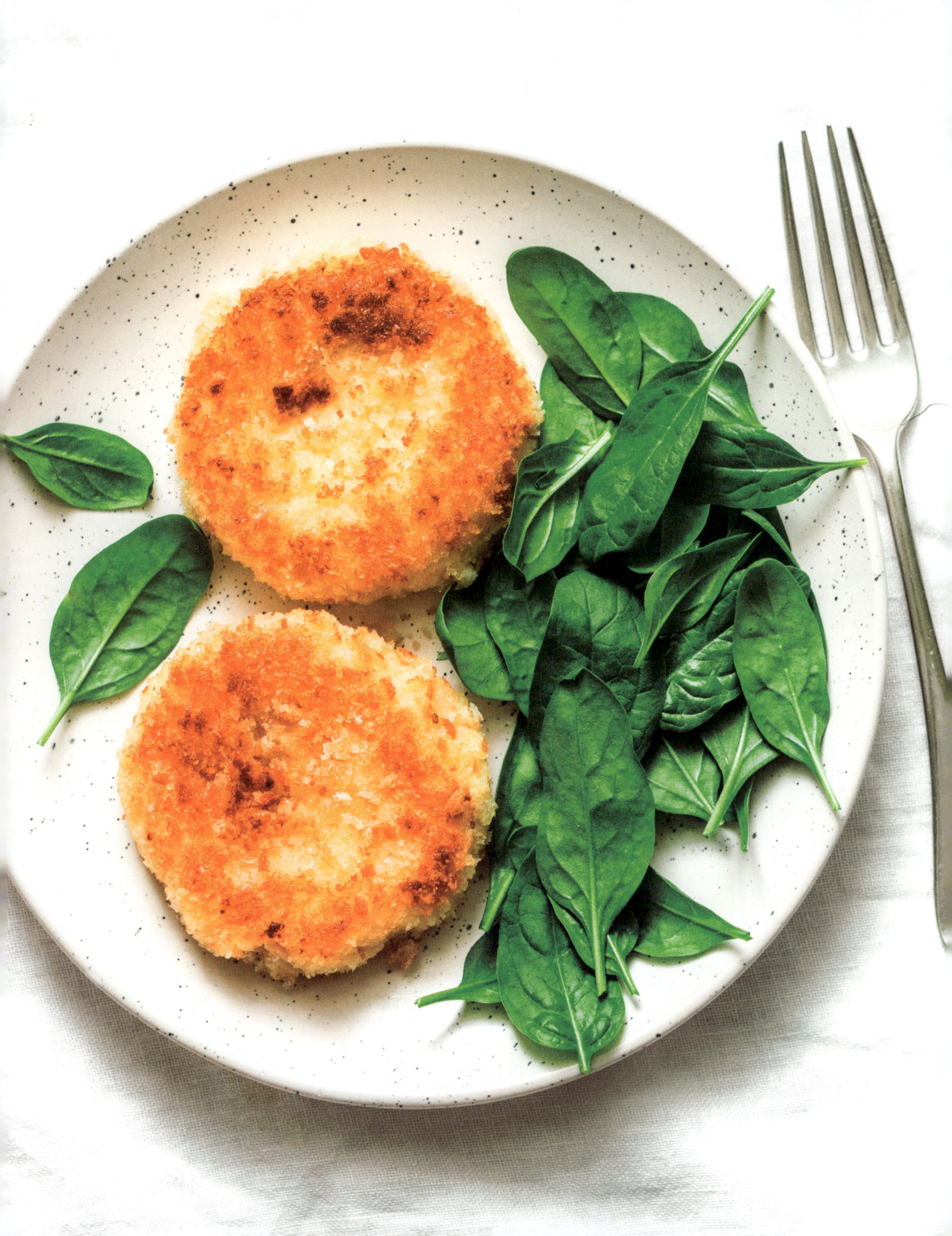

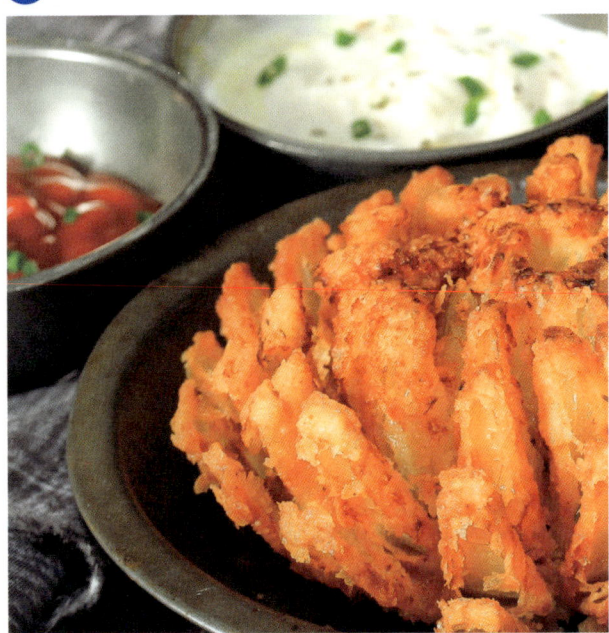

Blooming Onion

1 large onion

½ cup (60g) plain flour

1 tbsp salt

1 tsp garlic powder

1 egg

¼ cup (60ml) milk

Cut 1cm from the top (pointed end) of the onion, then peel off the outer skin. Place the onion on a chopping board cut-side down. Starting just beneath the root, make a downward cut all the way through to the board. Repeat until you have 16 evenly spaced cuts around the onion. Turn the onion over and using your fingers prise the outer pieces apart.

Preheat the air fryer to 190°C.

Combine the flour, salt and garlic powder in a bowl.

Beat the egg and milk together in a second bowl.

Place the onion cut-side up into the egg mixture and spoon over the egg mixture so that it is fully coated.

Then place the onion cut-side up into the flour mixture, again ensuring the flour coats the onion. When finished, shake the onion to remove excess flour.

Lightly spritz the onion with cooking spray and place into the basket of the air fryer.

Cook for 15 minutes until crispy and golden brown.

SERVES 2

Hasselback Potatoes

4 large potatoes

75g butter, melted

4 cloves garlic, thinly sliced

4 rashers bacon, cooked and sliced

1 cup (125g) mozzarella cheese, grated

2 spring onions, finely sliced

Scrub the potatoes and pat dry with a paper towel.

Cut slits along the potatoes approximately 1cm apart and down to 1cm from the base.

Preheat the air fryer to 180°C.

Brush the potatoes with butter, and inesert the slices of garlic in the slits. Place cut-side down in basket and cook for 30 minutes.

Remove from the basket and turn the potatoes over using tongs.

Top the potatoes with bacon, cheese and spring onion. Return to the air fryer and cook for a further 20 minutes until potatoes are tender and cheese has melted.

SERVES 4

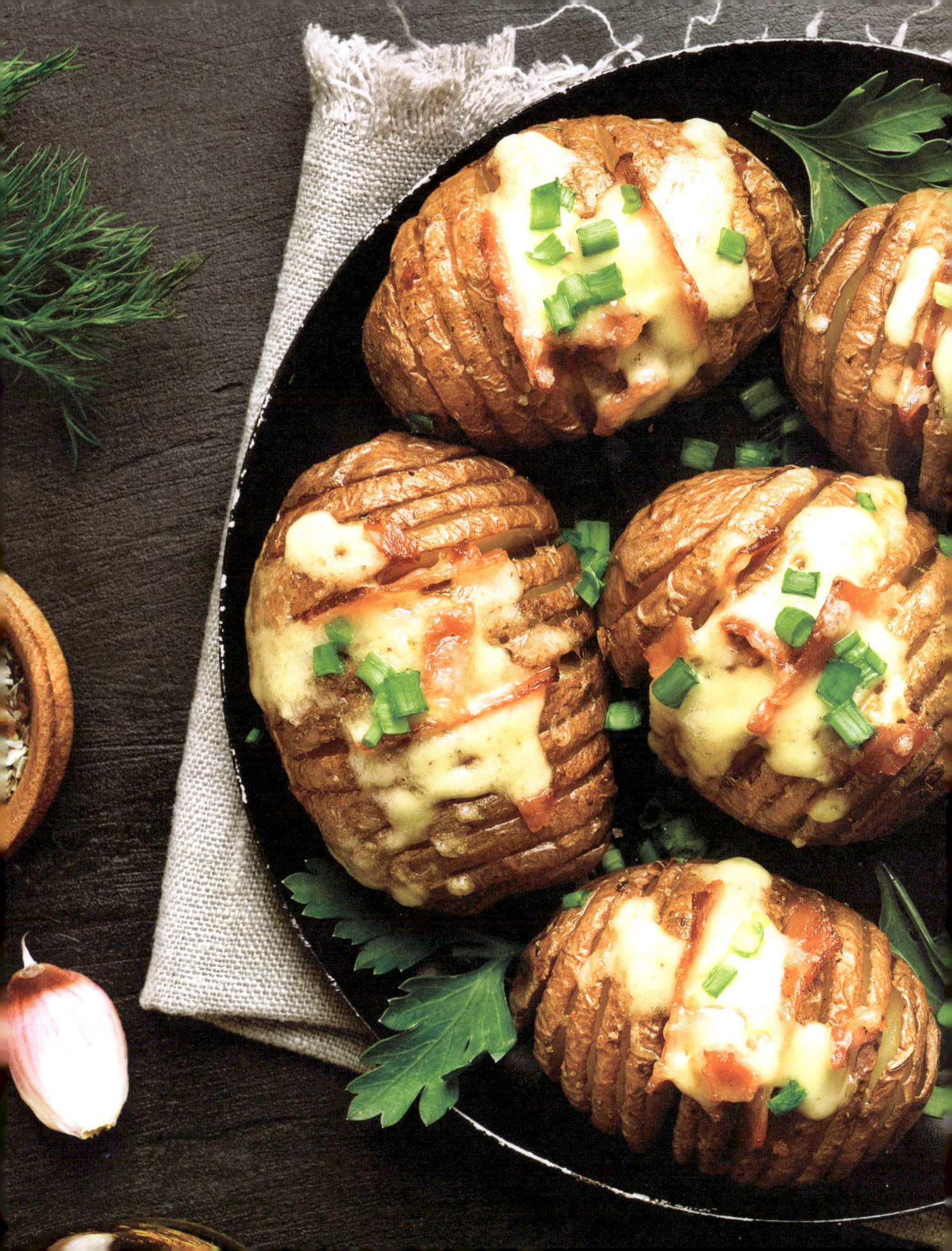

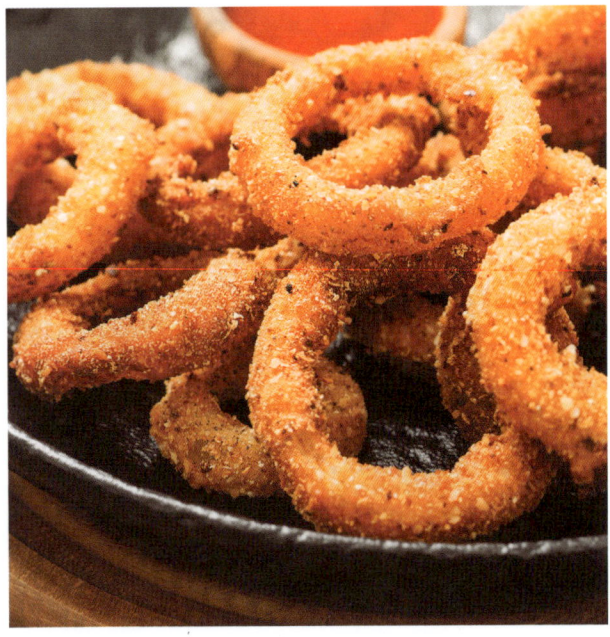

Breaded Onion Rings

1 large onion

½ cup (60g) plain flour

1 tbsp baking powder

1 tsp salt

1 egg

1 tsp pepper

1 cup (125g) breadcrumbs

Preheat the air fryer to 190°C.

Cut the onion into thick slices. Separate each slice into multiple rings.

Combine the flour, baking powder and salt together in a shallow bowl.

Beat the eggs and pepper together in another shallow bowl.

Place the breadcrumbs in a third shallow bowl.

Take each onion ring and dredge it in the flour mixture, then dip in the egg, shaking off any excess. Press into the breadcrumbs, ensuring it is evenly and fully coated.

Spritz the air fryer basket with cooking spray.

Lay the rings in the basket in an even layer (cook in batches if needed) and spray the tops with oil.

Cook for 7 minutes at 190°C.

SERVES 2

Gluten-Free Onion Rings

2 large onions

1 cup (250ml) buttermilk

1-2 eggs

½ cup (60g) gluten-free panko style breadcrumbs

1 cup (125g) gluten-free flour

1 tbsp Parmesan cheese, grated

1 tsp salt

1 tsp pepper

Cut the onion into thick slices. Separate each slice into multiple rings.

Combine the buttermilk and egg in a mixing bowl and beat together with a whisk.

Place the panko, flour, Parmesan, salt and pepper in a shallow bowl and mix together.

Dip each onion ring into the buttermilk mixture and then into the flour mixture. Place on the baking tray and transfer to the fridge to chill for 1 hour.

Preheat the air fryer to 200°C.

Spritz the air fryer basket with cooking spray.

Transfer the onion rings to the basket of the air fryer. (Be careful not to overcrowd the basket. Cook in batches or use a double layer accessory if needed.)

Cook for 5 minutes, turning halfway through cooking.

Repeat until all onion rings are cooked.

SERVES 4

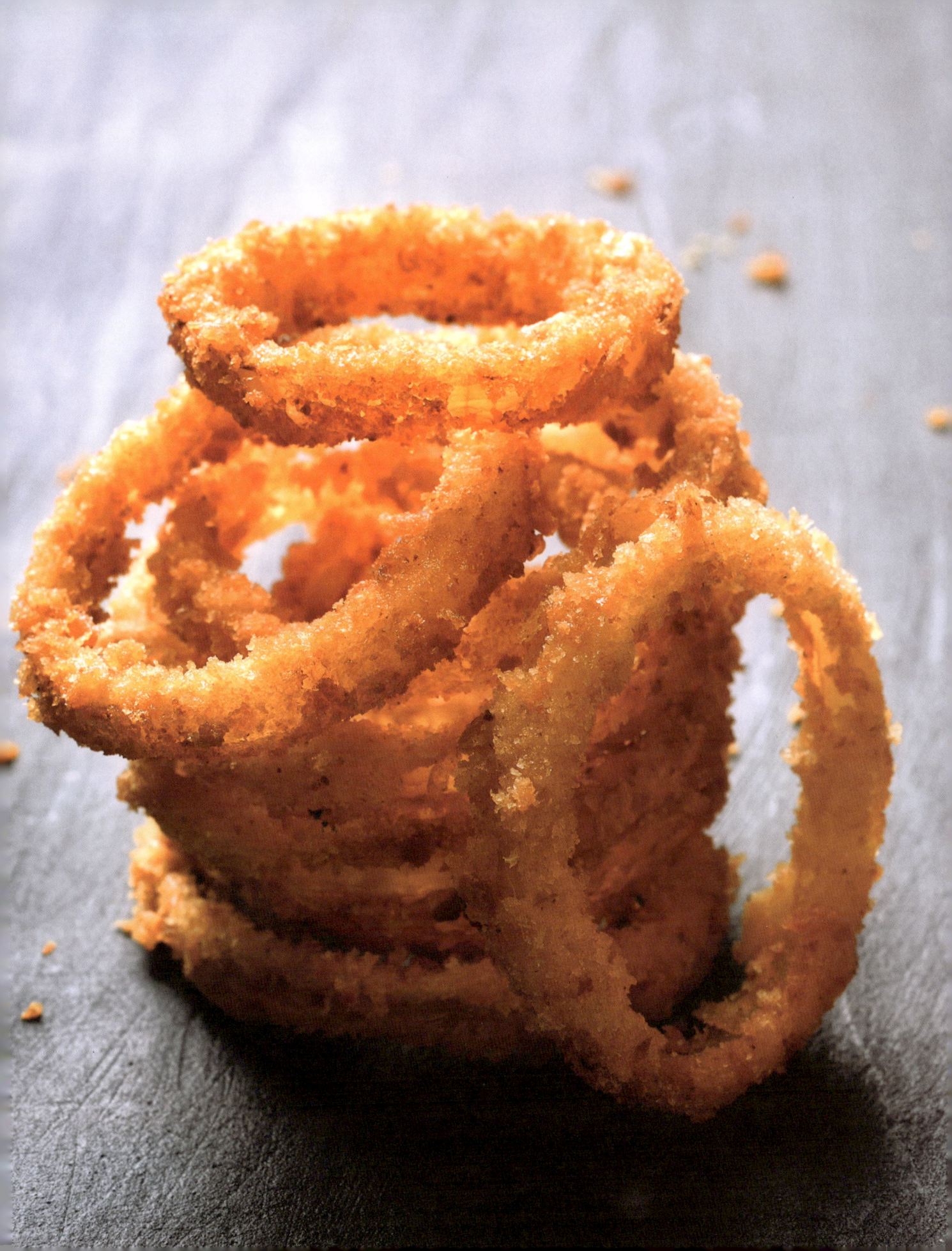

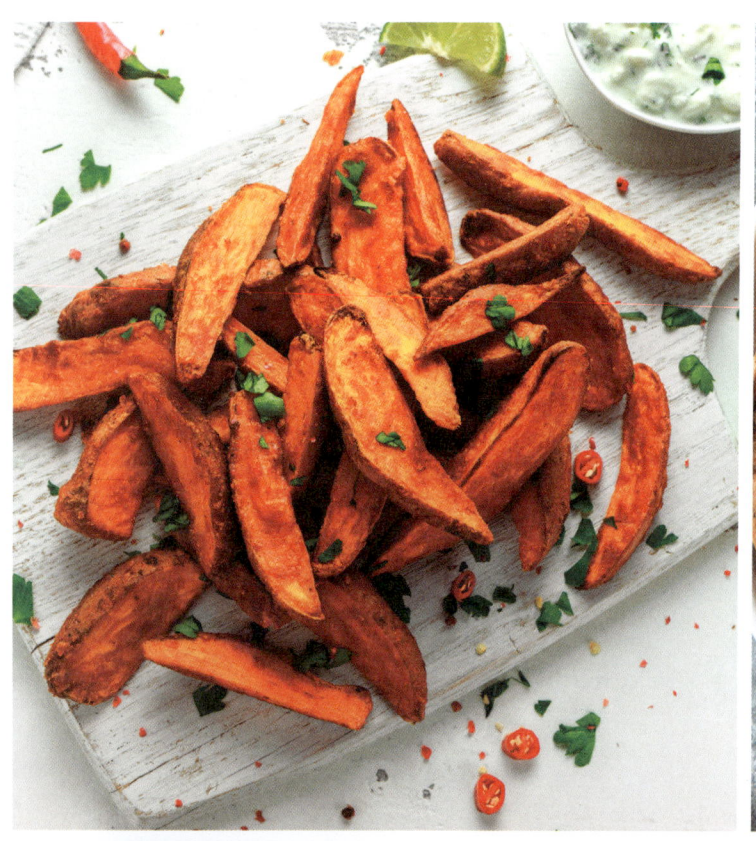
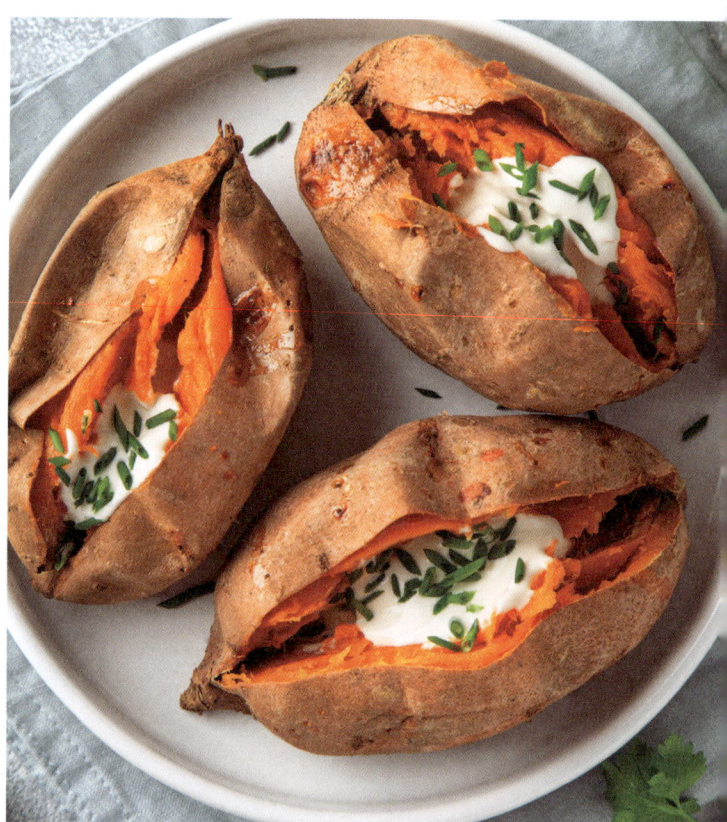
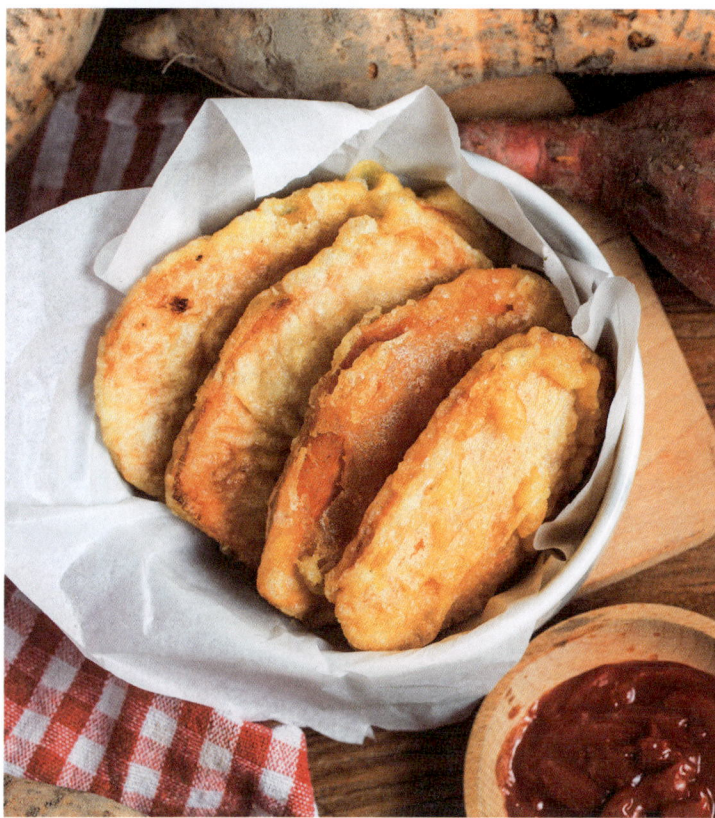
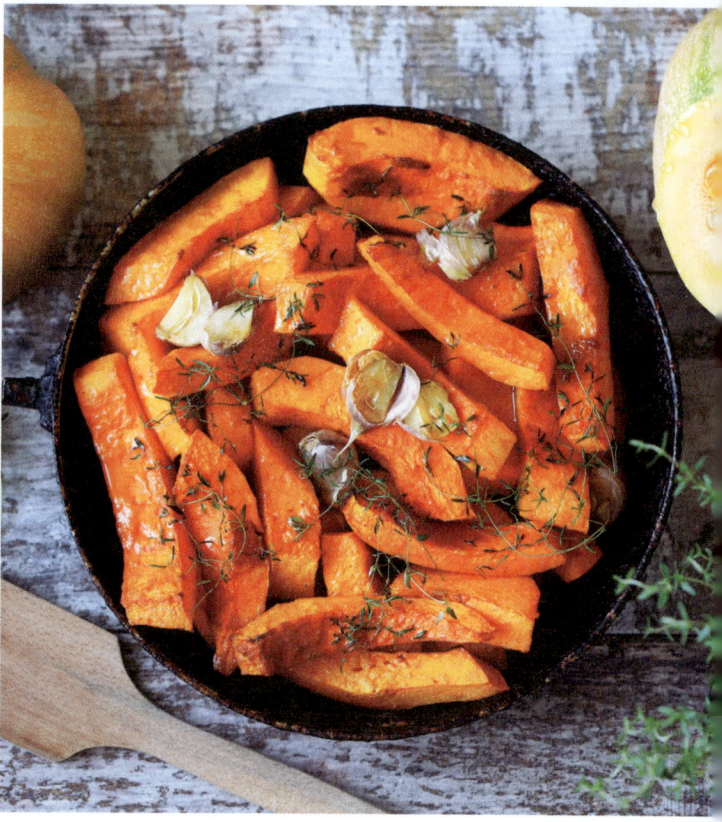

Sweet Potato Chips

2 sweet potatoes

Salt, to season (optional)

Peel the sweet potatoes, then slice into chips of a consistent size. Place into a large bowl.

Preheat the air fryer to 180°C.

Spray the potatoes with olive oil and then toss to coat. Sprinkle with salt if desired.

Place the sweet potatoes into the air fryer basket.

Cook for 20 minutes, shaking once during cooking.

SERVES 2

Baked Sweet Potatoes

3 sweet potatoes

1 tbsp olive oil

1 tsp salt

3 tbsps sour cream

1 tbsp fresh chives, chopped

Scrub potatoes and pat dry with paper towels. Prick a few times with a fork.

Sprinkle with olive oil and salt, and rub evenly into the potato skin.

Preheat the air fryer to 200°C.

Place potatoes into the air fryer basket.

Cook for 40 minutes until tender.

Serve with sour cream and chives on top.

SERVES 3

Sweet Potato Tempura

½ cup (75g) cornflour

¼ cup (30g) plain flour

1 egg

¼ cup (60ml) soda water

2 sweet potatoes, cut into slices

1 cup (125g) panko breadcrumbs

Preheat the air fryer to 200°C.

In a small mixing bowl, whisk together the cornflour, flour, egg and soda water.

Dip a sweet potato slice into the batter, shaking off any excess. Place it directly into the breadcrumbs, ensuring all sides are well coated. Repeat until all slices are coated.

Place the sweet potato slices into the fryer basket and spray with non-stick cooking spray.

Cook for 10 minutes, turning once during cooking.

SERVES 2

Pumpkin Slices with Thyme and Garlic

750g pumpkin

6 cloves garlic

8-10 sprigs thyme

Peel and cut the pumpkin into slices.

Preheat the air fryer to 180°C.

Place the pumpkin pieces into the air fryer basket.

Spritz the pumpkin with olive oil and add the thyme. Toss to coat.

Place basket into the air fryer.

Cook for 10 minutes until tender.

SERVES 4

Paprika Pumpkin Salad

800g pumpkin

1 tsp sweet paprika

1 tsp ground smoked paprika

4 tbsps pumpkin seeds

240g rocket

Peel and cut the pumpkin into cubes.

Preheat the air fryer to 180°C.

Place the pumpkin into the air fryer basket.

Spritz the pumpkin with olive oil and sprinkle with sweet and smoked paprika. Toss to coat.

Place basket into the air fryer.

Cook for 10 minutes until tender.

Place the rocket on serving plates and top with the spiced pumpkin and pumpkin seeds to serve.

SERVES 4

Sweet and Spiced Pumpkin Seeds

8 cups (2L) water

1½ cups (195g) pumpkin seeds

1 tbsp olive oil

1½ tsps salt

1 tsp cumin

1 tbsp brown sugar

Bring the water to a boil in a large pot. Add the pumpkin seeds and boil for 10 minutes. Line a baking tray or large plate with paper towel. Drain the pumpkin seeds and spread out on the prepared towels. Leave to dry for 15 minutes.

Preheat the air fryer to 180°C.

Toss the seeds with olive oil, salt, cumin and brown sugar.

Place the seeds in the air fryer basket. Cook for 35 minutes, shaking the basket every 5 minutes.

SERVES 4

Peppered Pumpkin Seeds

8 cups (2L) water

1½ cups (195g) pumpkin seeds

1 tbsp olive oil

1½ tsps salt

1 tsp four-colour pepper mix

Bring the water to a boil in a large pot. Add the pumpkin seeds and boil for 10 minutes. Line a baking tray or large plate with paper towel. Drain the pumpkin seeds and spread out on the prepared towels. Leave to dry for 15 minutes.

Preheat the air fryer to 180°C.

Toss the seeds with olive oil, salt and pepper mix.

Place the seeds in the air fryer basket. Cook for 35 minutes, shaking the basket every 5 minutes.

SERVES 4

Pumpkin and Feta Wedges

400g pumpkin

1 tsp mixed herbs

1 tbsp pumpkin seeds

50g feta cheese, crumbled

Cut the pumpkin into wedges (leaving the skin on).

Preheat the air fryer to 180°C.

Place the pumpkin pieces into the air fryer basket.

Spritz the pumpkin with olive oil. Add the mixed herbs and pumpkin seeds and toss to combine.

Place the basket into the air fryer.

Cook for 10 minutes until tender.

Sprinkle with feta cheese to serve.

SERVES 2

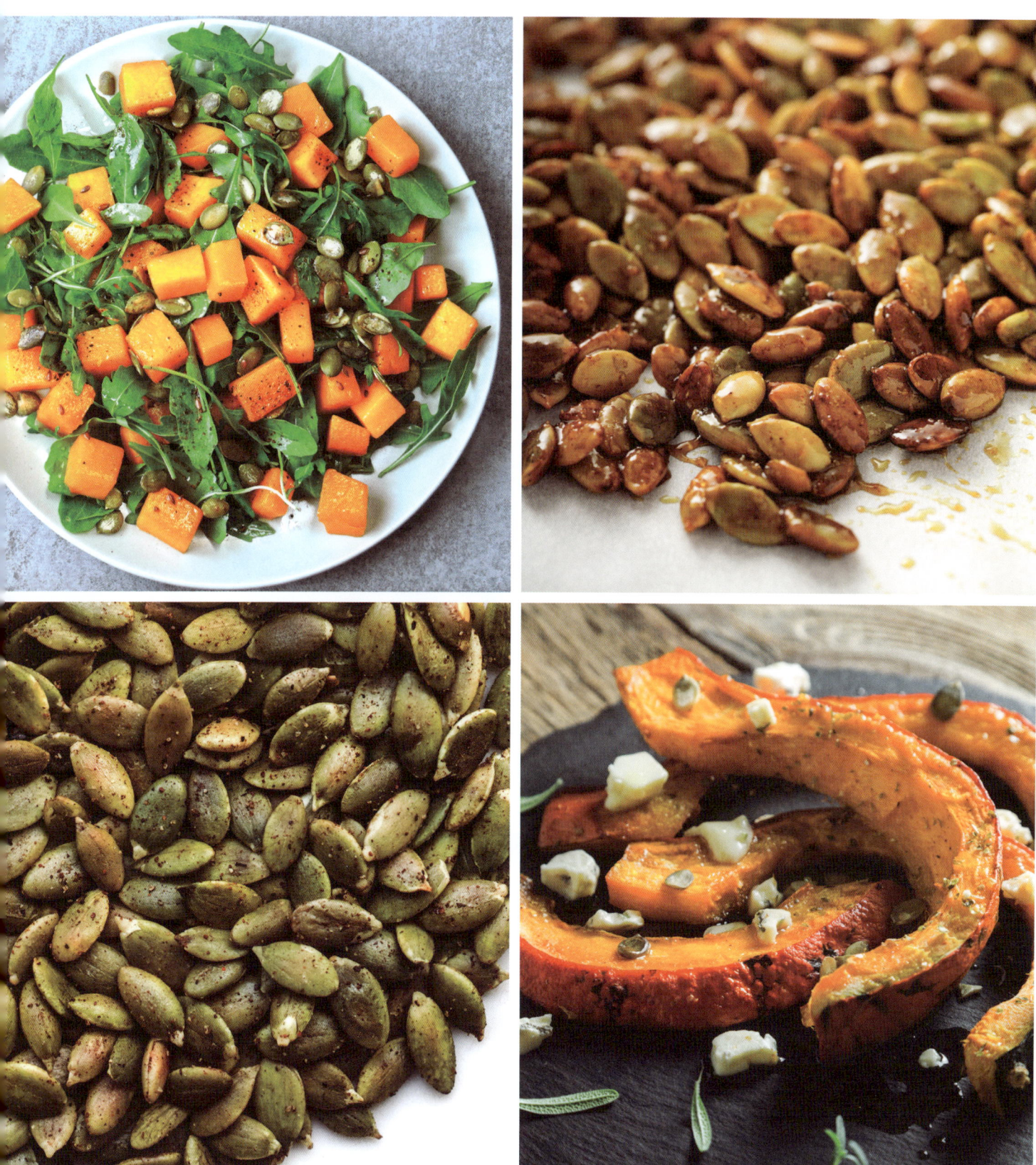

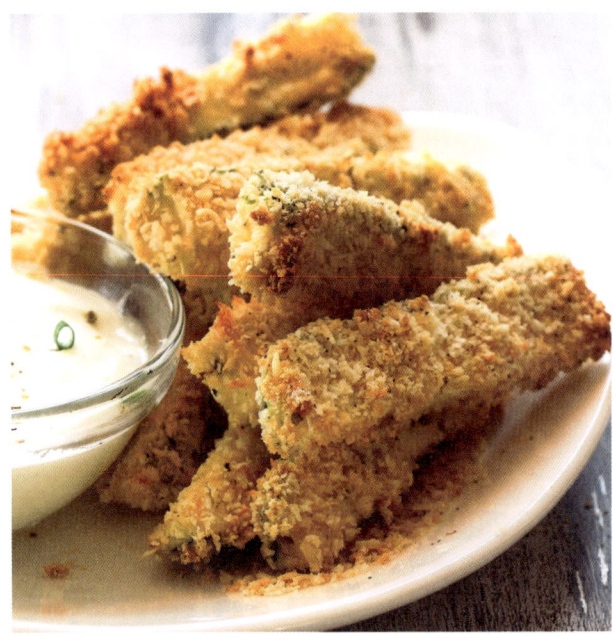

Baked Zucchini Fries

3 medium zucchinis

2 egg whites

Pinch of salt and pepper

½ cup (60g) panko breadcrumbs

¼ tsp garlic powder

¼ cup (25g) Parmesan cheese, grated

Cut the zucchinis into sticks.

Preheat the air fryer to 200°C. Spritz the air fryer basket with cooking spray.

Beat the egg whites in a small bowl and season with salt and pepper.

Place the panko, garlic powder and cheese into a second bowl and mix well.

Dip the zucchini sticks into the egg whites then into the panko and cheese mixture, a few at a time, ensuring that each is well coated.

Spray all sides of the zucchini sticks with oil.

Place the zucchini sticks in a single layer in the basket. (Be careful not to overcrowd the basket. Cook in batches or use a double layer accessory if needed.)

Bake for 20 minutes, or until crisp and golden.

SERVES 2

Vegetable Tots

½ cup (60g) plain flour

¼ tsp salt

1 tsp garlic powder

2 tsp dried basil

2 medium zucchinis

1 small onion, peeled

2 eggs + 1 egg white

½ cup (50g) Parmesan cheese, finely grated

Sweet chilli sauce, to serve

Preheat the air fryer to 200°C.

Grate the zucchinis and onion. Squeeze the liquid out by placing the grated vegetables in a tea towel, rolling up the towel and twisting it.

In a medium bowl, combine all the ingredients.

The mixture should be thick but quite soft. For best results, cover the bowl and place the mixture in the refrigerator to chill for 1 hour.

Form balls using wet hands, and place in the air fryer in a single layer. (Be careful not to overcrowd the basket. Cook in batches or use a double layer accessory if needed.)

Cook for 10 minutes.

Serve with sweet chilli sauce.

SERVES 2

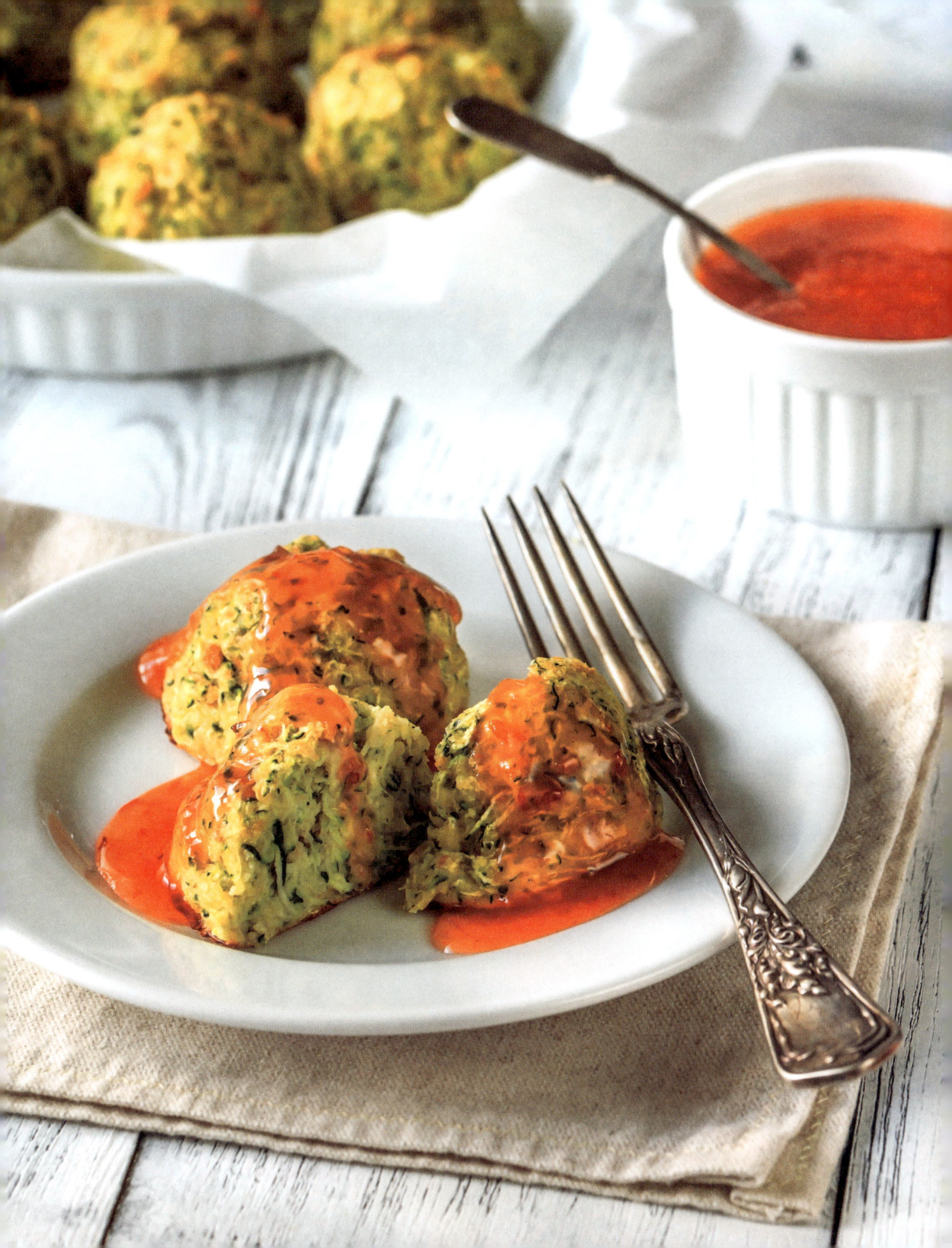

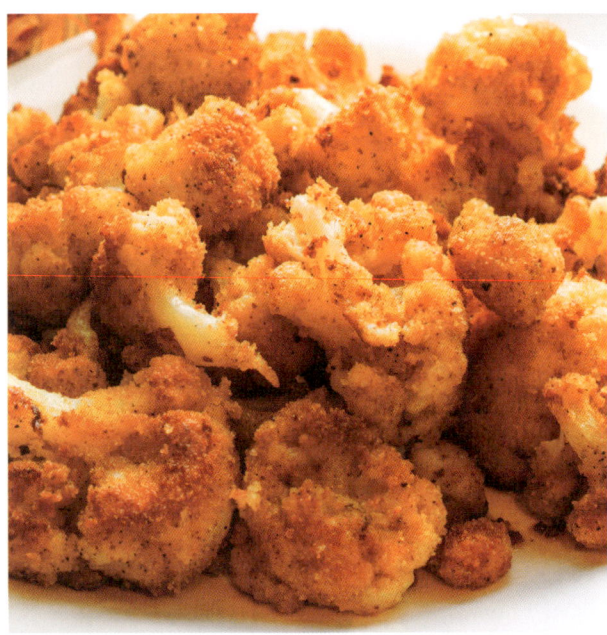

Breaded Cauliflower

1 small cauliflower

1 cup (125g) breadcrumbs

¼ cup (25g) Parmesan cheese, grated

¼ cup (30g) plain flour

2 eggs

Break the cauliflower into small florets.

Combine the breadcrumbs with the Parmesan in a shallow bowl.

Put flour in another shallow bowl. Place eggs in a third bowl and beat lightly.

Dredge the florets into the flour and then eggs, shaking off any excess. Next press into the breadcrumbs ensuring the florets are fully covered.

Preheat the air fryer to 190°C.

Cook for 12 minutes, shaking once or twice during cooking.

SERVES 4

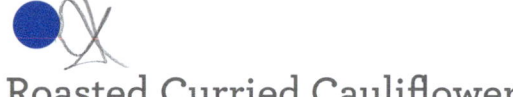

Roasted Curried Cauliflower

1 cauliflower

2 potatoes

4 tsps olive oil

1 tsp curry powder

¼ tsp salt

½ cup (125ml) yoghurt

Few sprigs of fresh parsley, to serve (optional)

Preheat the air fryer to 180°C.

Break the cauliflower into small florets. Peel and dice the potatoes into small chunks.

Add olive oil, curry powder and salt to the a mixing bowl and stir to coat.

Place the mixture into the air fryer basket.

Cook for 15 minutes. Check if tender and cook for another few minutes if necessary.

Serve with a dollop of yoghurt and fresh parsley, if desired.

SERVES 2

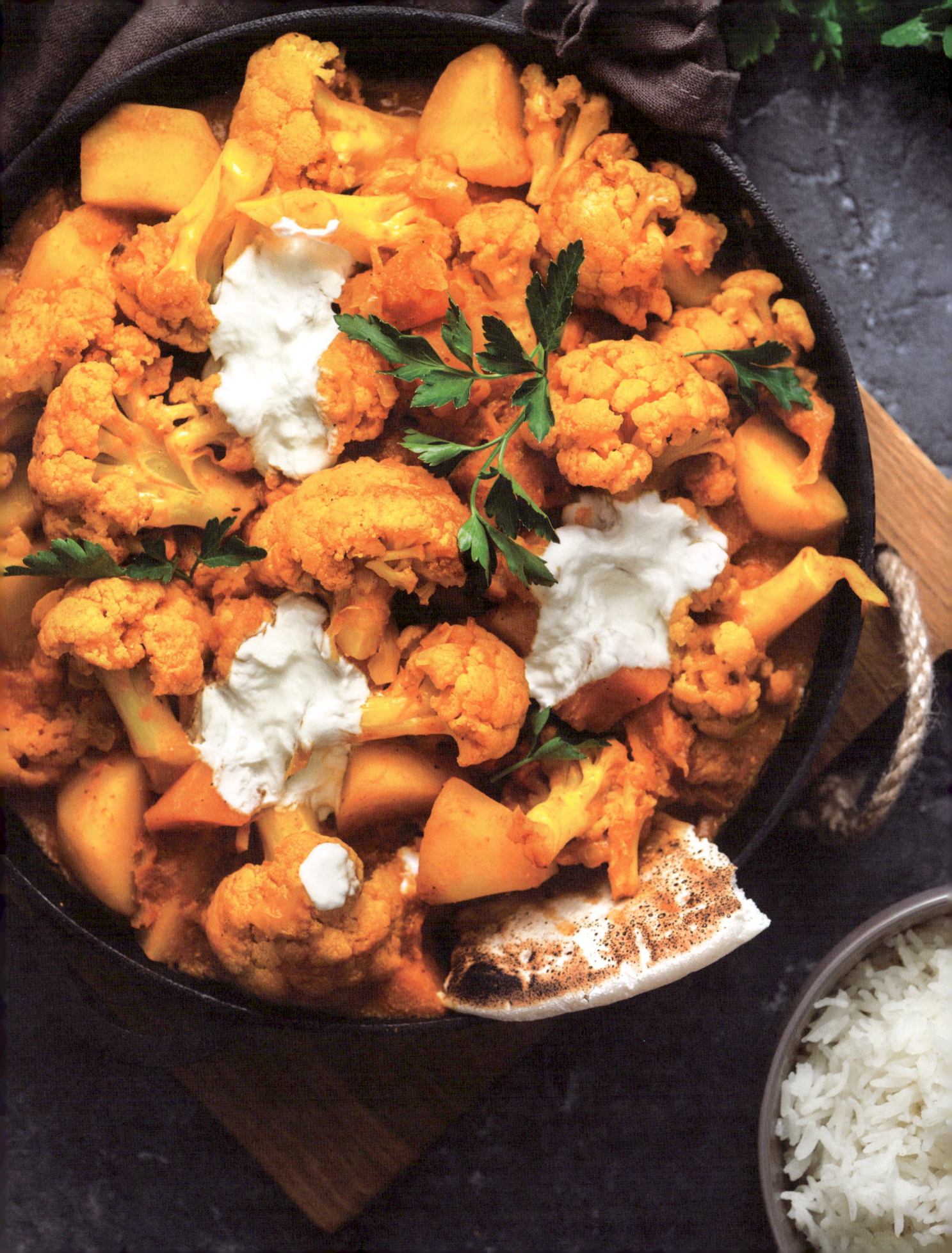

Cauliflower Bites

1 small cauliflower

2 large eggs

¼ cup (30g) breadcrumbs

¼ cup (25g) Parmesan cheese, grated

¼ tsp onion powder

1 tsp Italian herb mix

Grate the cauliflower using the large holes of a box grater or pulse in a food processor.

Preheat the air fryer to 200°C.

Combine all the ingredients in a bowl.

Spritz the air fryer basket with cooking spray.

Using wet hands, form small balls. Place in the air fryer as one layer.

Cook for 10 minutes, turning halfway.

SERVES 4

Zucchini Chips

2 medium zucchinis

1 tbsp olive oil

½ tsp garlic powder

Pinch of salt and pepper

Slice the zucchinis into thin chips.

Place zucchini into a large bowl and season with olive oil, garlic powder, salt and pepper.

Transfer to the basket of the air fryer. (Be careful not to overcrowd the basket. Cook in batches or use a double layer accessory if needed.)

Bake at 180°C for 14 minutes, turning halfway.

SERVES 2

Millet Patties

1½ cups (370g) cooked millet

1 small onion, finely chopped

1 large carrot, grated

2 cloves garlic, minced

1 tbsp ground coriander

1 tbsp mixed herbs

Salt and pepper, to season

Combine all the ingredients in a large mixing bowl and stir well.

Season with salt and pepper to taste.

Divide the mixture into medium-size balls and flatten using your hands to make patties.

Spray the patties with olive oil on both sides.

Transfer to the basket of the air fryer and cook for 20 minutes at 180°C, or until crisp and golden.

SERVES 4

Whole Roasted Cauliflower

1 cauliflower

⅓ cup (80ml) sour cream

¼ cup (25g) Parmesan cheese, finely grated

1 tsp salt

½ tsp pepper

1 clove garlic, minced

Remove the leaves from the head of cauliflower, and cut out the tough central stem as much as possible while still holding the cauliflower together.

Combine the sour cream, Parmesan, salt, pepper and garlic together. Spread the mixture over the cauliflower rubbing in well.

Place into the basket of the air fryer.

Cook for 15 minutes at 180°C, checking at the 10-minute mark to avoid it getting too brown.

SERVES 4

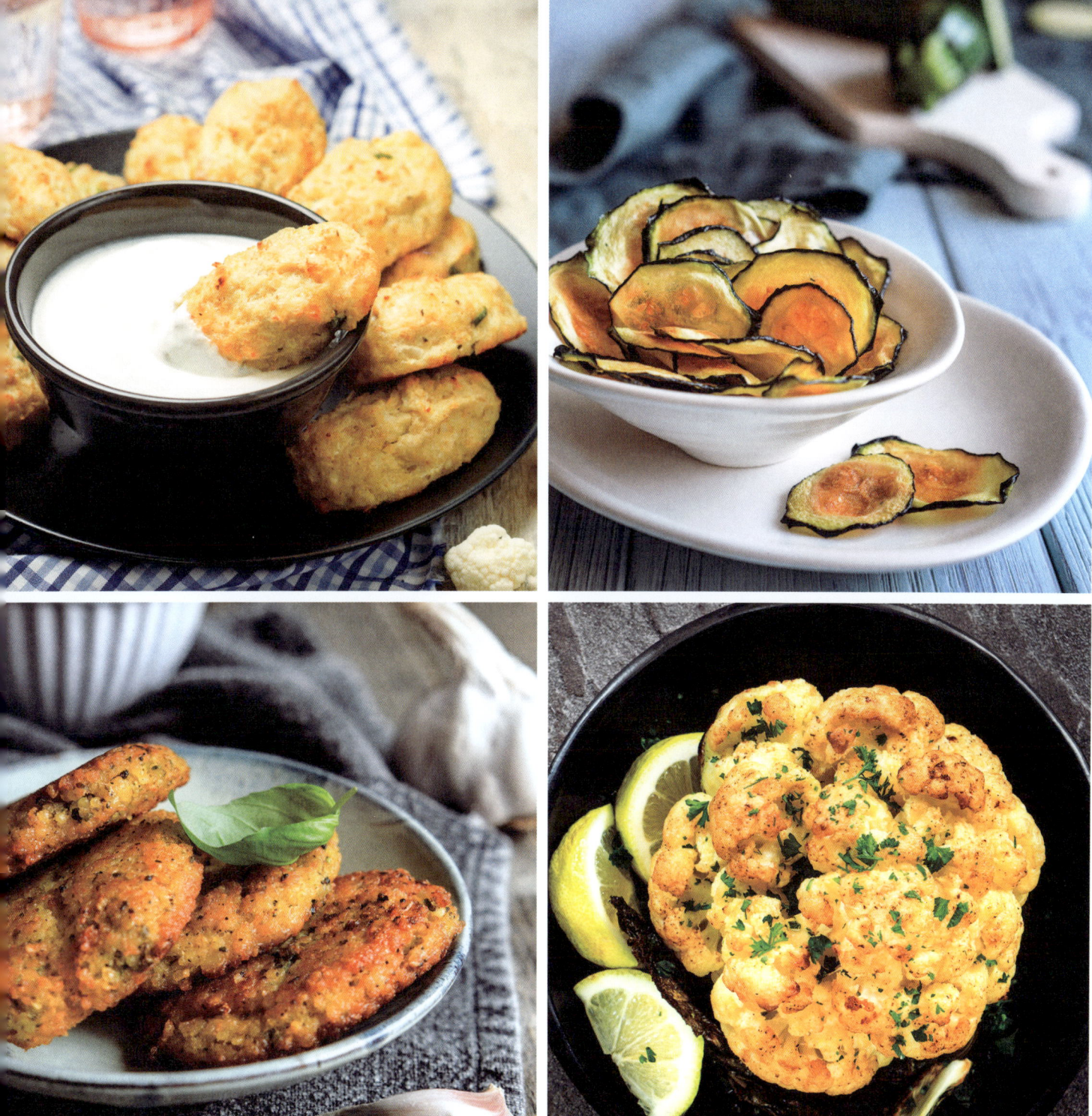

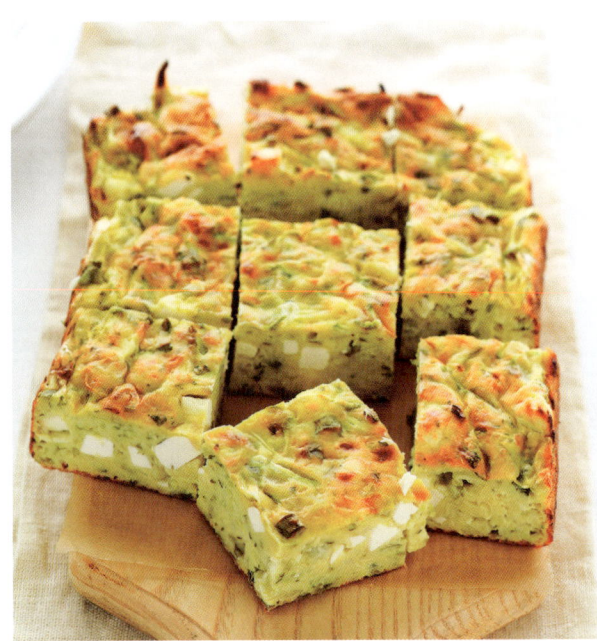

Zucchini and Feta Slice

5 eggs

1 cup (125g) self-raising flour

3 large zucchinis, grated

3 spring onions, chopped

80g soft feta, cut into small pieces

½ cup (125ml) oil

Pinch of salt and pepper

½ cup (60g) tasty cheese, grated

Cake tin

Preheat the air fryer to 180°C.

Whisk the eggs in large bowl. Add the flour and beat until smooth, then add the zucchini, spring onion, feta, oil, salt and pepper and stir to combine.

Pour the mixture into the cake tin and sprinkle with the tasty cheese. Transfer to the air fryer.

Cook for 30 minutes.

SERVES 4

Note: When cooked, a skewer inserted in the centre should come out clean.

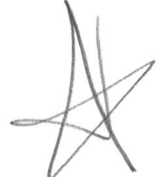

Ratatouille

1 eggplant, cut into cubes

2 red capsicums, de-seeded and sliced into chunks

3 tomatoes, roughly chopped

1 large zucchini, sliced

2 squash, chopped

1 onion, chopped

3 cloves garlic, minced

1 tbsp mixed herbs

¼ cup (5g) fresh oregano

1½ tbsps olive oil

1 tbsp white wine vinegar

Salt and pepper, to taste

Baking dish

Preheat the air fryer to 200°C.

Place all the ingredients into a mixing bowl including salt and pepper to taste. Toss to combine and coat well with the seasonings.

Empty the mixture into the baking dish and transfer to the air fryer. Cook for 15 minutes, stirring halfway.

SERVES 2

Note: You can omit the oregano if you don't have any, or substitute with a herb of your choice.

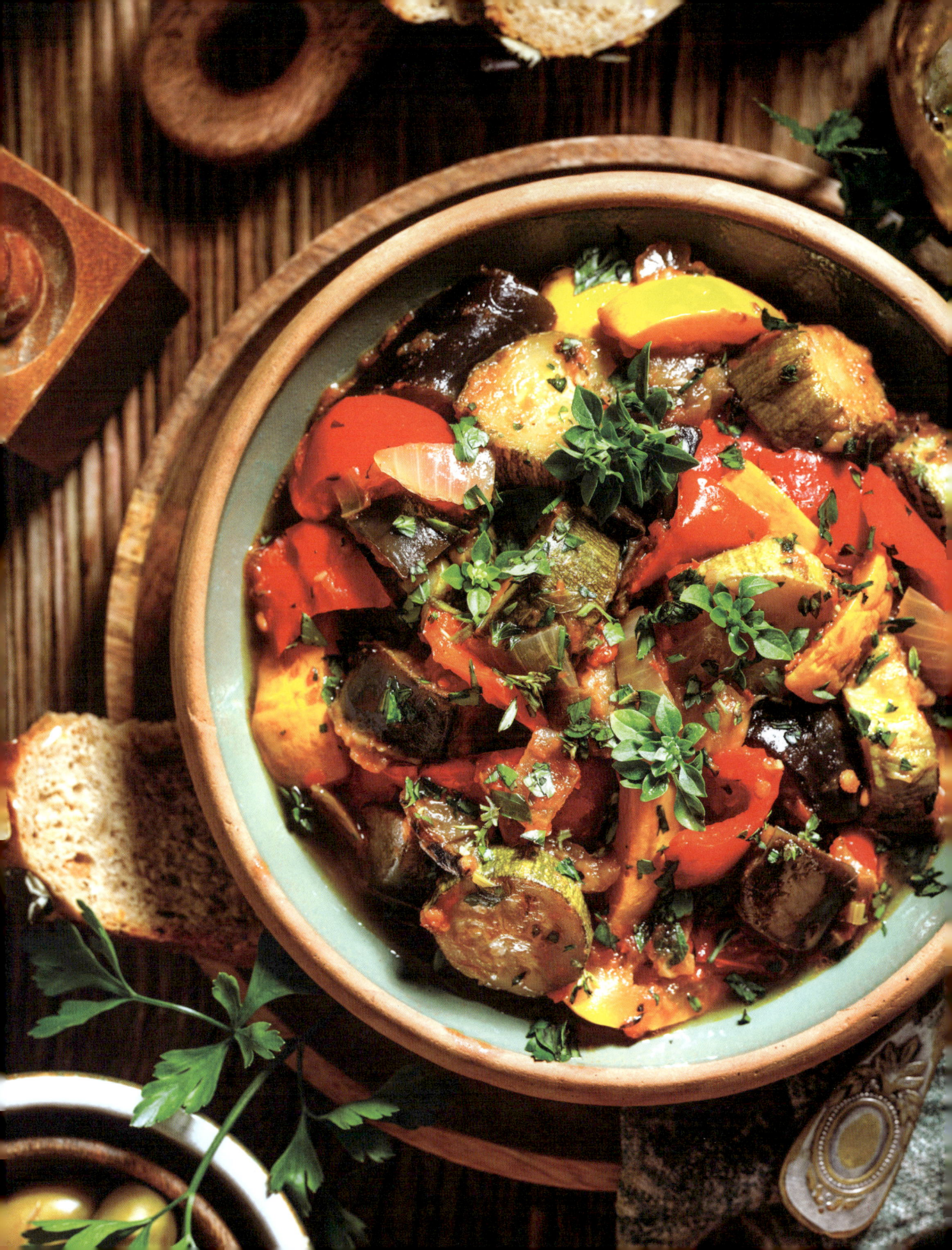

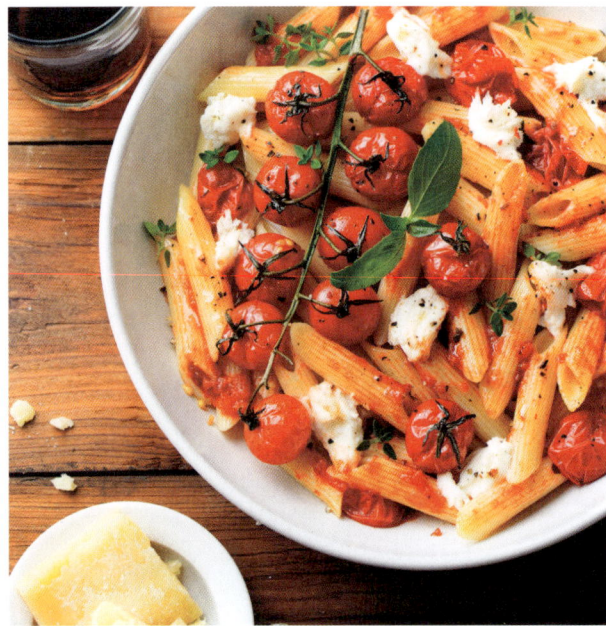

Tomato and Feta Pasta

500g cherry tomatoes on the vine

2 tbsps olive oil

1 tbsp white wine vinegar

1 clove garlic, minced

1 tsp Italian herbs

1 tbsp fresh basil, chopped

Salt and pepper, to taste

250g penne pasta, cooked

Soft feta, to serve

Preheat the air fryer to 200°C.

Place the tomatoes, olive oil, vinegar, garlic, Italian herbs and basil in a large mixing bowl. Season with salt and pepper and toss to combine.

Transfer the ingredients to basket of the air fryer.

Cook for 20 minutes. During cooking remove from the air fryer a few times to stir with a wooden spoon, crushing some of the tomatoes to create the sauce.

When cooked, toss the cooked pasta with the tomato sauce.

Pour over any liquid from the bottom drawer of the air fryer that has leaked through the basket.

Sprinkle with soft feta to serve.

SERVES 2

Cheesy Vegetable Tart

1 savoury pie crust, chilled (see note)

2 eggs

¼ cup (60ml) milk

Pinch of salt and pepper

½ cup (90g) zucchini, chopped

½ cup (75g) onion, chopped

¼ cup (50g) tomato, chopped

2 button mushrooms, sliced

¼ cup (30g) mozzarella cheese, grated

¼ cup (30g) Cheddar cheese, grated

Tart pan

Preheat the air fryer to 180°C.

Line the tart pan with the crust and trim off any excess. Prick the base a few times with a fork.

Beat the eggs with an electric mixer until they are pale and fluffy. Add milk, salt and pepper, zucchini, onion, tomato, mushroom and mozzarella cheese. Stir well to combine.

Transfer the mixture into the prepared crust. Don't fill it quite to the top, so there is room for the tart to rise.

Place the tart into the basket of the air fryer. Cook for 15 minutes then remove and sprinkle the top of the tart with the Cheddar cheese. Return to the air fryer to cook for a further 4 minutes until golden and cheese has melted.

SERVES 4

Note: Purchase a pre-made pie crust or make your own. The crust should be big enough to line a 16cm tart pan.

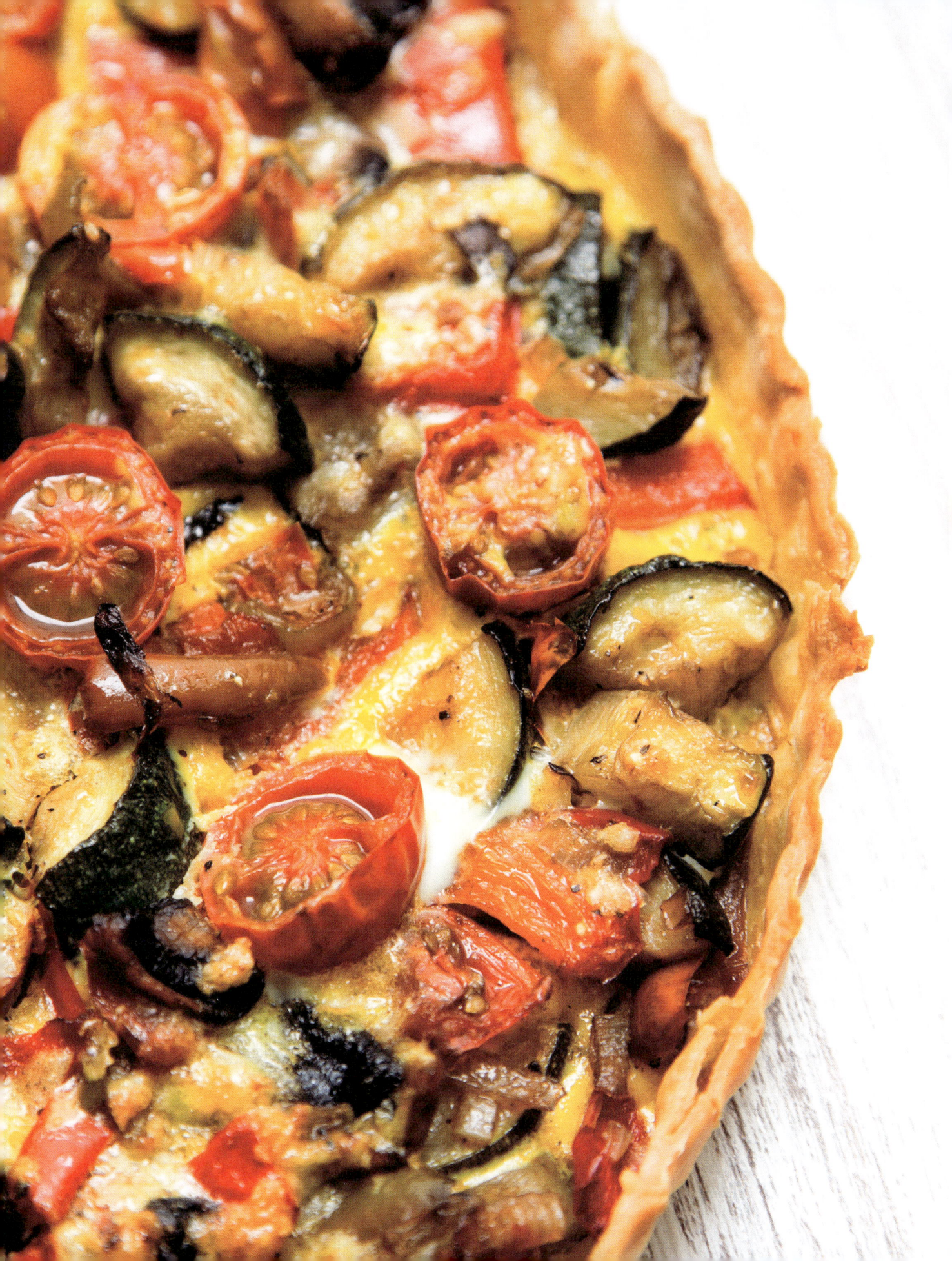

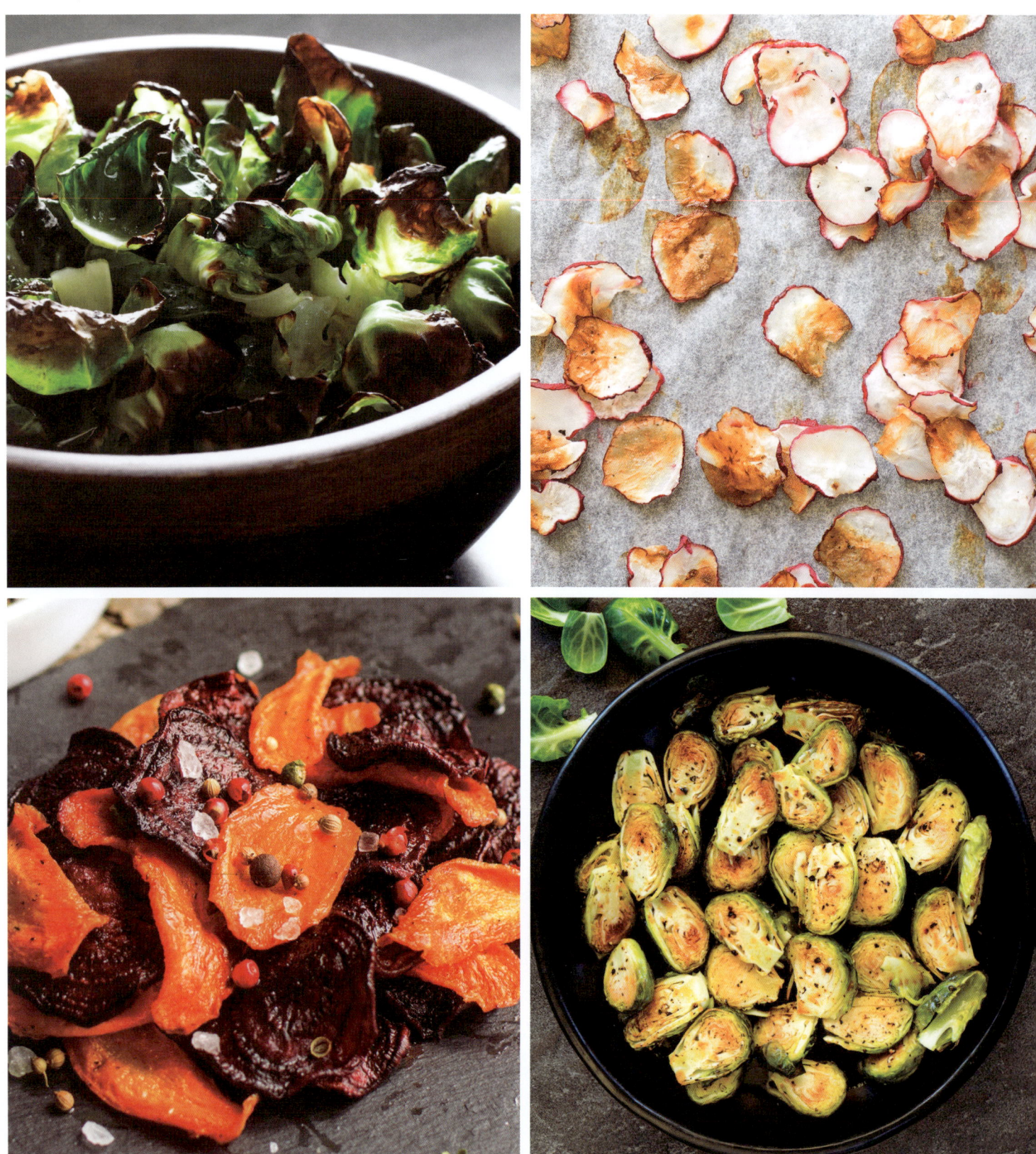

Brussels Sprouts Chips

500g Brussels sprouts

2 tbsps olive oil

1 tbsp balsamic vinegar

Pinch of salt and pepper

Remove the ends of the Brussels sprouts and separate the leaves.

Place the leaves in a large bowl and drizzle with oil and balsamic vinegar, and season with salt and pepper. Toss to fully coat.

Transfer to the air fryer basket. For crispy sprouts, cook at 180°C for 20 minutes, shaking gently halfway through cooking.

SERVE 4

Radish Chips

6 radishes

1 tbsp balsamic vinegar

½ tsp salt

Wash and pat dry radishes. Using a sharp knife or mandolin, finely slice.

Place the radishes in the air fryer basket and spread out in an even layer. (Be careful not to overcrowd the basket. Cook in batches or use a double layer accessory if needed.)

Lightly spritz with olive oil, drizzle over the balsamic vinegar and sprinkle with salt.

Cook in the air fryer for 10 minutes at 190°C, shaking the basket halfway through.

Spritz with a little more oil and cook for a further 6 minutes, again shaking the basket halfway through.

SERVES 2

Beetroot and Carrot Chips

1 small beetroot, peeled

1 large carrot, peeled

½ tsp pepper

1 tsp salt

½ tsp cumin (optional)

Using a sharp knife or mandolin, slice the beetroot and carrot into thin slices.

Spritz the air fryer basket with cooking spray. Preheat the air fryer to 180°C.

Place the vegetable chips in single layer in the air fryer. (Be careful not to overcrowd the basket. Cook in batches or use a double layer accessory if needed.)

Cook for 15 minutes, turning a few times during cooking.

SERVES 2

Toasted Brussels Sprouts

500g Brussels sprouts

2 tbsps olive oil

1 tsp all-purpose seasoning

Pepper, to taste

Clean the sprouts and remove the tough outer leaves.

Place the sprouts in a large bowl and add the oil, seasoning and pepper. Toss to coat.

Transfer to the air fryer basket. Cook for 12 minutes at 200°C, shaking the basket halfway through.

SERVES 4

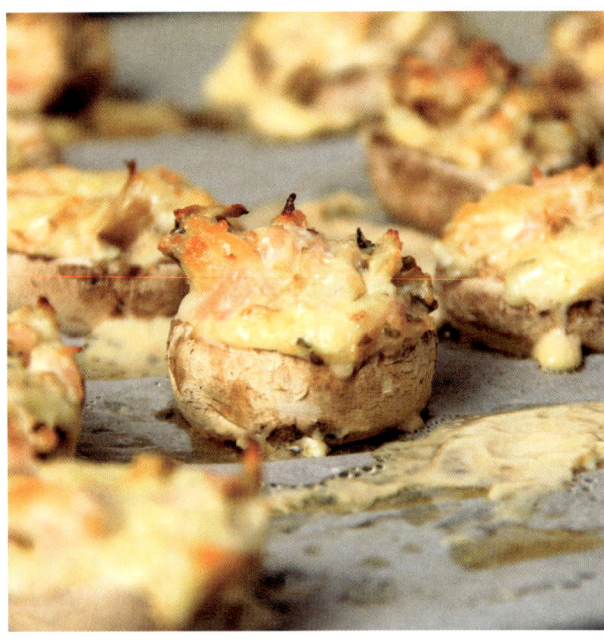

Button Mushroom Melt

20 button mushrooms, rinsed and stems removed

Pinch of salt and pepper

1 tsp mixed herbs

1 tbsp olive oil

¼ cup (60ml) cream

¼ cup (30g) mozzarella cheese

Rub the mushrooms clean with a paper towel and pat dry with a fresh towel.

Season with salt and pepper and herbs.

Preheat the air fryer to 180°C.

Poke a few holes in a sheet of baking paper and place it in the base of the air fryer basket.

Place the mushrooms on top of the baking paper and with the rounded side down. Drizzle olive oil and cream evenly into each mushroom, then sprinkle with cheese.

Cook for 8 minutes.

SERVES 4

Garlic Crumbed Mushrooms

20 white button mushrooms

1 cup (125g) breadcrumbs

¼ cup (25g) Parmesan cheese, finely grated

½ tsp paprika

½ tsp salt

½ tsp pepper

2 eggs

3 cloves garlic, minced

½ cup (60g) plain flour

Rub the mushrooms clean with a paper towel and pat dry with a fresh towel.

Combine the breadcrumbs, Parmesan, paprika, salt and pepper in a shallow bowl.

Beat the egg together with the minced garlic and place in a second shallow bowl.

Place the flour in a third bowl.

Dip each mushroom into the flour then through the egg mixture, shaking off any excess. Then press into the breadcrumb mixture, ensuring it is evenly and fully coated.

Lightly spritz the crumbed mushrooms with cooking spray.

Cook for 15 minutes on 190°C until golden brown.

SERVES 4

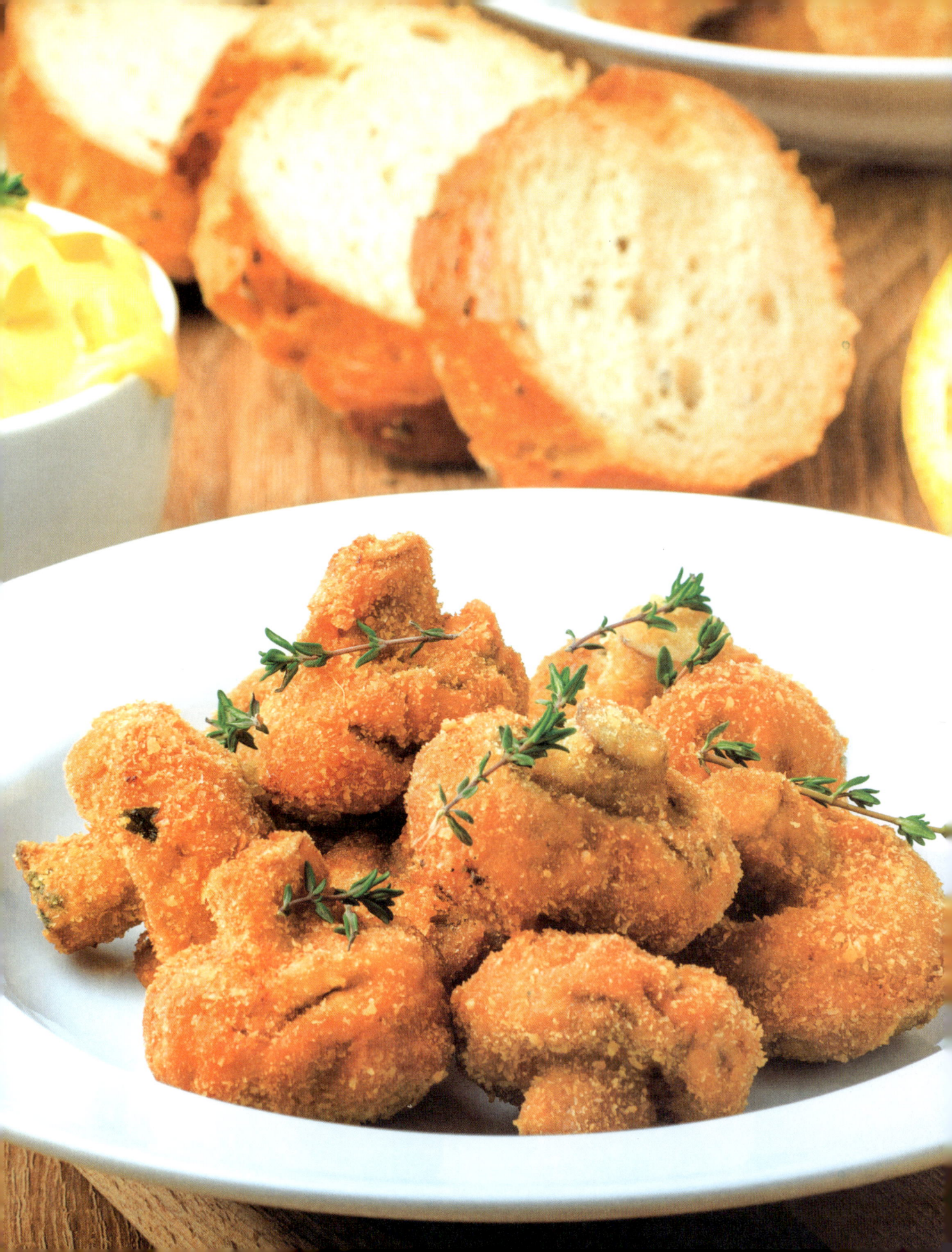

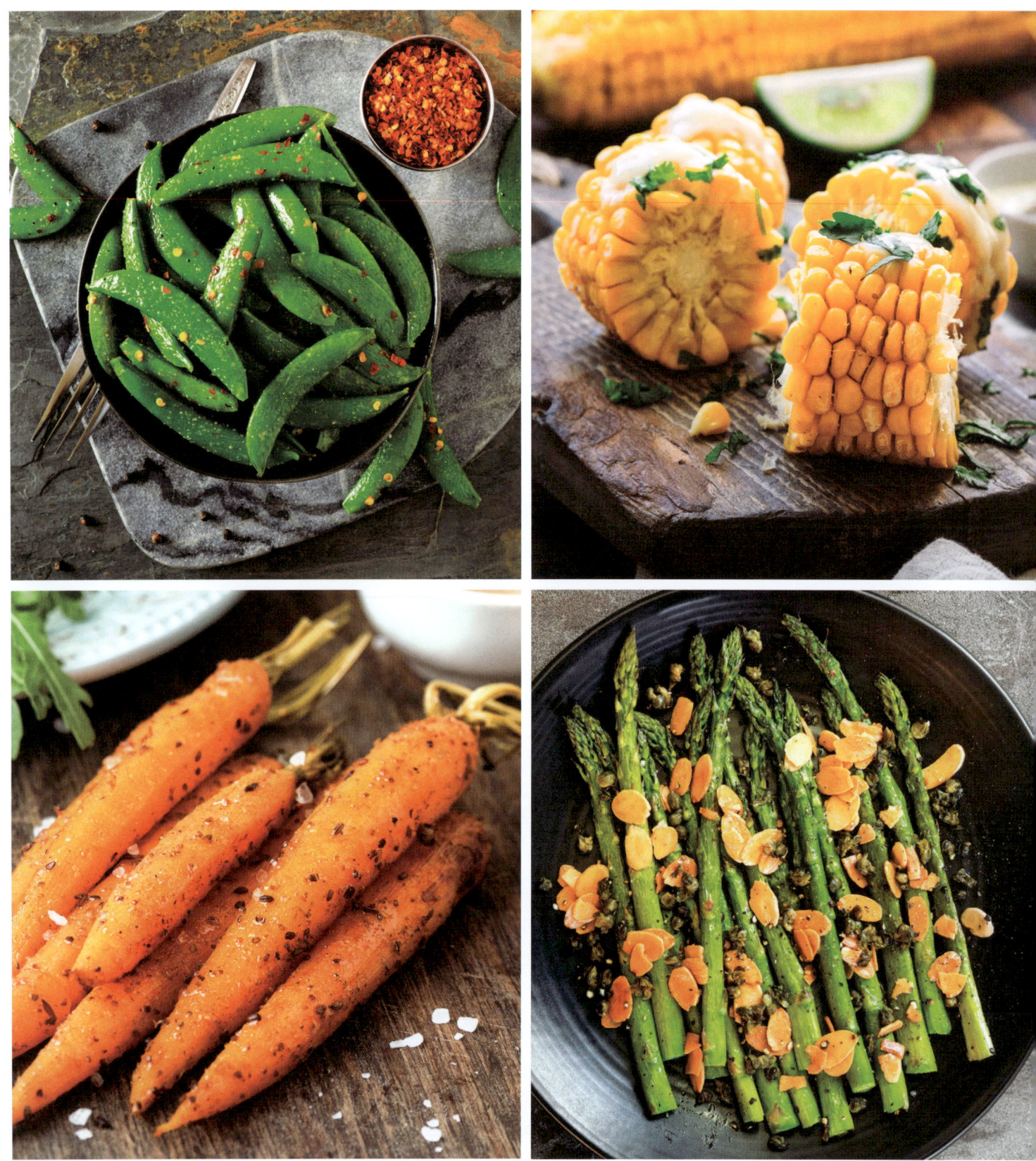

Chilli Snap Peas

250g fresh sugar snap peas

½ tsp sesame oil

1 tsp olive oil

1 tsp chilli flakes

Preheat the air fryer to 190°C.

Combine all the ingredients in a bowl and toss to coat.

Transfer the mixture into the air fryer basket.

Cook for 6 minutes, shaking halfway through cooking.

SERVES 2

Corn on the Cob

2 corn cobs

Pinch of salt and pepper

Fresh parsley, chopped, to garnish

Dehusk the corn cobs and break each one into three pieces. Spray with oil and season with salt and pepper.

Transfer into the basket of the air fryer and cook for 10 minutes at 190°C, shaking twice during cooking.

SERVES 3-4

Honey Carrots

Bunch of baby carrots

1 tbsp honey

1 tbsp olive oil

Pinch of salt and pepper

Scrub clean the carrots and trim the ends if needed.

Combine the carrots, honey and olive oil in a shallow mixing bowl and toss to fully coat. Season with salt and pepper.

Preheat the air fryer to 200°C.

Transfer the carrots into the air fryer basket and slide into the air fryer. Cook for 12 minutes.

SERVES 4

Asparagus, Almonds and Capers

1 bunch asparagus

2 tbsps balsamic vinegar

2 tbsps olive oil

2 tbsps capers

Pinch of salt and pepper

⅓ cup (40g) sliced almonds

Place the asparagus on a plate and drizzle with the balsamic vinegar and oil. Sprinkle with capers, salt and pepper. Turn the spears around through the mixture so that each one is well coated.

Transfer the asparagus to the basket of the air fryer and spread out in a single layer. Sprinkle the sliced almonds on top.

Preheat the air fryer to 180°C.

Cook for 5 minutes, shaking halfway through cooking.

SERVES 4

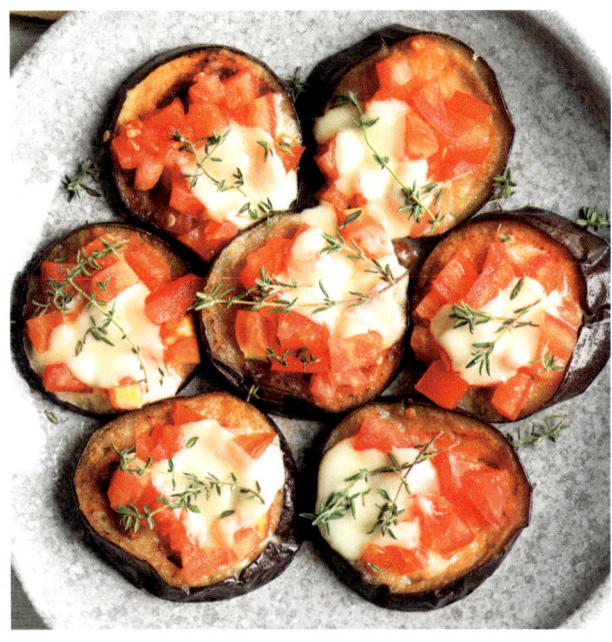

Eggplant Slices with Tomato and Cheese

1 large eggplant

1 tsp salt

1 tbsp mixed herbs

2 medium tomatoes, chopped

¼ cup (30g) mozzarella cheese slices

Fresh thyme, to garnish

Cut eggplant into thick slices. Sprinkle salt over both sides of the eggplant slices. Set aside for 15 minutes then dab off any excess moisture using a paper towel.

Preheat the air fryer to 180°C.

Lightly spray the eggplant slices with olive oil and then transfer to the air fryer basket. (Be careful not to overcrowd the basket. Cook in batches or use a double layer accessory if needed.)

Cook for 6 minutes. Remove basket and sprinkle eggplant with the mixed herbs, then place the chopped tomatoes and cheese on top of the eggplant slices. Return to the air fryer to cook for a further 4 minutes.

Sprinkle with fresh thyme to serve.

SERVES 4

Eggplant Schnitzels

1 eggplant

1 tsp salt

1 cup (125g) breadcrumbs

1 tsp Italian herbs

¼ cup (60ml) olive oil

2 eggs

½ cup (60g) plain flour

Slices the eggplant lengthwise into 4 or 5 even slices. Place the eggplant in a colander over a bowl and sprinkle with the salt. Allow to drain for 45 minutes. Discard water in the bowl.

Combine the breadcrumbs, herbs and olive oil together in a shallow bowl.

Beat the eggs in a shallow bowl.

Place the flour in a shallow bowl.

Dip the eggplant slices first in the flour and then in the egg mixture, shaking off any excess.

Then dip into the breadcrumb mixture pressing in to ensure they are evenly covered.

Preheat the air fryer to 200°C.

Place a single layer of breaded eggplant into the basket of the air fryer and cook for 14 minutes, turning halfway during cooking.

SERVES 2

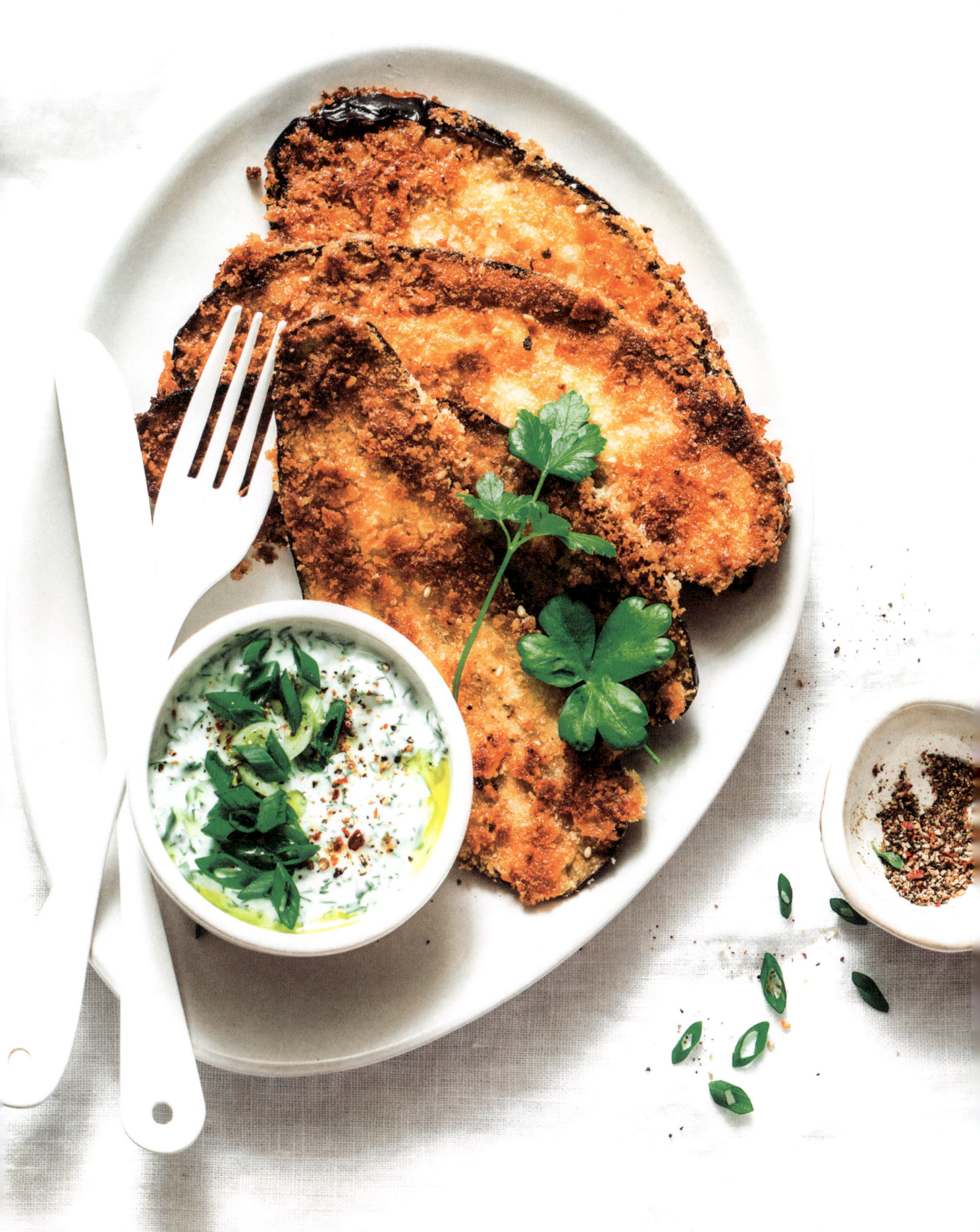

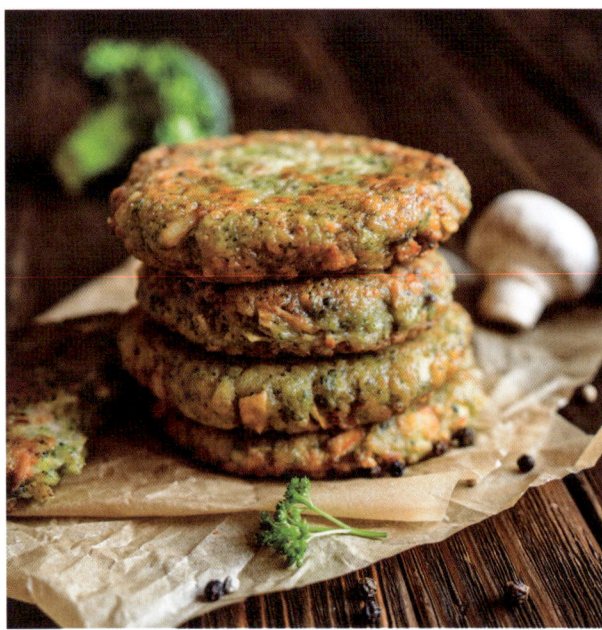

Broccoli and Mushroom Burgers

1 large head broccoli

1 cup (160g) canned chickpeas, rinsed

2 Swiss mushrooms, finely chopped

1 small onion, finely chopped

1 tbsp lemon herb and garlic seasoning

½ tsp salt

2 eggs, beaten

¾ cup (75g) Parmesan cheese, grated

½ cup (60g) panko breadcrumbs

Bring a large pan of water to the boil and cook the broccoli until soft (approximately 6 minutes). Drain and set in a large bowl. Mash roughly with a potato masher.

Add the chickpeas to the bowl and roughly mash. Next add the mushrooms, onion, seasoning and salt. Stir until just combined. Add the eggs, cheese and breadcrumbs and mix gently until combined.

Cover and transfer to the fridge to chill for 1 hour.

Roll into balls and then press to form patties.

Preheat the air fryer to 190°C.

Spritz the burgers with olive oil on both sides and transfer to the basket of the air fryer. Cook for 12 minutes, turning halfway.

SERVES 3

Ricotta Balls

1 cup (250g) ricotta

2 tbsps flour

1 egg, separated

½ tsp salt

¼ tsp pepper

½ cup (20g) basil, chopped

2 spring onions, chopped

3 slices stale white bread (or use breadcrumbs)

1/4 cup olive oil

1 x 700g jar passata (or homemade tomato sauce, see page 124)

300g spaghetti, cooked

¼ cup (25g) Parmesan cheese, grated, to garnish

Combine the ricotta in a bowl with the flour, egg yolk, salt and pepper. Stir through the basil and spring onions.

Divide the mixture into 20 equal portions and shape into balls using wet hands. Set aside.

Place the bread into the bowl of a food processor and pulse until finely ground. Add the olive oil and pulse until just combined. Shake the mixture into a bowl.

Beat the egg white in a second bowl.

Preheat the air fryer to 200°C.

Dip the ricotta balls into the egg mixture, shaking off any excess. Gently roll through the breadcrumb mixture.

Place 10 balls in the basket of the air fryer and slide into the air fryer.

Cook for 8 minutes. Remove from the air fryer and pour over half of the passata. Return to the air fryer for 3 minutes. Remove and keep warm.

Repeat with the second batch of ricotta balls.

Serve ricotta balls in tomato sauce on top of freshly cooked spaghetti and garnished with Parmesan.

SERVES 2-3

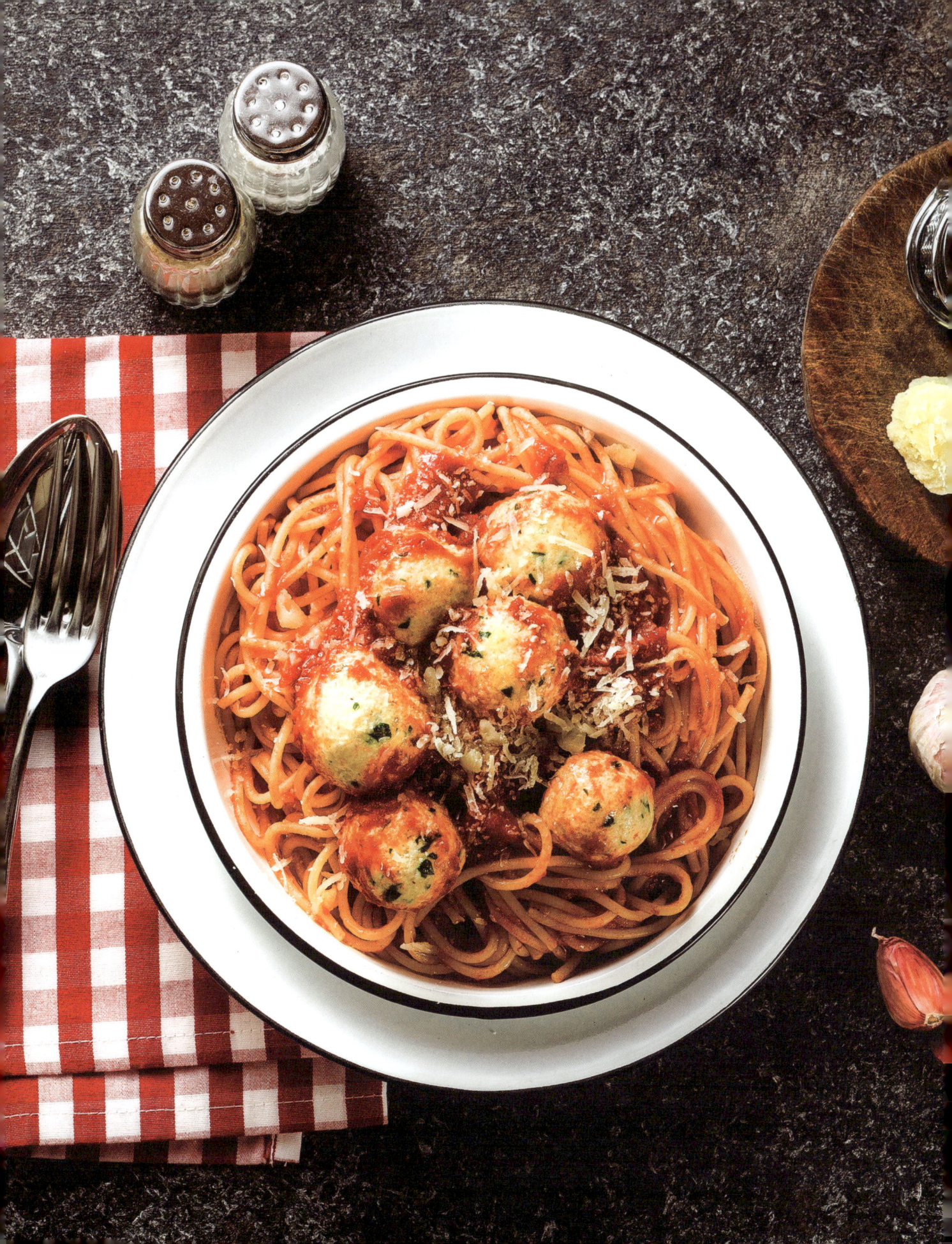

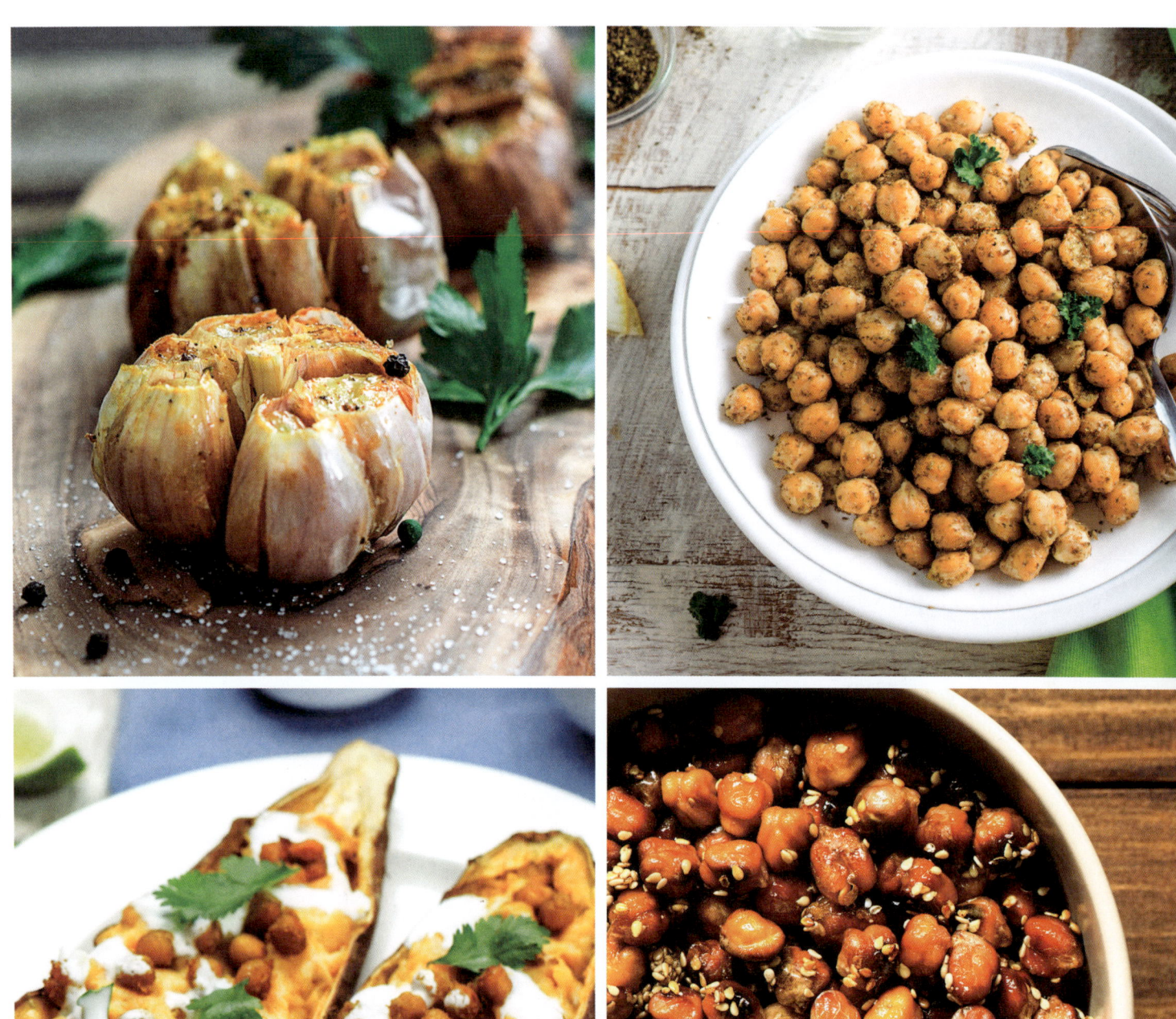

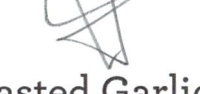
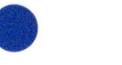
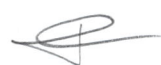

Roasted Garlic

4 heads garlic

1 tbsp olive oil

Slice the tops off of the garlic heads, exposing the individual cloves.

Place on a square of foil large enough to cover the heads.

Drizzle with oil. Fold foil around garlic and seal.

Place in the packet in the air fryer basket.

Cook at 200°C for 25 minutes. Remove from the air fryer and take off the foil. Return to the air fryer to cook for a further 2 minutes until garlic is golden.

Serve immediately on crackers, or squeeze the garlic out of the cloves into a small jar for use later.

Spiced Chickpeas

1 x 400g can chickpeas

2 tsps olive oil

1 tsp ground coriander

1 tsp garlic powder

1 tsp ground cumin

Pinch of ground ginger

½ tsp salt

Drain and rinse the chickpeas. Place into a large bowl and add all the remaining ingredients. Toss to coat.

Preheat the air fryer to 190°C.

Transfer the mixture into the air fryer basket and cook for 20 minutes, removing the basket and stirring three times at regular intervals during cooking. Continue to cook at 1 minute intervals until the chickpeas are golden and crunchy.

SERVES 2

Sweet Potatoes with Spiced Chickpeas and Greek Dressing

1 tbsp lime juice

1 clove garlic, minced

1 cup (250ml) plain yoghurt

2 tbsps fresh coriander, chopped

½ tsp salt

2 sweet potatoes

1 cup (160g) spiced chickpeas (see top right)

To make the dressing combine lime juice, garlic, yoghurt, coriander and salt in a sealable jar. Close the lid tightly and shake to combine.

Preheat the air fryer to 200°C.

Scrub clean and pat dry the sweet potatoes. Spritz lightly with cooking spray. Pierce sweet potato skin with a fork and transfer to the air fryer. Cook 40 minutes until tender.

To serve, cut open the potatoes and top with spiced chickpeas and yoghurt dressing.

SERVES 2

Honey Sesame Chickpeas

1 x 400g can chickpeas

1 tsp olive oil

1 tsp sesame oil

1 tbsp honey

1 tsp ground cumin (optional)

¼ tsp salt

2 tbsps sesame seeds

Drain and rinse the chickpeas. Place into a large bowl and add all the remaining ingredients. Toss to coat.

Preheat the air fryer to 190°C.

Transfer the mixture into the air fryer basket and cook for 20 minutes, removing the basket and stirring three times at regular intervals during cooking. Continue to cook at 1 minute intervals until the chickpeas are golden and crunchy.

SERVES 2

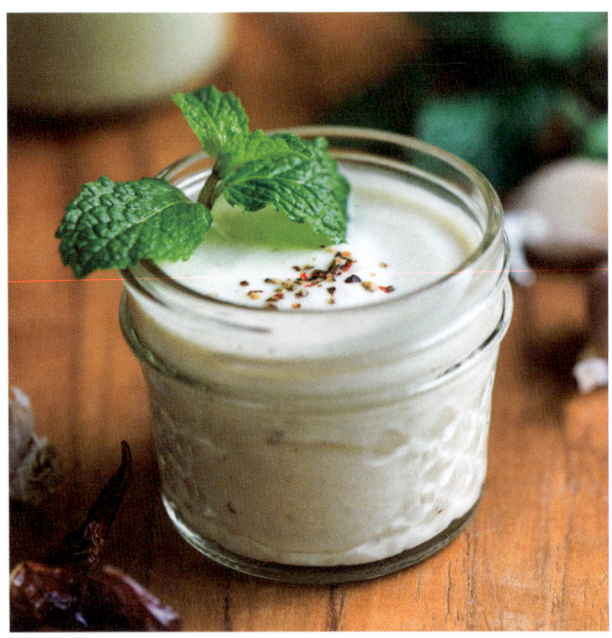

Tahini Yoghurt Sauce

1 cup (250ml) yoghurt

1 lemon, juiced

Pinch of salt

1 tbsp olive oil

1 tsp minced garlic

2 tbsps tahini paste

Add all the ingredients to a bowl and stir until well combined.

Taste and adjust any of the elements to your preference.

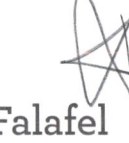

Falafel

1½ cups (250g) dried chickpeas, soaked overnight (or use canned)

2 cloves garlic, minced

1 red onion, chopped

¼ cup (10g) fresh coriander, roughly chopped

3 tbsps olive oil

1 tsp ground coriander

1 tsp ground cumin

Pinch of allspice (optional)

½ tsp salt

½ tsp baking powder

4 tbsps almond meal

Place the chickpeas, garlic, onion and chopped coriander in the bowl of a food processor and whiz until a rough paste forms. Slowly add the olive oil and continue to process until smooth and combined.

Transfer the mixture to a bowl. Add the ground coriander, cumin, allspice, if using, salt, baking powder and almond meal and mix well.

Cover and place in the fridge for 1 hour (minimum).

Roll the mixture into small balls using wet hands, and transfer to a plate.

Place the falafel in the air fryer basket, ensuring they do not touch. (Be careful not to overcrowd the basket. Cook in batches or use a double layer accessory if needed.)

Cook at 190°C for 15 minutes until crisp and golden, shaking air fryer basket halfway through cooking.

Serve with tahini yoghurt sauce (see opposite).

SERVES 2

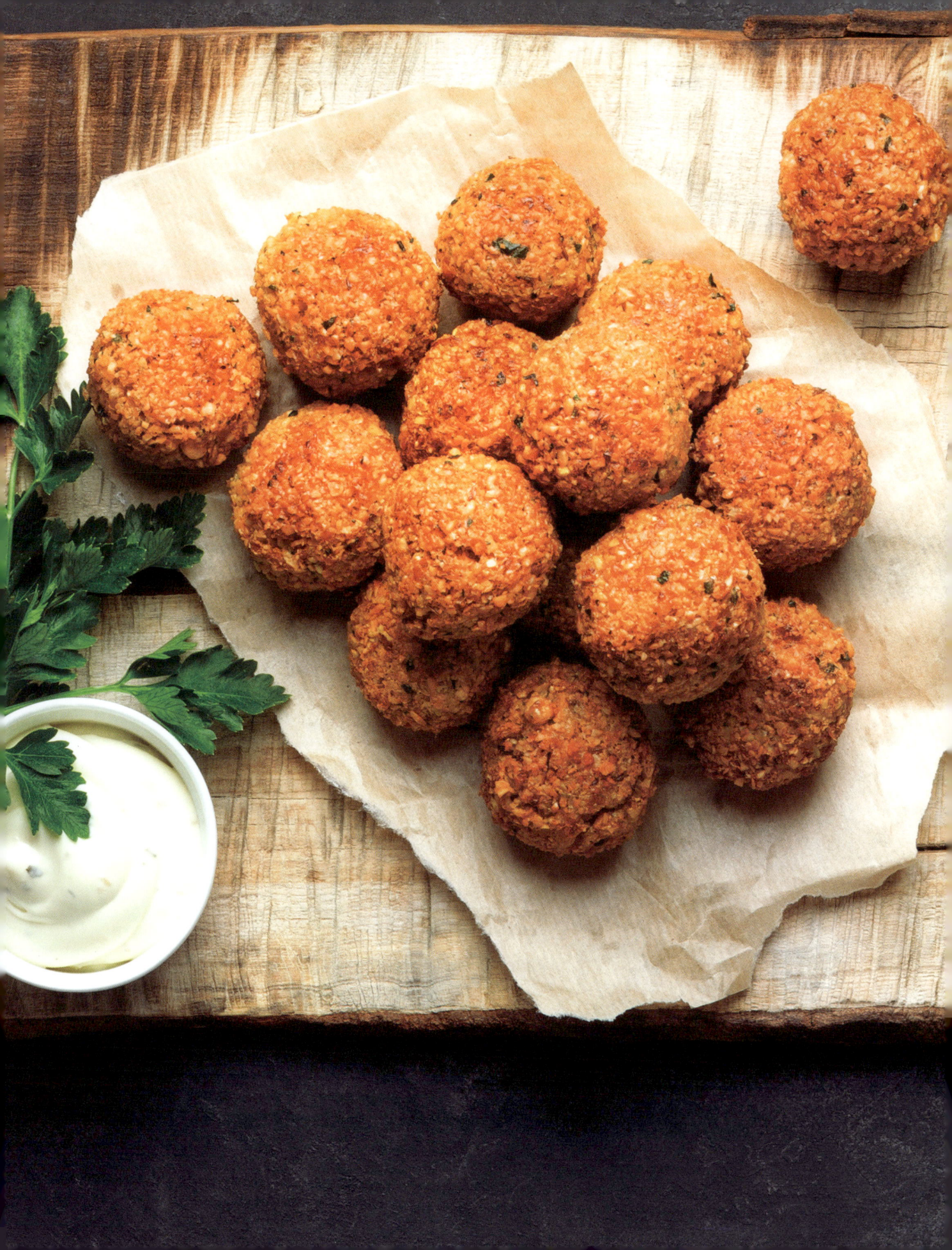

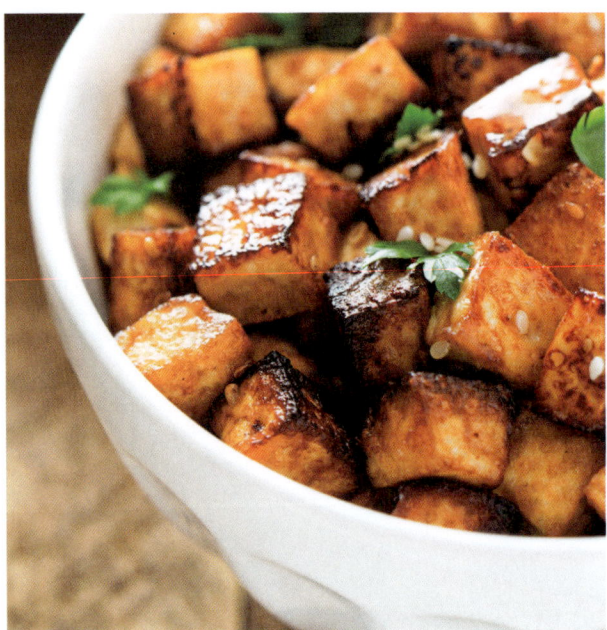

Crispy Tofu

450g firm tofu

2 tbsps soy sauce

1 tbsp rice wine vinegar

1 tsp sesame oil

1 tbsp potato starch (or cornflour)

First press the tofu to remove excess moisture: Cut the tofu into thick slices. Place them evenly on a flat surface lined with paper towels or a clean dishcloth. Cover with a layer of paper towels, set a baking tray on top and then place a cookbook (or other heavy object) on top. Press like this for 15 minutes. Cut the slices into small squares.

Whisk the soy sauce, rice wine vinegar and sesame oil together in a mixing bowl.

Add the tofu cubes to the bowl and gently toss to coat the pieces. Cover and transfer to the fridge to marinate for 30 minutes or longer, if you have the time.

When ready to cook, preheat the air fryer to 200°C and lightly spritz the air fryer basket with oil. Toss the tofu in the potato starch.

Place the tofu in the air fryer basket and spray the tops with oil. (Be careful not to overcrowd the basket. Cook in batches or use a double layer accessory if needed.)

Cook for 20 minutes, or until golden and crispy, shaking the basket a few times during cooking.

SERVES 2

Tofu in Ginger Soy Sauce

450g firm tofu

¼ cup (30g) arrowroot flour

½ tsp smoked paprika

½ tsp ground cumin

1 tsp salt

3 tbsps soy sauce

1 tbsp brown sugar

2 tbsps honey

1 tbsp sesame oil

1 tbsp ginger, freshly grated

1 tbsp garlic, minced

1 tsp white sesame seeds

1 spring onion, chopped, for garnish

Press and prepare the tofu according to the instructions in the recipe opposite.

Place the arrowroot flour, paprika, cumin and salt in a large mixing bowl and stir to combine. Place the tofu cubes into the bowl and gently toss to coat the pieces.

When ready to cook, preheat the air fryer to 190°C and lightly spritz the air fryer basket with oil. Place the tofu cubes in the basket of the air fryer and spray the tops with oil. (Be careful not to overcrowd the basket. Cook in batches or use a double layer accessory if needed.)

Cook for 25 minutes, turning once during cooking.

Meanwhile, make the sauce. Place the soy sauce, brown sugar, honey, sesame oil, ginger, garlic and sesame seeds in a large mixing bowl and whisk well.

Remove tofu from air fryer and allow to cool slightly, then transfer to the bowl with the sauce. Toss gently to coat the tofu in sauce and transfer to serving bowls.

Sprinkle with spring onion and extra sesame seeds to serve.

SERVES 2

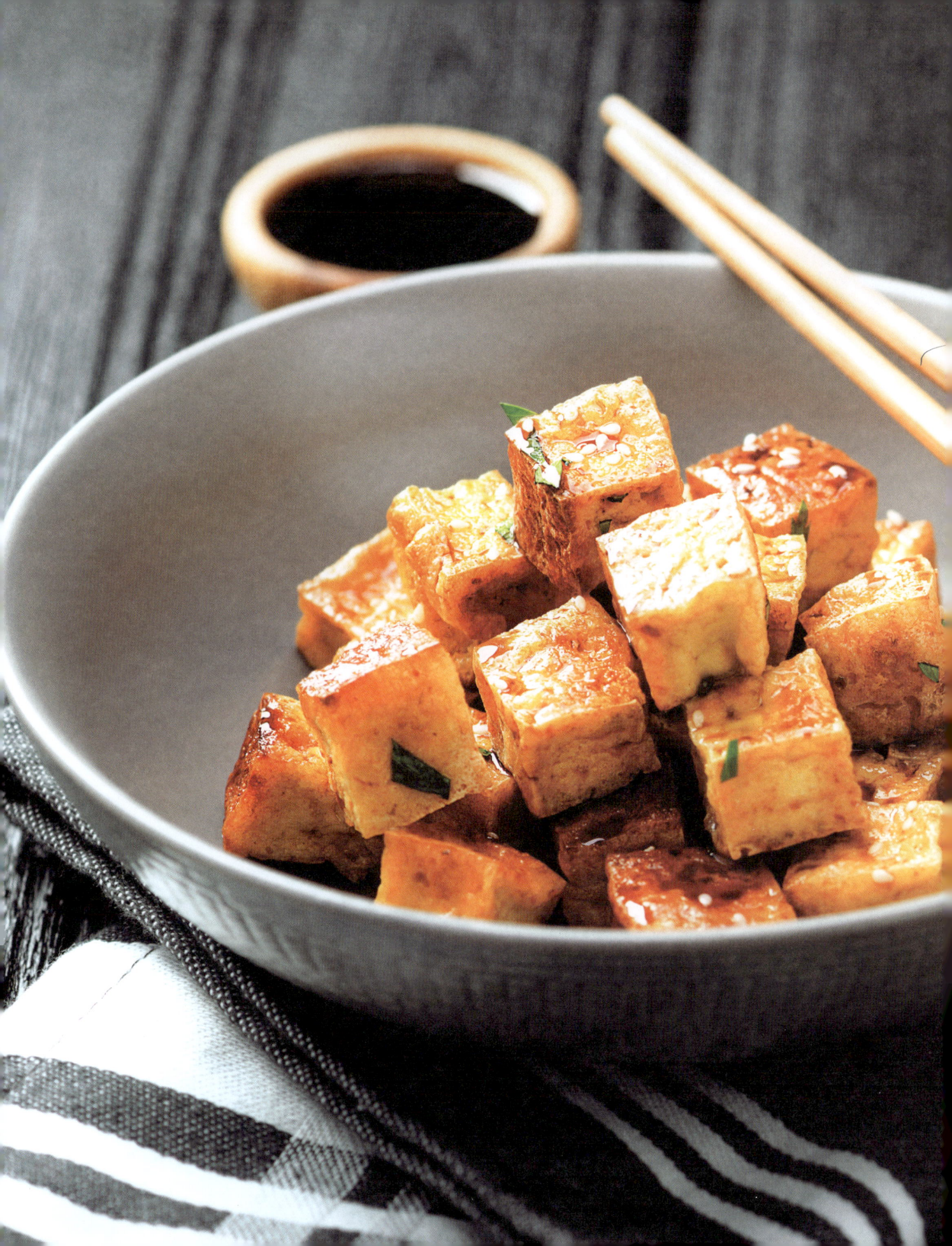

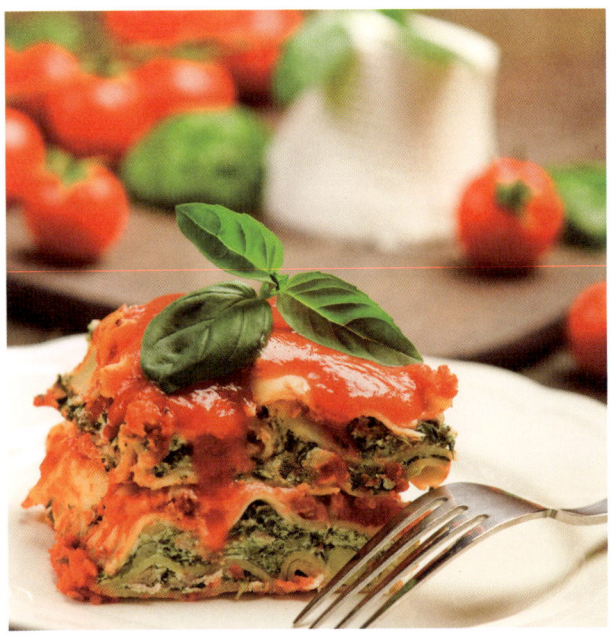

Spinach and Ricotta Lasagne

4 sheets lasagne noodles

1 cup (225g) passata

¾ cup (200g) ricotta

1 cup baby spinach leaves, chopped

½ zucchini, grated

½ cup basil, chopped

Loaf tin

Cook the lasagne sheets according to the directions on the packet. Drain and set aside to cool slightly.

Line the bottom of the loaf tin with 2 tablespoons of passata and place a lasagne sheet over the top. Next add a similar amount each of the ricotta, spinach and zucchini. Place another lasagne sheet on top. Continue like this until all ingredients have been used up, finishing with a layer of the passata.

Cover the loaf tin with foil and transfer to the air fryer.

Cook for 10 minutes on 200°C, then remove the foil and return to the air fryer to cook for a further 3 minutes.

Transfer to a plate to serve.

SERVES 2

Note: A large air fryer can accommodate two loaf tins.

Fried Ravioli

¾ cup (90g) panko breadcrumbs

½ cup (50g) Parmesan cheese, grated

1 tsp mixed herbs

Pinch of salt and pepper

2 eggs

280g ravioli (fresh or frozen)

Place the panko, Parmesan, mixed herbs, salt and pepper in a shallow bowl and mix until combined.

Beat the eggs in a second shallow bowl.

Dip each ravioli in the egg mixture, shaking off any excess. Then dip into the panko mixture, pressing in to ensure it is well covered.

Preheat the air fryer to 190°C.

Place the ravioli in a single layer in the air fryer. (Be careful not to overcrowd the basket. Cook in batches or use a double layer accessory if needed.) Lightly spritz the ravioli with cooking spray.

Cook for 8 minutes, turning over carefully with tongs halfway through cooking.

SERVES 2

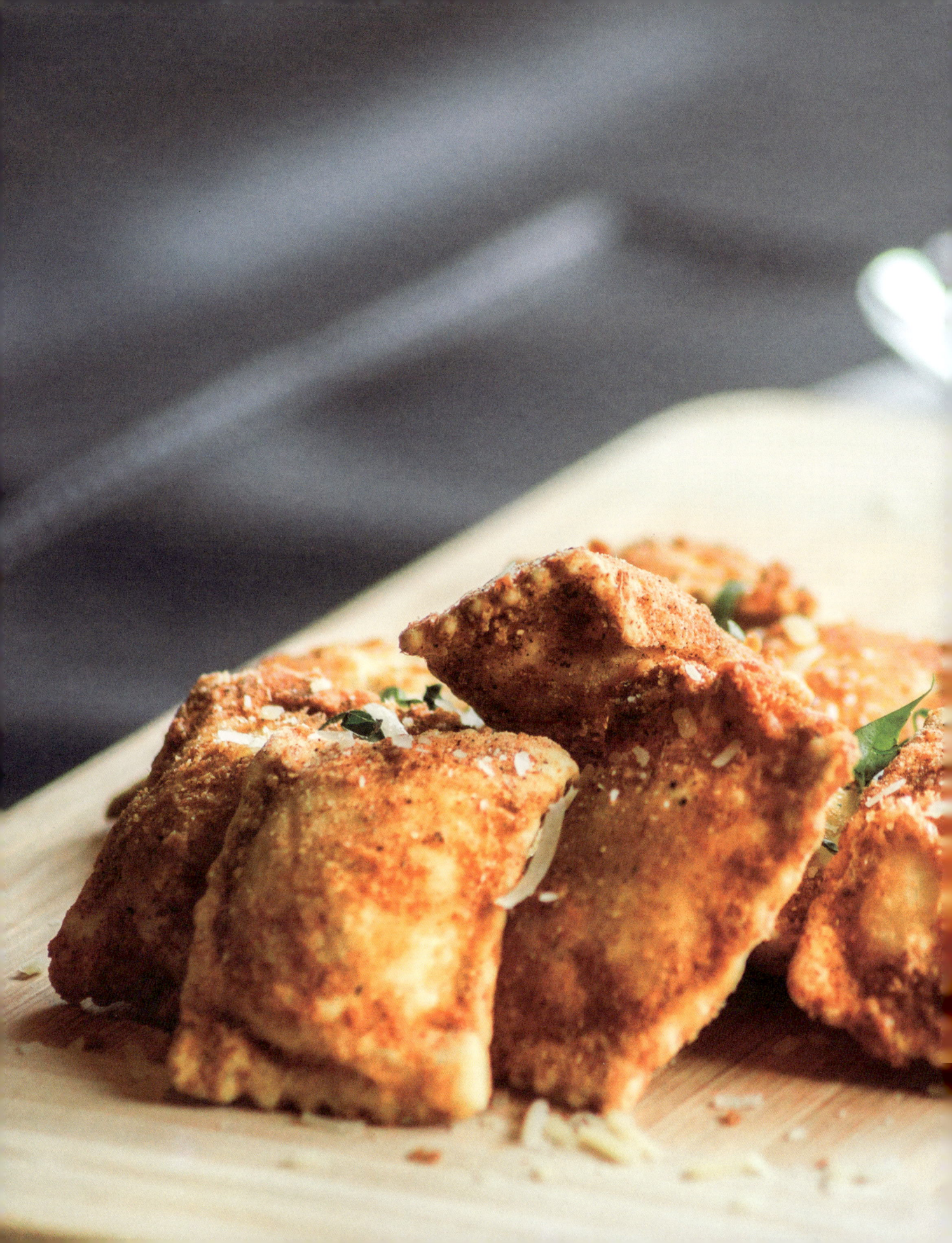

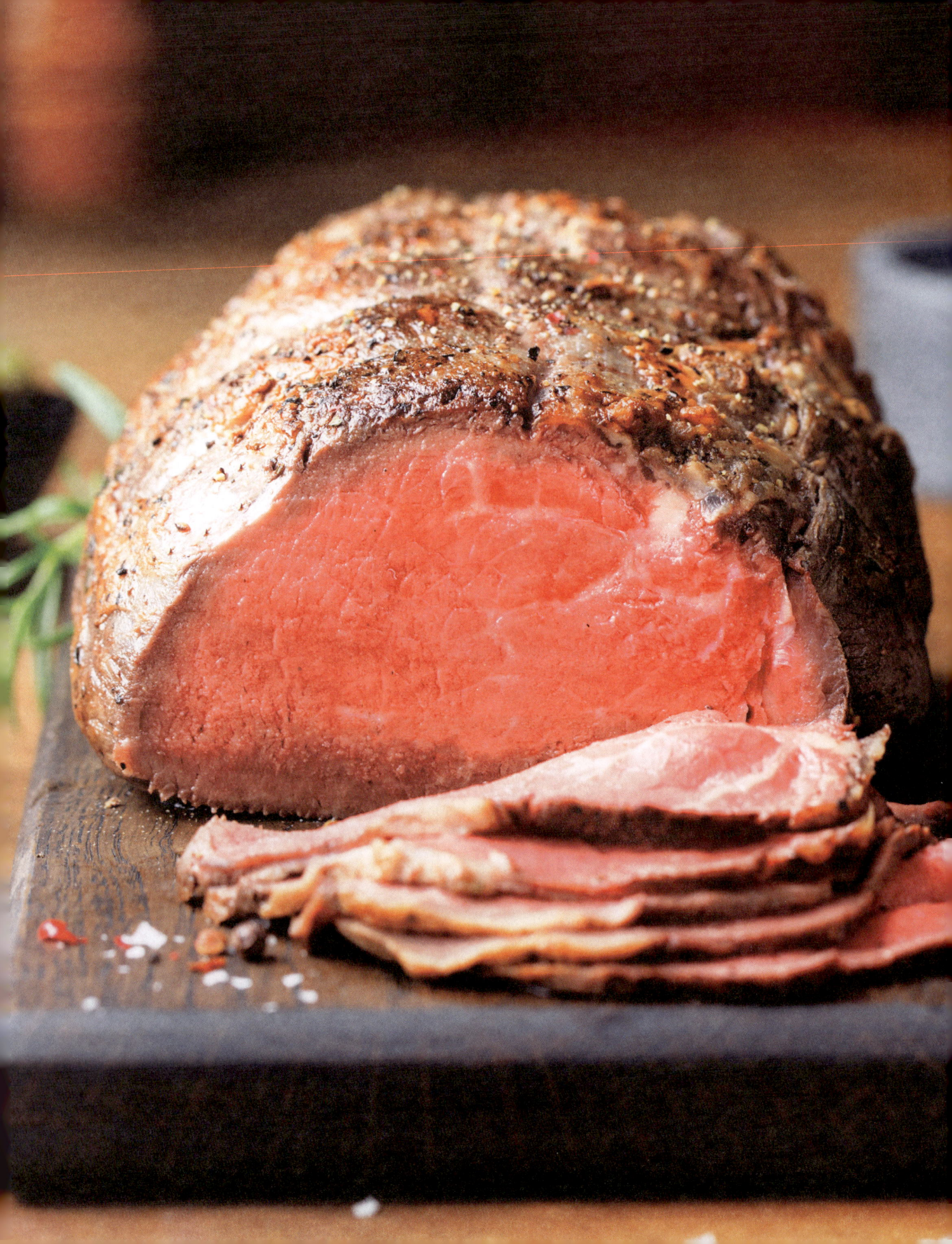

Meat

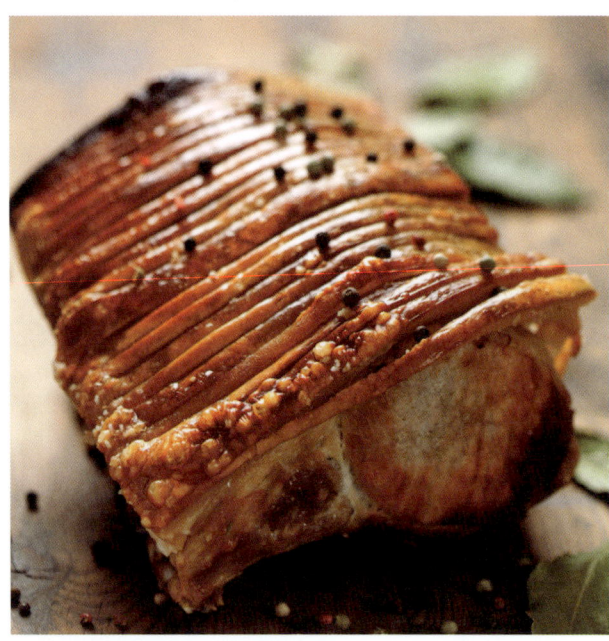

Crispy Pork Rack

6 chop pork loin rack

1 tbsp salt

4 tbsps olive oil

Preheat the air fryer to 200°C.

Cut the rack in half, if needed, to fit into the air fryer basket.

Dry the skin of the pork using paper towels.

Rub salt all over skin then drizzle with the oil. Continue to rub into the skin until well covered.

Place in the air fryer basket skin-side up.

Cook for 40 minutes.

SERVES 2

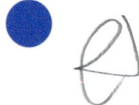

Pork Belly Roast

750g pork belly

1 tbsp salt

2 tbsps olive oil

Preheat the air fryer to 200°C.

Dry the skin of the pork using paper towels.

With a sharp knife, score the skin about halfway towards the meat at regular intervals.

Sprinkle salt into the cuts, rubbing it in well.

Drizzle with the oil and rub well into the skin, ensuring it is completely covered.

Place in the air fryer basket skin-side up.

Cook for 30 minutes.

Reduce the heat to 180°C, and cook for a further 45 minutes.

SERVES 4

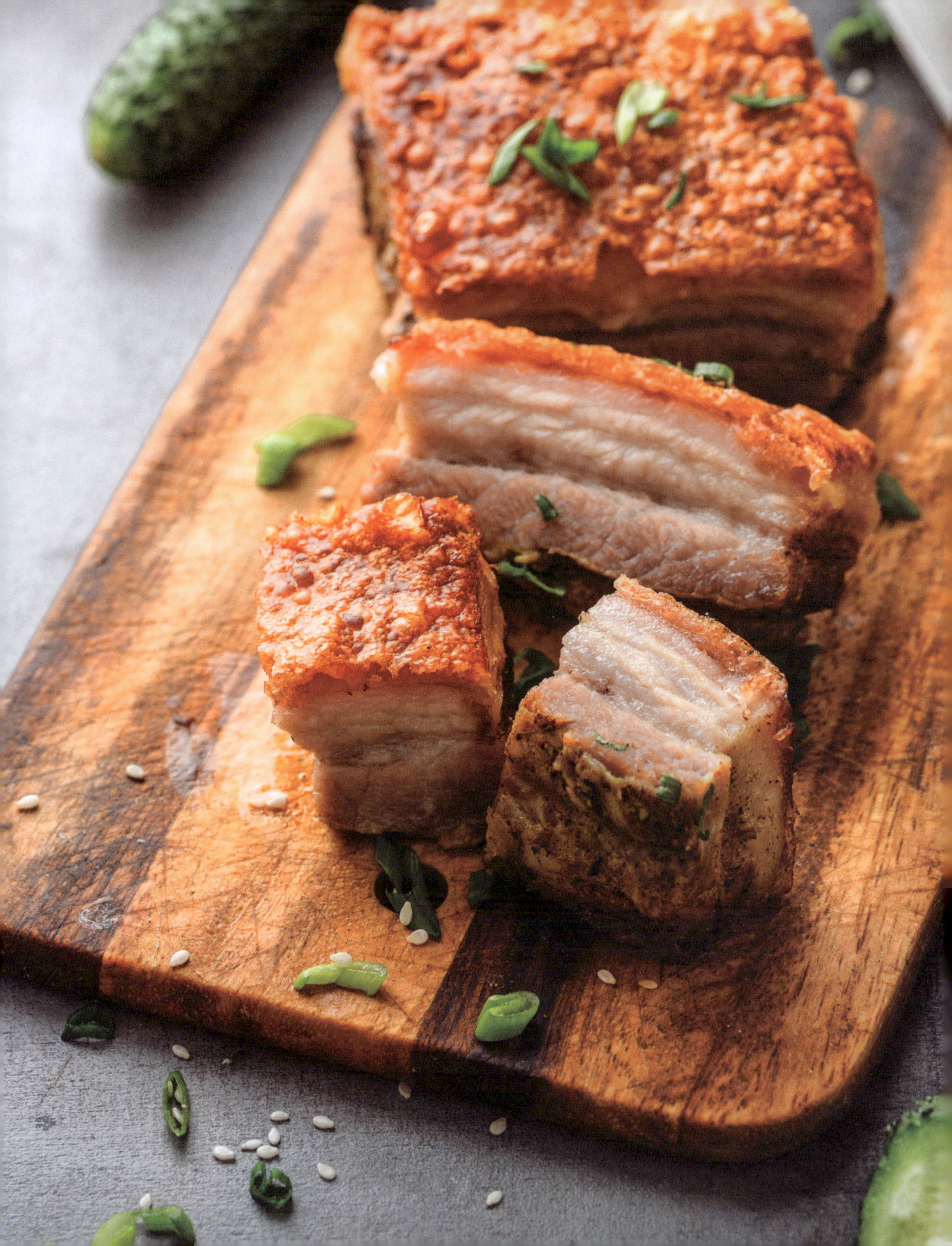

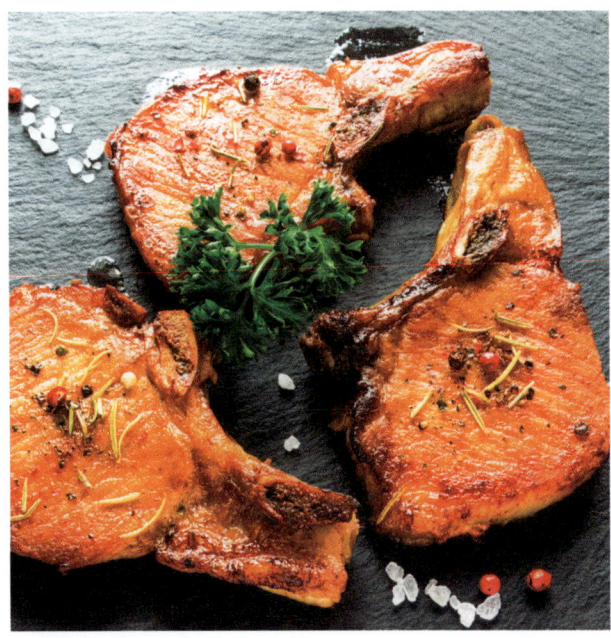

Pork Chops

1 tsp olive oil

1 tsp maple syrup

1 tsp Dijon mustard

1 tsp dried rosemary

⅛ tsp salt

½ tsp pepper

2 pork chops

Preheat the air fryer to 200°C.

Whisk together the oil, syrup, mustard, rosemary, salt and pepper in a medium bowl. Drizzle the chops with the mixture and rub in gently.

Place the pork chops into the air fryer basket. Be careful not to overcrowd the basket. Cook in batches or use a double layer accessory if needed.

Cook for 12 minutes, turning once.

SERVES 2

Sweet and Sour Pork

500g pork belly

1 tbsp potato starch

3 tbsps soy sauce, divided

1 tsp five-spice powder

1 tsp pepper

2 tbsps oil

⅔ cup (100g) red onion, chopped

1 red capsicum + 1 yellow capsicum, seeded and diced

⅓ cup (75g) tomato puree

1 tbsp apple cider vinegar

⅓ cup (80ml) water

2 tbsps sugar

4 tomatoes, diced

Ovenproof bowl

Remove the skin from the pork belly, cut into chunks and place into a large bowl. Add potato starch, 1 tablespoon soy sauce, five-spice powder and pepper, and stir until well coated. Cover and transfer to the fridge; marinate for 45 minutes.

Preheat the air fryer to 200°C and spritz the air fryer basket with cooking spray.

Transfer the pork to the air fryer basket and cook for 5 minutes. Take out and set aside.

Place the oil, onion and capsicums in the bowl and cook in the air fryer for 5 minutes.

In a small bowl, prepare the sauce. Mix together the tomato puree, vinegar, water, sugar and remaining soy sauce.

Pour the sauce into the bowl with the onion and capsicum. Add tomatoes, stir well and return to the air fryer to cook for 8 minutes.

Add the pork cubes and cook for a final 2 minutes.

SERVES 4

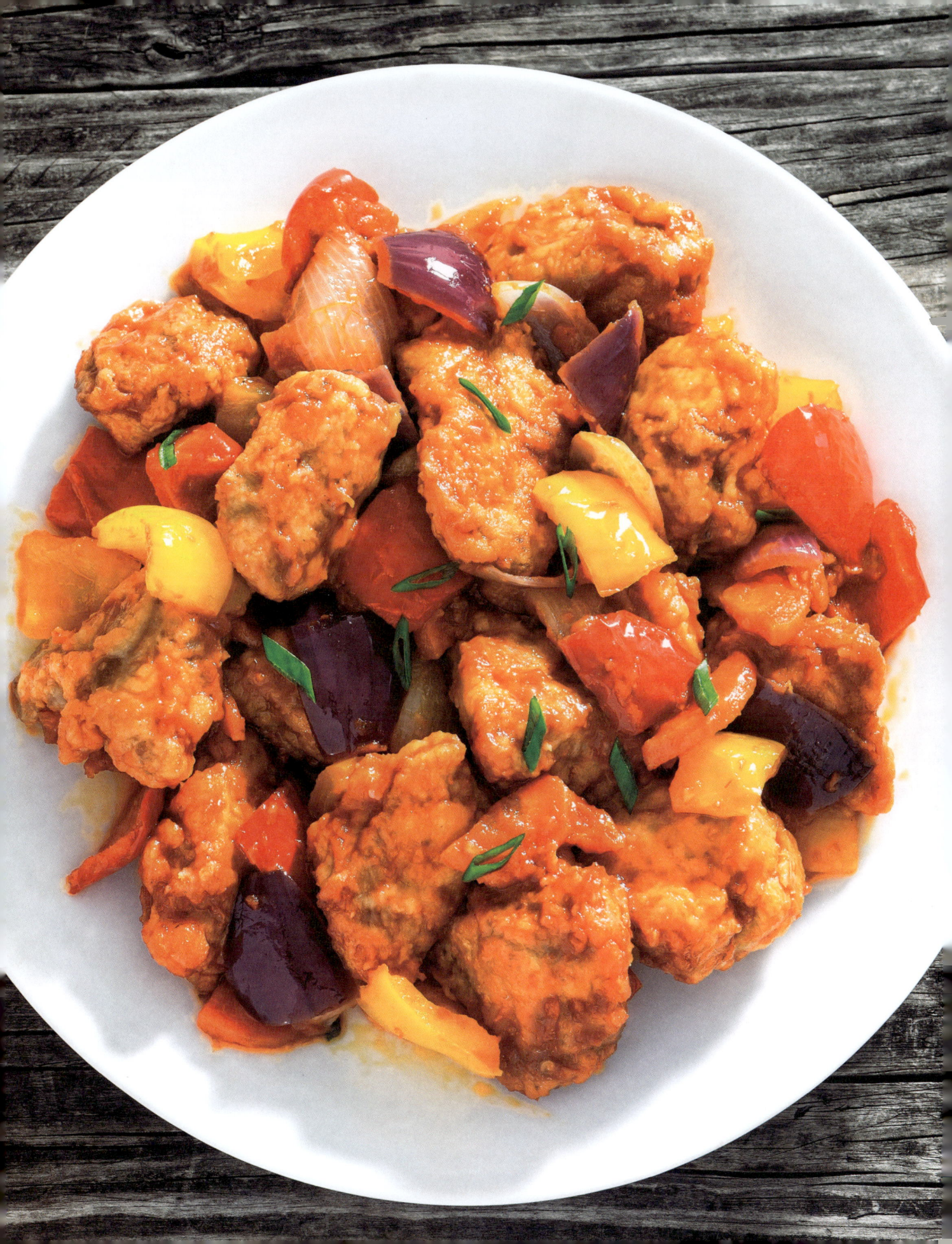

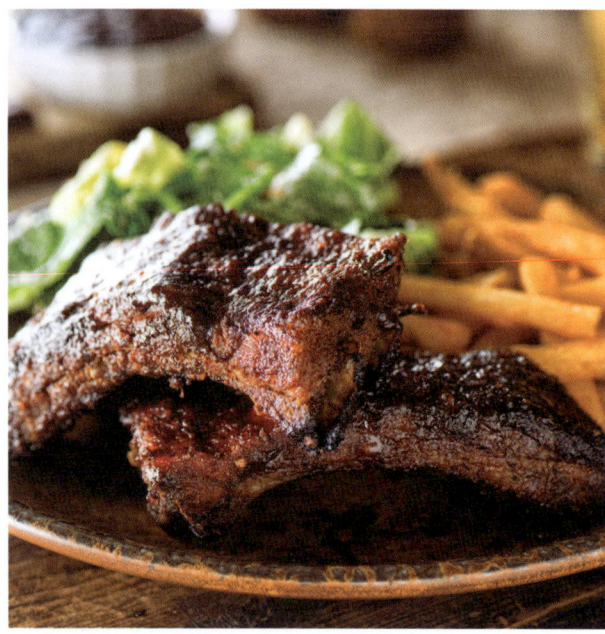

Dry Spice Ribs

1 tbsp salt

1 tbsp dark brown sugar

1 tbsp sweet paprika

1 tsp garlic powder

1 tsp onion powder

½ tsp mustard powder

½ tsp pepper

800g pork spare ribs

Place all the seasonings in a large bowl and stir to combine.

Place the ribs in the bowl and coat with the seasonings using your hands to rub them well into the skin.

Preheat the air fryer to 180°C.

Arrange the ribs so that they are upright and leaning against the edges of the air fryer basket.

Cook for 35 minutes until tender.

SERVES 2

Ribs with Homemade BBQ Sauce

3 tbsps olive oil

5 cloves garlic, minced

Salt and pepper, to taste

⅔ cup (160ml) chicken stock

⅓ cup (50g) brown sugar

¼ cup (60ml) apple cider vinegar

¼ cup (60ml) tomato sauce

3 tbsps yellow mustard

2 tbsps soy sauce

1kg pork ribs

Place the olive oil in a saucepan over medium heat. Add garlic and fry until just brown. Add the remaining ingredients except the ribs and stir to combine. Simmer on low for 15 minutes, or until the sauce starts to thicken. Set aside to cool.

Preheat the air fryer to 200°C.

Season the ribs with salt and pepper. Peel away the membrane from the underside of the ribs.

Smother the ribs with the sauce and then transfer them to the air fryer basket.

Cook for 16 minutes, turning halfway through cooking.

Remove from the air fryer. Brush with a little extra sauce if desired.

SERVES 4

Notes: Use a thermometer to determine if the meat is cooked as the size of ribs can vary quite a lot.

You can easily substitute store-bought BBQ sauce to make this recipe super quick and easy.

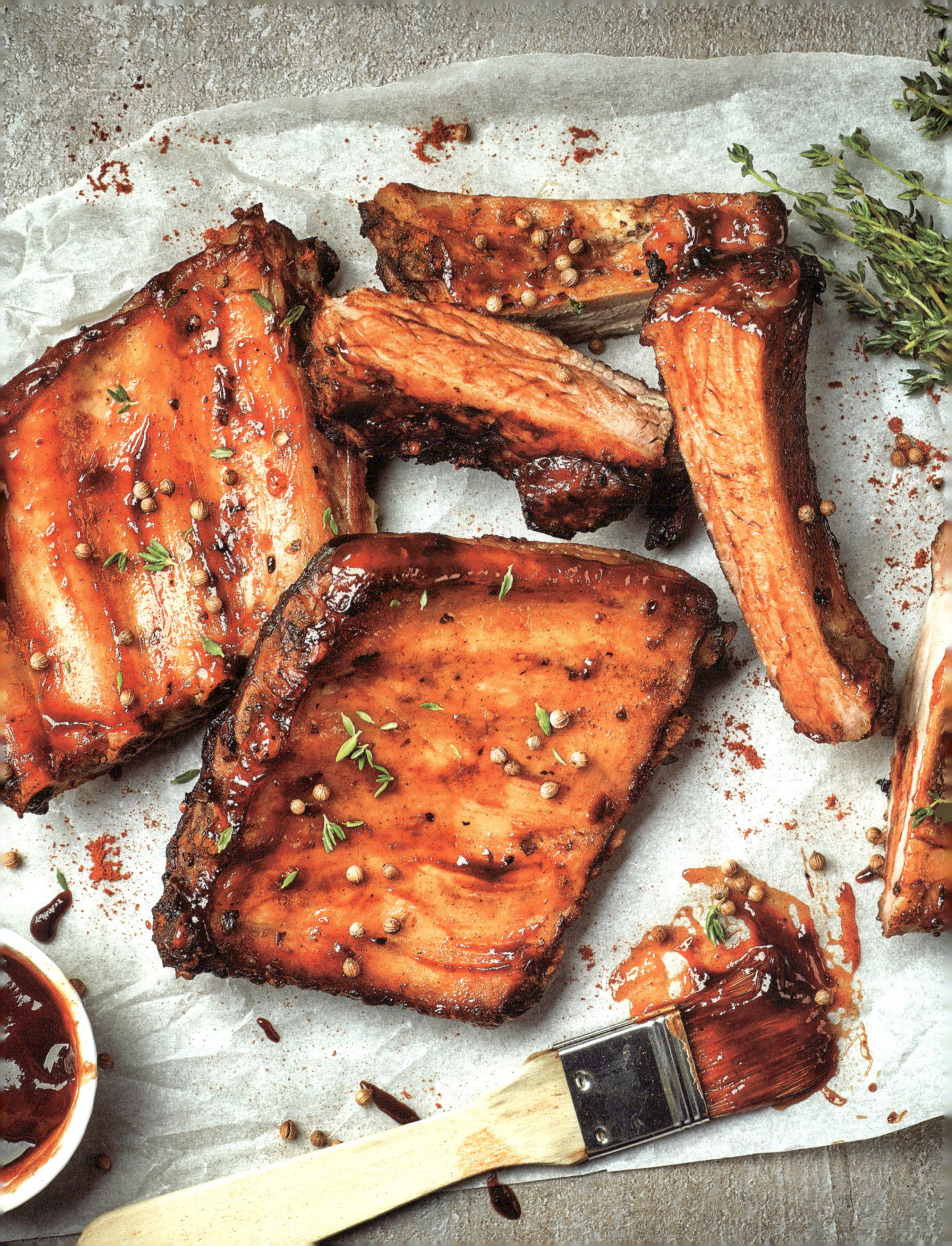

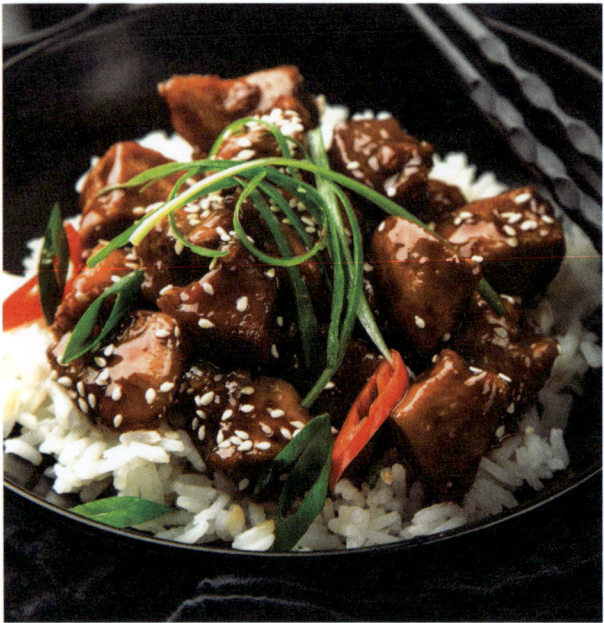

Pork Satay with Peanut Sauce

2 tbsps garlic, crushed

1 tbsp fresh ginger, minced

2 tsps hot chilli sauce, divided

2 tbsps kecap manis

2 tbsps vegetable oil, divided

400g lean pork chops, cut into cubes

1 spring onion, finely chopped

1 tsp ground coriander

¾ cup (200ml) coconut milk

⅓ cup (100g) unsalted peanut butter

1 tbsp soy sauce

Skewer rack

Whisk together the garlic, ginger, 1 teaspoon hot chilli sauce, kecap manis and 1 tablespoon of the oil in a large bowl. Add the meat and stir to combine. Cover and place in the fridge to marinate for 30 minutes.

Thread the pork cubes onto skewers. Place the kebabs on the skewer rack and spritz with oil.

Preheat the air fryer to 190°C. Spritz the air fryer basket with cooking spray.

Place the skewer rack in the air fryer. Cook for 12 minutes until golden and cooked through, turning halfway during cooking.

To make the peanut sauce, heat 1 tablespoon of the oil in a saucepan. Add the spring onion and coriander and stir-fry for a minute. Pour in the coconut milk, peanut butter, soy sauce and remaining chilli sauce and bring to the boil. Cook for 5 minutes, stirring constantly. Add a little water if the sauce is too thick. Serve sauce on the side as an accompaniment to the satay.

SERVES 3

Note: You can easily substitute store-bought satay marinade to make this recipe super quick and easy.

Teriyaki Pork

450g pork shoulder, trimmed and cut into pieces

½ cup (125ml) + 1 tbsp teriyaki sauce

2 tbsps water

1 tbsp honey

Cooked rice, to serve

2 tbsps sesame seeds

1 small red chilli, sliced (optional)

Toss the pork in the ½ cup of teriyaki sauce and water, and then cover and transfer to the fridge to marinate for 45 minutes.

Preheat the air fryer to 220°C.

Transfer the pork into the basket of the air fryer and cook for 15 minutes, removing the basket and shaking three times during cooking.

Whisk together the remaining tablespoon of teriyaki sauce with the honey.

Pour the sauce over the cooked pork to serve. Serve with cooked rice and garnish with sesame seeds and sliced chilli, if desired.

SERVES 2

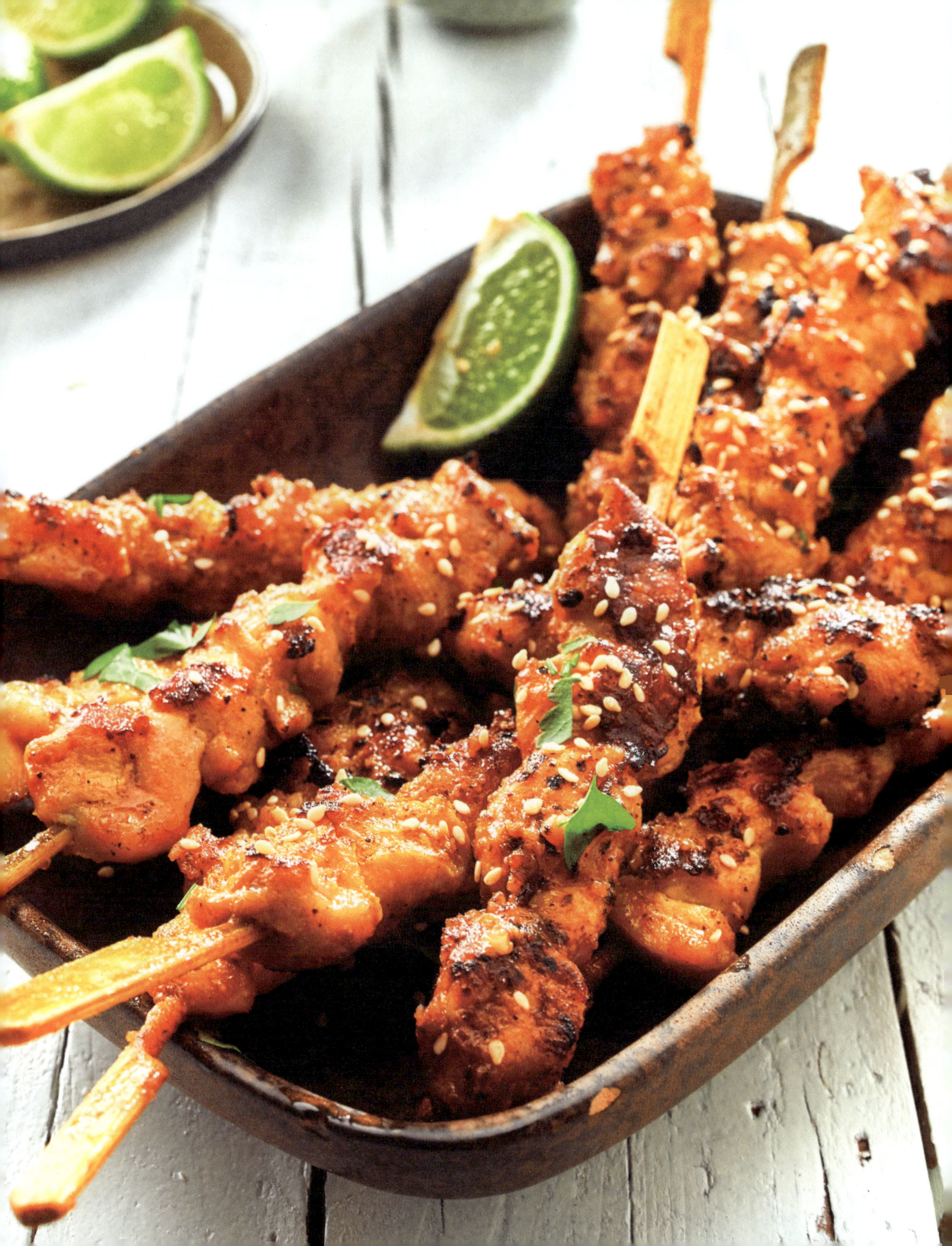

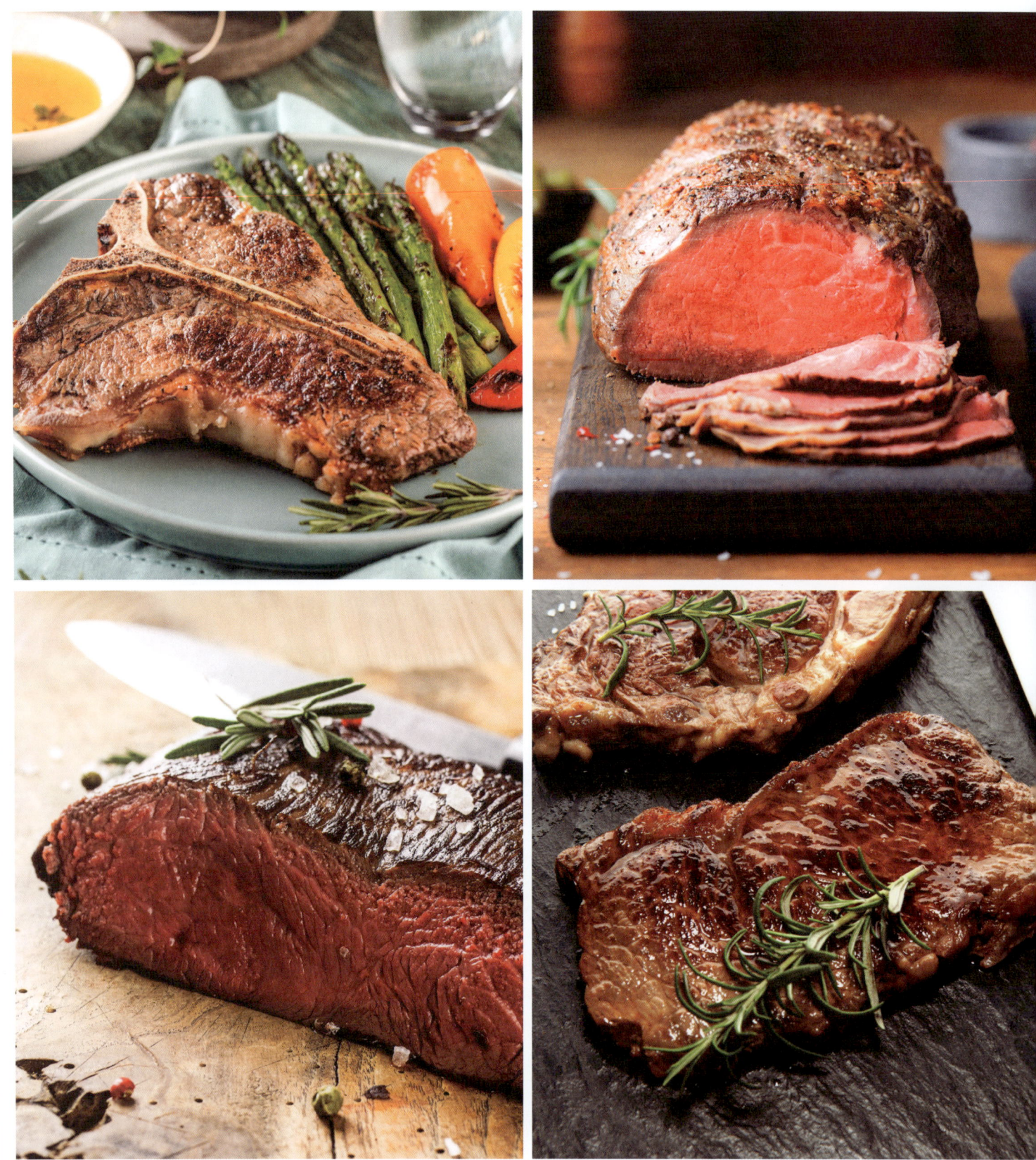

T-Bone Steak

2 T-bone steaks

2 tsps olive oil

1 tbsp steak seasoning

Cake tin (optional)

Remove the steak from the fridge and bring to room temperature (approximately 30 minutes out of the fridge).

Rub olive oil into the steaks and season on both sides.

Preheat the air fryer to 200°C.

If using a cake tin, transfer steaks to it and slide into the air fryer.

For medium rare steak, cook for 7 minutes, turning once halfway through cooking.

Rest on a plate for a few minutes before serving.

SERVES 2

Medium-Rare Roast Beef

1 tsp salt

1 tsp pepper

1 tsp dried rosemary

1 tbsp olive oil

1.3kg beef roast

Preheat the air fryer to 180°C.

Place the salt, pepper, rosemary and oil on a plate. Take the beef roast and turn it around through the mixture to ensure even coating.

Place the beef in the basket of the air fryer and cook for 45 minutes. To confirm meat is cooked to medium rare, check with a meat thermometer. The meat should be at 55°C.

Cook for longer if you prefer meat more well done.

Remove from the air fryer, cover with foil and rest for 10 minutes before serving.

SERVES 4

Scotch Fillet

375g Scotch fillet

Pinch of salt and pepper

Preheat the air fryer to 180°C.

Season the fillet with salt and pepper and spritz all over with olive oil.

Place in the air fryer basket and for medium rare, cook for 7 minutes, turning once during cooking.

If you prefer your fillet well done, add 2 further minutes cooking time. For rare meat, reduce cooking time by 2 minutes.

SERVES 2

Porterhouse Steak

2 medium porterhouse steaks

Herbs and spices, to taste

Pinch of salt and pepper

Preheat the air fryer to 190°C.

Season the steak with your favourite herbs and spices, as well as some salt and pepper, and spritz all over with olive oil.

Place the steak in the air fryer basket and slide in. Cook for approximately 7 minutes for medium.

To cook rare air fryer fillet steak, subtract 2 minutes, for well done, add 2 minutes.

SERVES 2

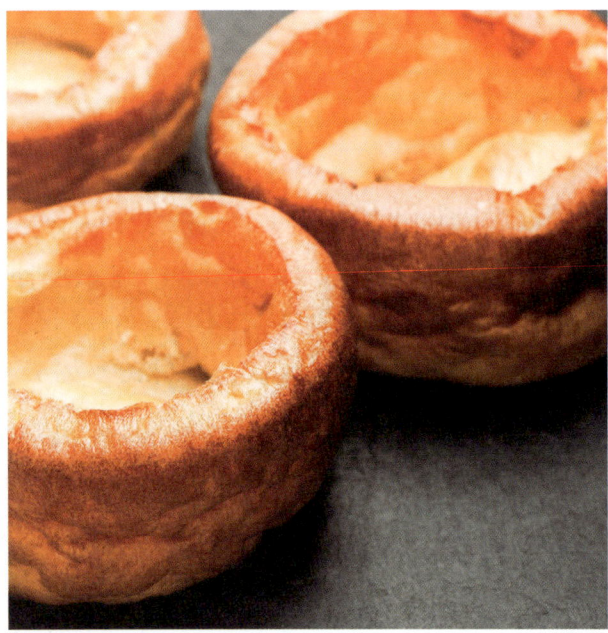

Yorkshire Pudding

½ cup (60g) plain flour

Pinch of salt and pepper

1 egg

⅔ cup (150ml) milk

Muffin tray

Preheat the air fryer to 200°C.

Combine the plain flour and the salt and pepper in a bowl.

Gradually stir in the egg and then the milk. Beat well until it forms bubbles on top of the batter.

Lightly spritz the muffin tray with oil and place in the air fryer for 5 minutes until oil is just shimmering.

Reduce the temperature to 180°C.

Pour the mixture halfway up each muffin hole and return to the air fryer. Cook for 15 minutes.

SERVES 4

Beef Wellington

1 tsp oil

450g beef fillet

2 sheets puff pastry

150g pâté

2 egg yolks

Pinch of salt and pepper

Grill pan

Preheat a frying pan until very hot.

Rub oil over the beef fillet and transfer it to the hot pan. Quickly sear on all sides. Remove and set aside to cool slightly.

Arrange the puff pastry sheets into a rectangular shape that is wider and longer than the size of the fillet.

Spread the pâté over the cooled beef, then place it on top of the pastry, and roll the meat until it is covered with the pastry. Brush a little of the egg yolk at the edge of the pastry and join it together.

Place the Wellington in the air fryer grill pan. Brush the surface with the remaining egg yolk and transfer to the fridge to chill for 15 minutes.

Preheat the air fryer to 180°C.

Score the surface of the chilled Wellington in a criss-cross pattern to allow steam to escape during cooking.

Cook for 30 minutes.

Rest for 10 minutes before serving.

SERVES 2

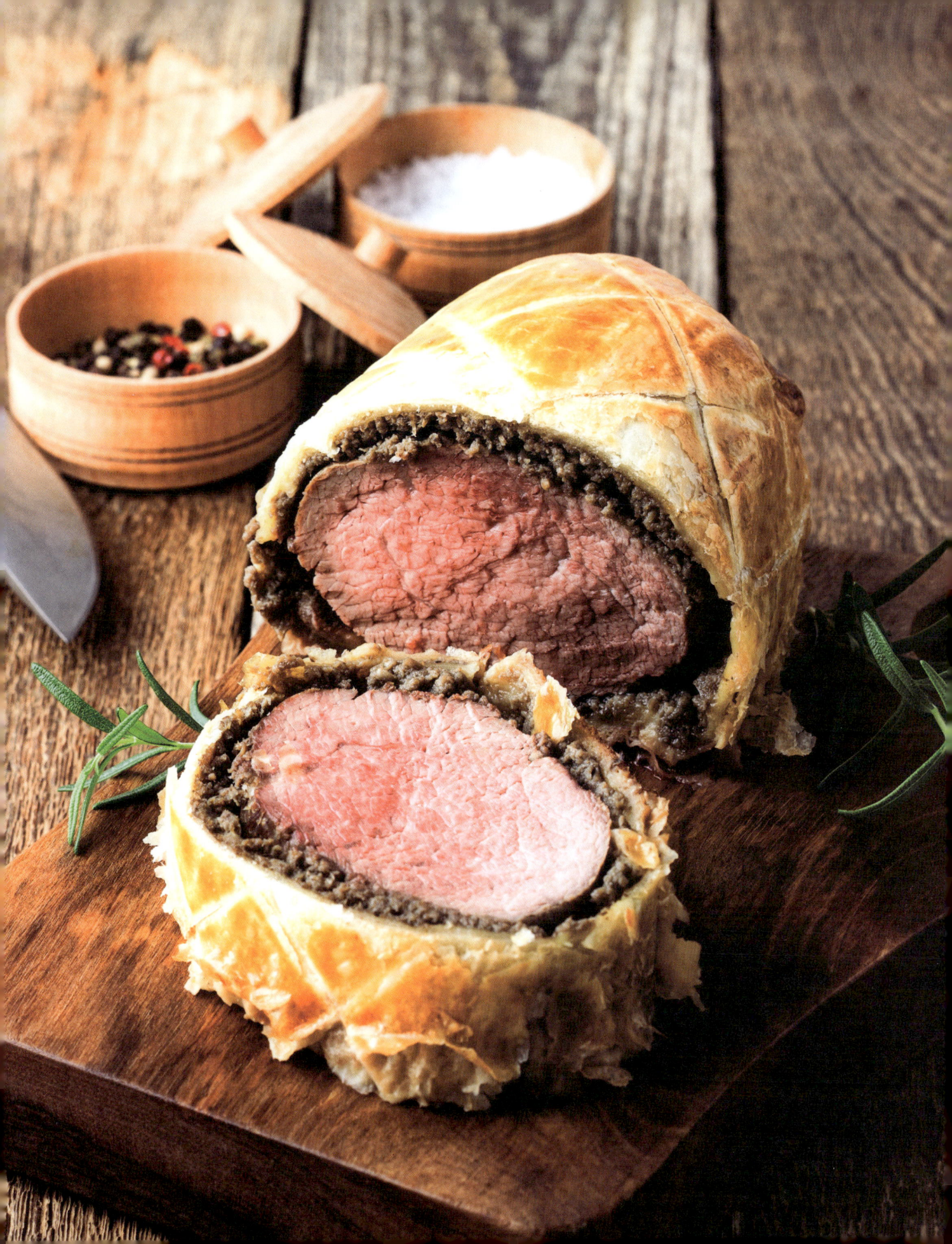

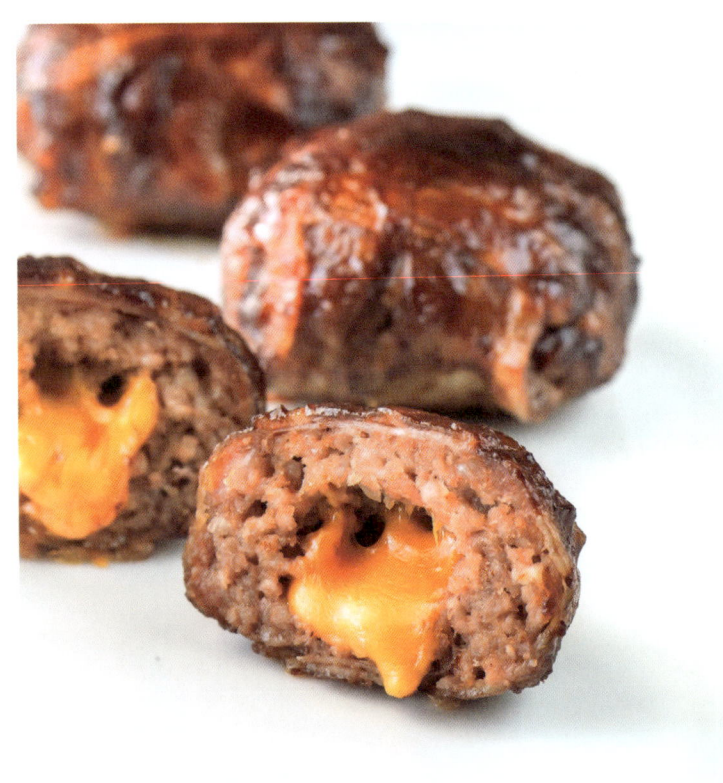

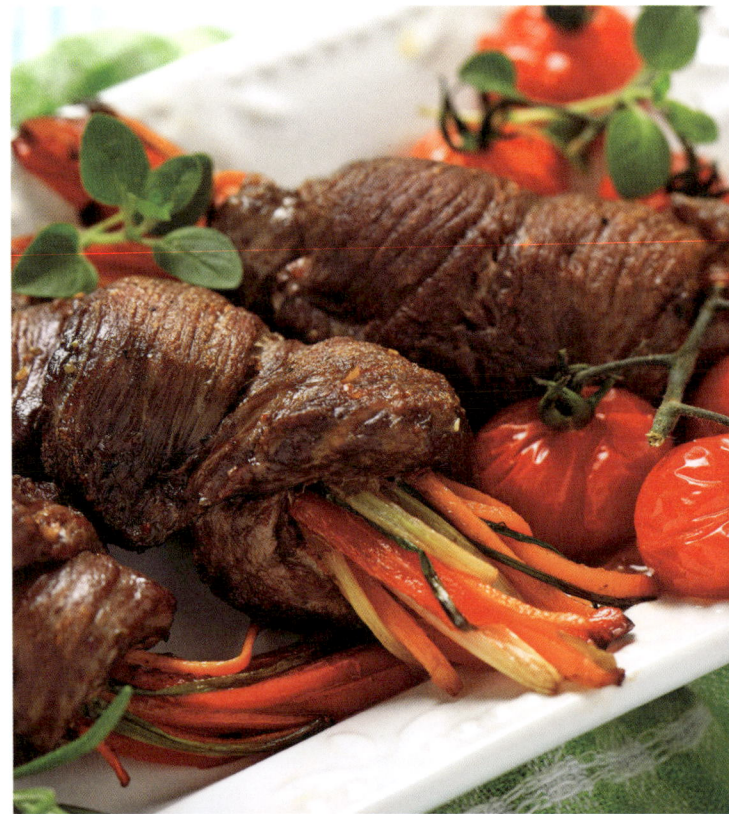

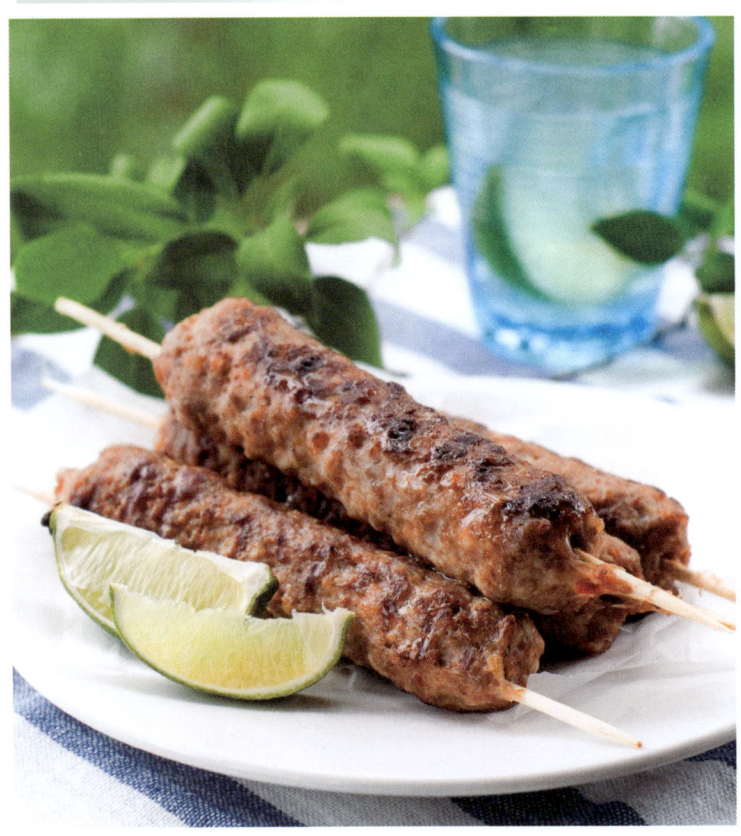

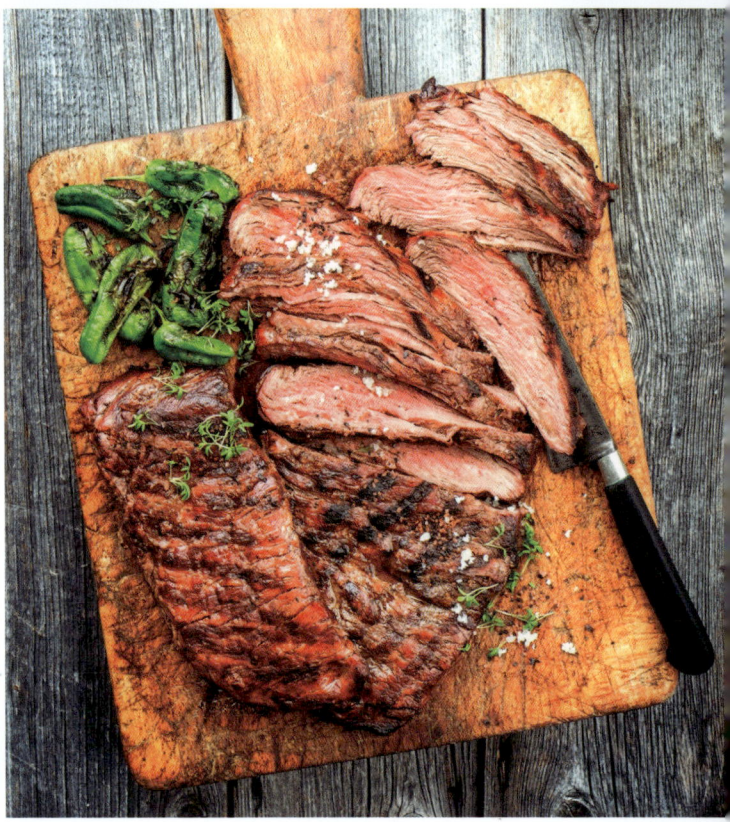

Cheesy Meatballs

500g beef mince

1½ tsps Italian herbs

½ cup (60g) breadcrumbs

1 tsp ground paprika

2 tsps garlic powder

100g Cheddar cheese, cut into chunks

Combine all the ingredients, except the cheese, together in a large bowl.

Using damp hands, rolls the mixture into golf-ball-size balls.

Push a chunk of cheese into the middle of each portion and then gently roll again to re-form meatballs.

Preheat the air fryer to 180°C. Spritz the air fryer basket with cooking spray.

Place the meatballs in the air fryer basket and lightly spray the tops. Be careful not to overcrowd the basket. Cook in batches or use a double layer accessory if needed.

Cook 18 minutes.

SERVES 4

Beef Kofte

1 tbsp oil

500g beef mince

4 tbsps parsley, chopped

2 cloves garlic, minced

1 tbsp all-purpose seasoning

1 tsp salt

Skewer rack

Combine all the ingredients in a large mixing bowl.

Cover and transfer to the fridge to chill for 30 minutes (or longer if convenient).

Form the kebabs into sausage shapes using your hands. When roughly done insert a skewer in the centre and then gently roll to reshape if needed.

Place kebabs on the skewer rack and spritz with olive oil.

Preheat the air fryer to 190°C. Cook for 10 minutes or to an internal temperature of 71°C with a thermometer.

SERVES 4

Steak Rolls with Vegetables

4 flank steaks, cut in half

Pinch of salt and pepper

½ cup (125ml) soy sauce

2 cloves garlic, crushed

1 carrot, julienned

1 red capsicum, seeded and julienned

1 stalk celery, julienned

Season steaks with salt and pepper. Place in a large ziplock bag. Add the soy sauce and garlic. Massage steaks to coat well. Transfer to fridge to marinate for 1 hour.

When ready to cook, remove steaks and discard marinade.

Equally divide and then place carrots, capsicum and celery in the middle of each piece of steak. Roll steak around vegetables and secure with toothpicks.

Preheat the air fryer to 200°C.

Place the bundles into the basket of the air fryer and spray with olive oil spray. Cook for 5 minutes.

Rest for 5 minutes prior to serving.

SERVES 4

Beef Flank Steak

400g flank steak

Preheat the air fryer to 190°C.

Spray the meat with olive oil and place it in the basket of the air fryer.

Cook for 20 minutes until tender.

SERVES 2

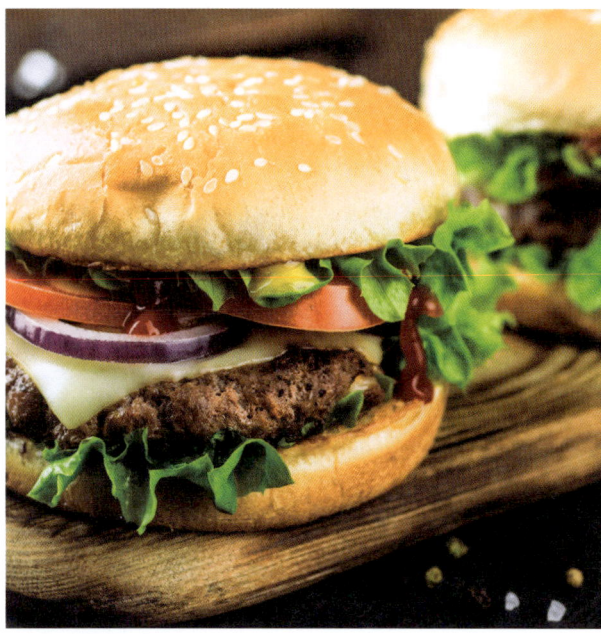

Burger Patties

500g beef mince

1 tbsp Worcestershire sauce

1 tsp BBQ sauce

½ tsp garlic powder

½ tsp onion powder

½ tsp salt

½ tsp pepper

½ tsp oregano

Preheat the air fryer to 180°C.

Place all the ingredients together in a large mixing bowl and mix well to combine.

Shape the mixture into four burger patty shapes, using your hands.

Spritz the patties on both sides with cooking spray and place into the air fryer basket.

Cook for 10 minutes.

MAKES 4

Italian Meatballs

2 tbsps olive oil

1 spring onion, finely chopped

1 tbsp minced garlic

1 cup (125g) breadcrumbs

¼ cup (60ml) milk

450g beef mince

1 egg

1 tsp Italian herbs

1 tbsp Dijon mustard

½ tsp salt

Heat the olive oil in a frying pan over medium heat. Add spring onion and cook for 2 minutes, until softened. Add the garlic and cook for a further minute. Remove from heat and set aside.

Place the breadcrumbs in a large bowl and sprinkle over the milk. Stir once, cover and let stand for 5 minutes.

Add the onion and garlic mixture to the breadcrumbs and stir. Add the mince, egg, herbs, mustard and salt. Stir to combine.

Preheat the air fryer to 200°C.

Using hands, shape mixture into about 12 meatballs. Transfer balls into the air fryer basket. (Be careful not to overcrowd the basket. Cook in batches or use a double layer accessory if needed.)

Cook for 12 minutes, turning once halfway through cooking.

SERVES 4

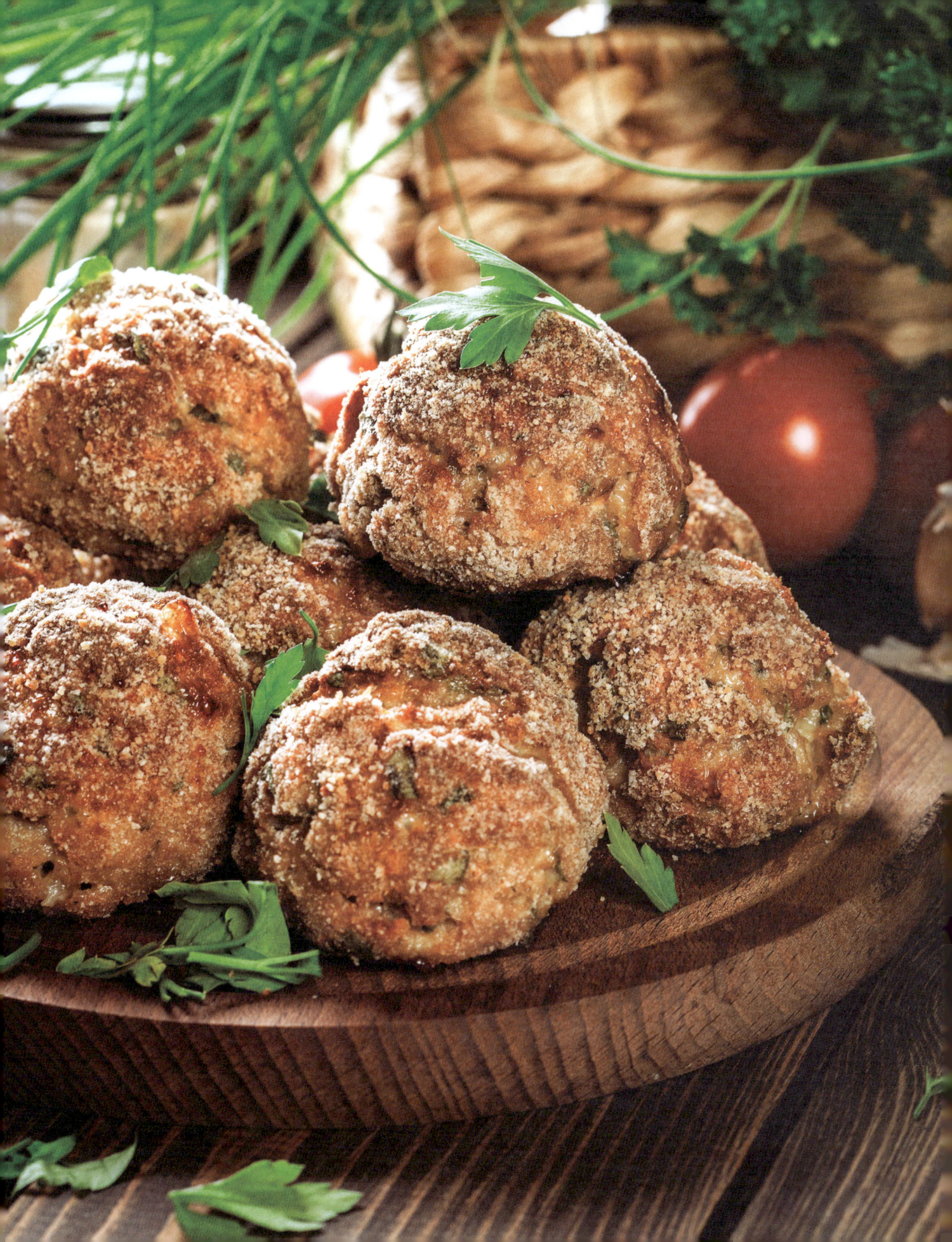

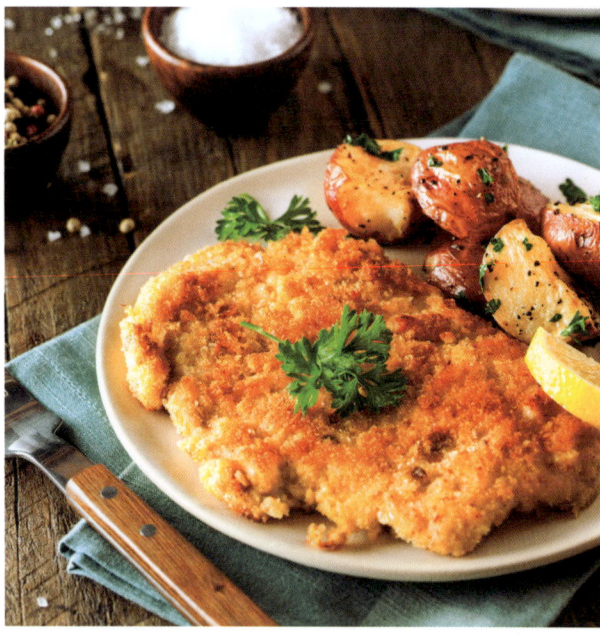

Crumbed Veal Schnitzel

3 tbsps vegetable oil

1⅔ cups (200g) breadcrumbs

½ tsp salt

1 egg

6 thin veal schnitzels

Preheat the air fryer to 180°C.

Combine the oil and the breadcrumbs together until a crumbly mixture forms. Place on a plate or in a shallow bowl.

Beat the egg in another shallow bowl.

Dip the schnitzel into the egg, shaking off any excess. Then dip the schnitzel into the crumb mix, pressing in to ensure it is evenly and fully covered.

Place in the air fryer basket (Be careful not to overcrowd the basket. Cook in batches or use a double layer accessory if needed.)

Cook for 8 minutes until golden, turning once during cooking.

SERVES 2

Air Fryer Pot Roast

1 tbsp rosemary, chopped

½ onion, finely chopped

3 tbsps olive oil

1 tbsp balsamic vinegar

1 tsp salt

½ tsp pepper

1.2kg beef chuck roast, thawed

Place the rosemary, onion, olive oil, vinegar, salt and pepper in a small bowl and whisk to combine.

Pour the mixture over the roast, cover and transfer to the fridge to marinate for 8 hours.

Preheat the air fryer to 200°C.

Place roast in the air fryer basket.

Cook for 30 minutes, flipping roast halfway through.

Allow to rest for at least 5 minutes.

Slice into thick cuts to serve.

SERVES 4-6

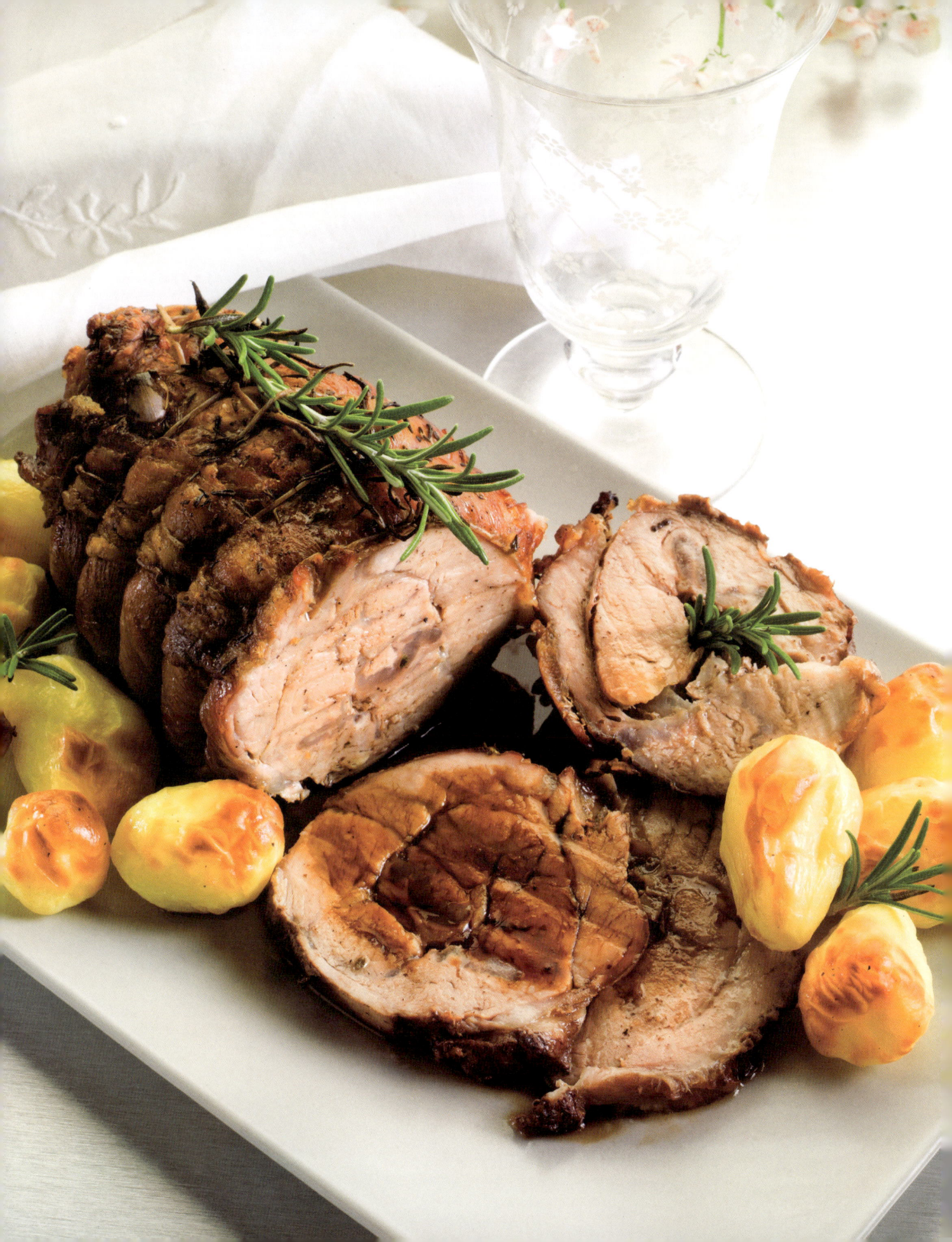

6 Lovely Lamb Marinades

Lamb is a versatile meat which goes well with many flavour combinations. Use the recipes in the following lamb section as a guide for cooking times and improvise with your favourite marinades – or choose from the ideas on this page.

To make a marinade simply combine the ingredients in a small bowl and whisk well. Use what you need and store the rest in a sealed container in the fridge for use later.

Marinate meat in a covered container in the fridge for a minimum of 30 minutes and maximum of 24 hours. The longer you leave it, the stronger the flavour.

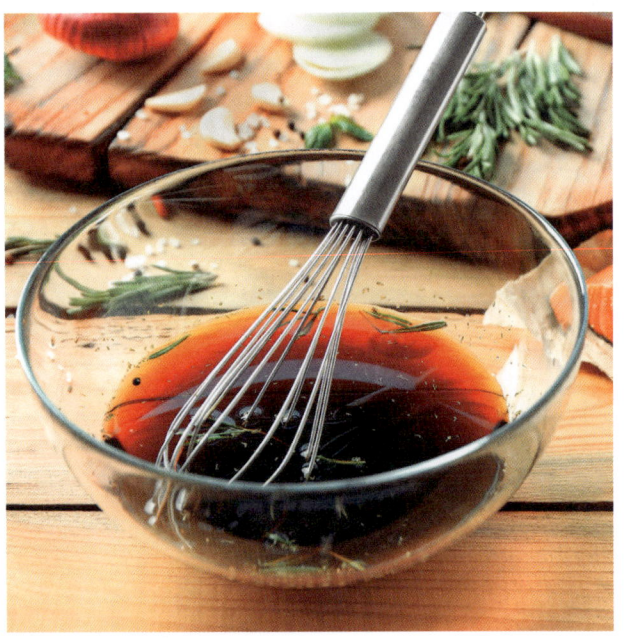

LEMON AND OREGANO

1 lemon

1 tsp salt

½ tsp pepper

½ tbsp dried oregano

3 cloves garlic, minced

MINT PESTO

½ cup (125ml) olive oil

1 tbsp lemon juice

1 cup (45g) fresh mint, chopped

1 tsp salt

½ cup (70g) pine nuts (processed into a paste)

SATAY

1 tbsp sesame oil

¼ cup (65g) crunchy peanut butter

½ cup (125ml) coconut milk

1 clove garlic, minced

2 tsps kecap manis

2 tsps fresh lime juice

2 tsps fresh ginger, minced

½ tsp ground cumin

½ tsp ground coriander

¼ tsp chilli powder

CLASSIC MEDITERRANEAN

3 cloves garlic, minced

½ cup (115g) tomato paste

½ cup (125ml) olive oil

2 tsps fresh oregano, chopped (or 1 tbsp dried)

¼ cup (60ml) red wine

HONEY, MUSTARD AND ROSEMARY

1 tbsp olive oil

1 tbsp red wine vinegar

2 tbsps mustard

2 tbsps fresh rosemary (or 1 tbsp dried)

1 tbsp honey

1 tbsp lemon juice

SIMPLE SOY AND GINGER

3 tbsps soy sauce

3 tbsps olive oil

1 tbsp brown sugar

2 tbsps ginger, minced

1 clove garlic, minced

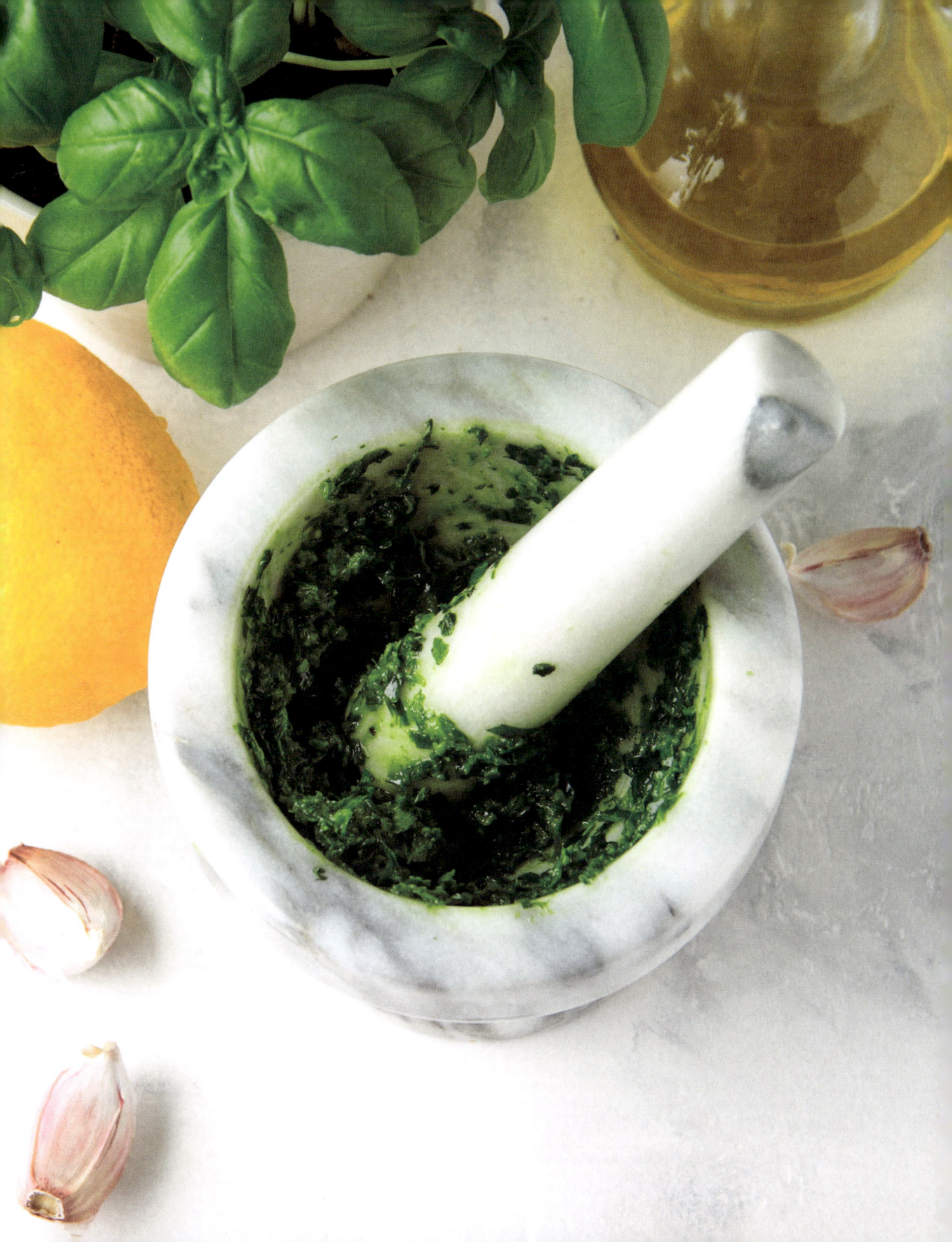

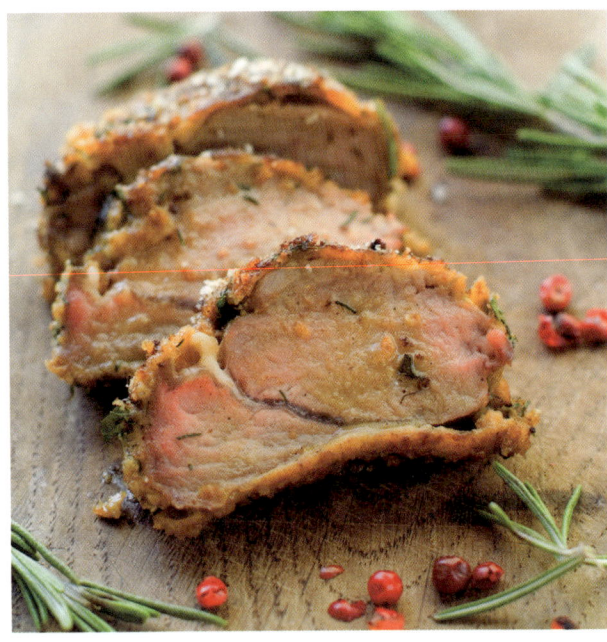

Herbed Lamb Steaks

4 boneless leg steak

1 clove garlic, chopped

¼ onion, finely chopped

1 tsp mixed herbs

½ tsp ground fennel

1 tsp salt

1 tbsp olive oil

1 tbsp breadcrumbs

Place the lamb steaks on a cutting board and use a sharp knife to lightly score across them,

Combine all the other ingredients in a mixing bowl. Stir to create a paste.

Rub the herb paste around and into the edges of the lamb and, if time allows, transfer to the fridge to marinate for 45 minutes. Otherwise transfer to the air fryer basket.

Cook on 180°C for 15 minutes, turning the steaks over halfway through cooking.

SERVES 2

Rack of Lamb with Macadamia and Rosemary Crust

2 tbsps olive oil

2 cloves garlic, minced

750g rack of lamb

½ tsp salt

Pinch of pepper

¾ cup (90g) macadamia nuts

½ cup (60g) breadcrumbs

1 tbsp rosemary, finely chopped (or use dried)

1 egg

Combine the olive oil and garlic in a small bowl. Using a pastry brush, coat the lamb rack with garlic oil and season with salt and pepper.

Grind the nuts in a spice grinder or blender into a coarse crumble. Transfer to a shallow bowl and add the breadcrumbs and rosemary.

Beat the egg in another bowl.

Preheat the air fryer to 180°C.

Dip the meat into the egg mixture, shaking off any excess. Then roll the lamb through the macadamia crumb, ensuring the top side is well coated.

Place the lamb rack in the air fryer basket.

Cook for 10 minutes. Increase the temperature to 200°C and cook for a further 5 minutes.

Remove the meat and cover with foil. Rest for 5-10 minutes before serving.

SERVES 4

Note: Increase cooking time for well done meat.

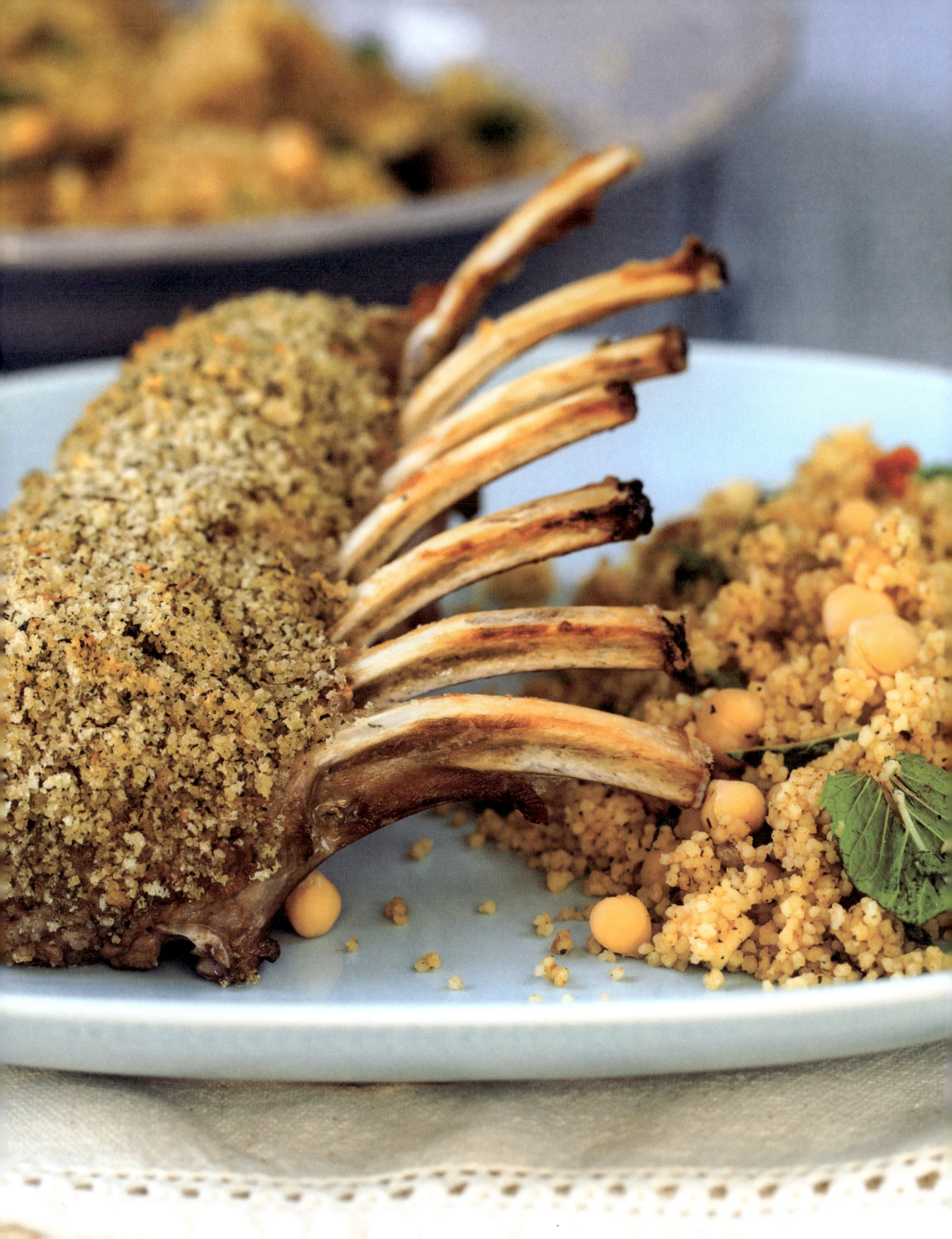

Spiced Roast Lamb

1 tbsp ginger, minced

2 tbsps garlic, minced

1 tsp garam masala

1 tsp ground fennel

1 tsp ground cinnamon

1 tsp cayenne

1 tsp salt

1 tbsp olive oil

1.1kg lamb roast

Place all the ingredients apart from the lamb into a spice grinder or blender and pulse until a paste forms.

Clean and pat dry the lamb. Lightly score the skin with a sharp knife. Rub the spice paste into the skin of the lamb well until completely coated.

Place the lamb into the air fryer basket and cook for 15 minutes at 200°C . Reduce the temperature to 160°C and cook for a further 1 hour, 15 minutes.

SERVES 4

Note: Reduce cooking time for rarer meat.

Thyme and Lemon Lamb Shanks

1 lemon

10 sprigs thyme (or 2 tsps dried thyme)

1 tbsp garlic, minced

1 tbsp brown sugar

1 tbsp olive oil

2 lamb shanks

Cut a few slices from the lemon and set aside. Juice and zest the remaining lemon.

Combine the lemon juice, zest, thyme, garlic, sugar and olive oil in a small bowl.

Brush mixture over shanks, retaining some for use later.

Transfer lamb to the basket of the air fryer and cook for 10 minutes at 180°C.

Remove and apply more glaze, then return to cook for a further 10 minutes. Remove and turn shanks over, apply more glaze and add the lemon slices to the basket. Cook for a further 20 minutes.

SERVES 2

Lamb Cutlets

4 lamb cutlets

2 tbsps olive oil

1 tsp garlic, minced

Pinch of salt and pepper

Preheat the air fryer to 180°C.

Rinse and pat dry lamb cutlets with a paper towel.

Whisk together oil, garlic, salt and pepper.

Rub the mixture generously over the cutlets and transfer to the air fryer basket.

Cook for 12 minutes, turning once halfway through cooking.

SERVES 2

Lamb Chops

8 loin chops

2 tbsps wholegrain mustard

½ tsp olive oil

1 tsp rosemary (or any dried herb of your choice)

1 tbsp lemon juice

Pinch of salt and pepper

Preheat the air fryer to 200°C.

Whisk together the mustard, olive oil, rosemary, lemon juice, salt and pepper in a small bowl.

Rinse and pat dry lamb chops with a paper towel.

Rub the mixture generously over the chops and transfer to the air fryer basket, leaving space between the chops. Cook in batches if needed.

For medium rare, cook for 15 minutes, turning the chops over halfway through cooking.

SERVES 4

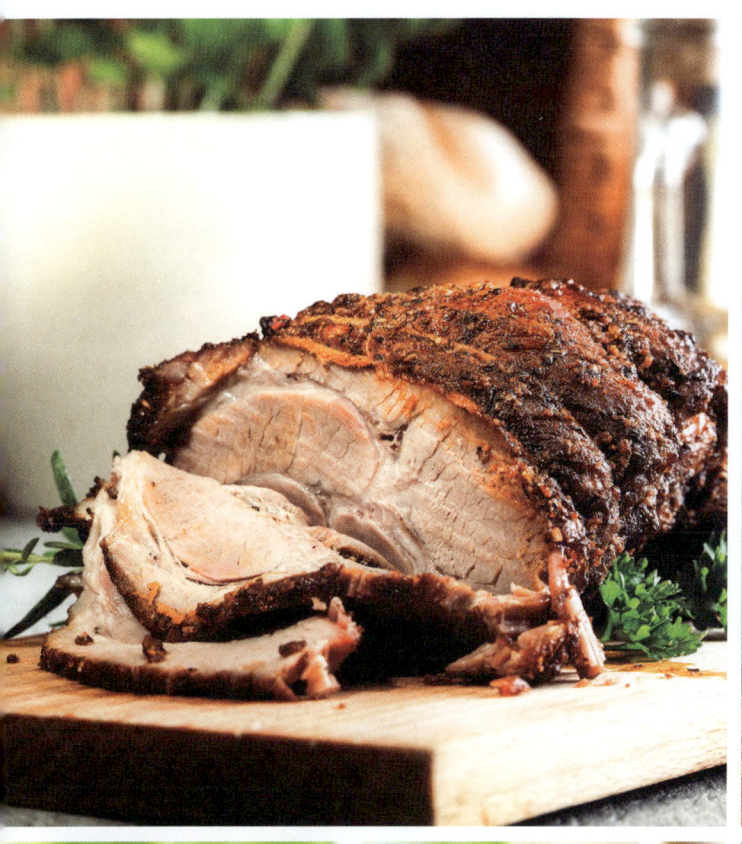

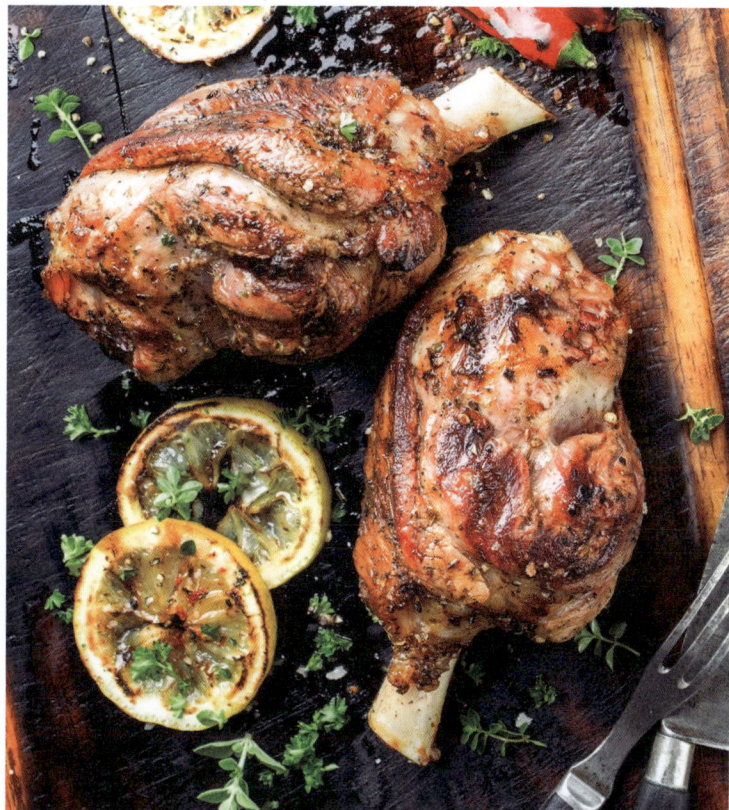

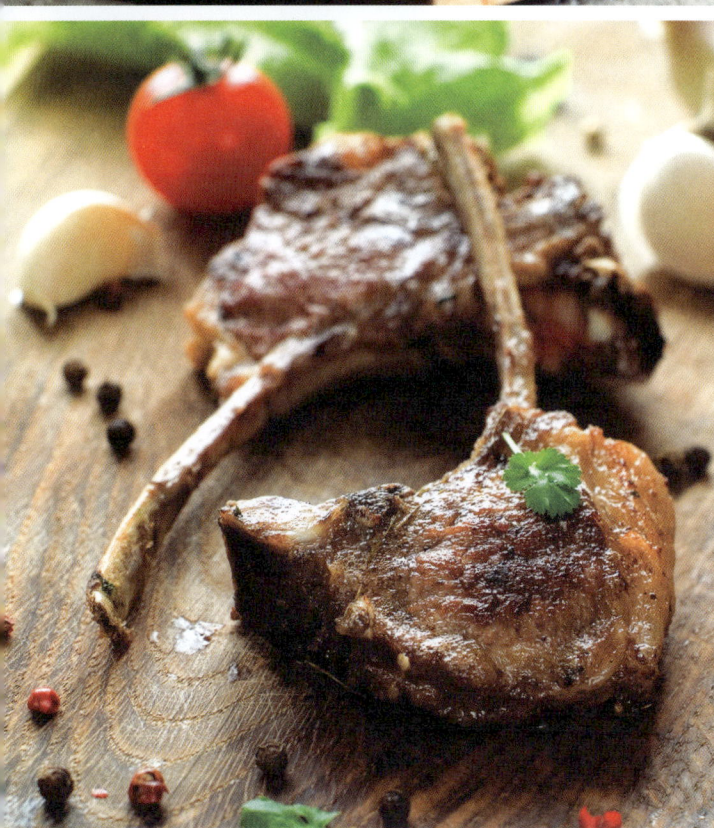

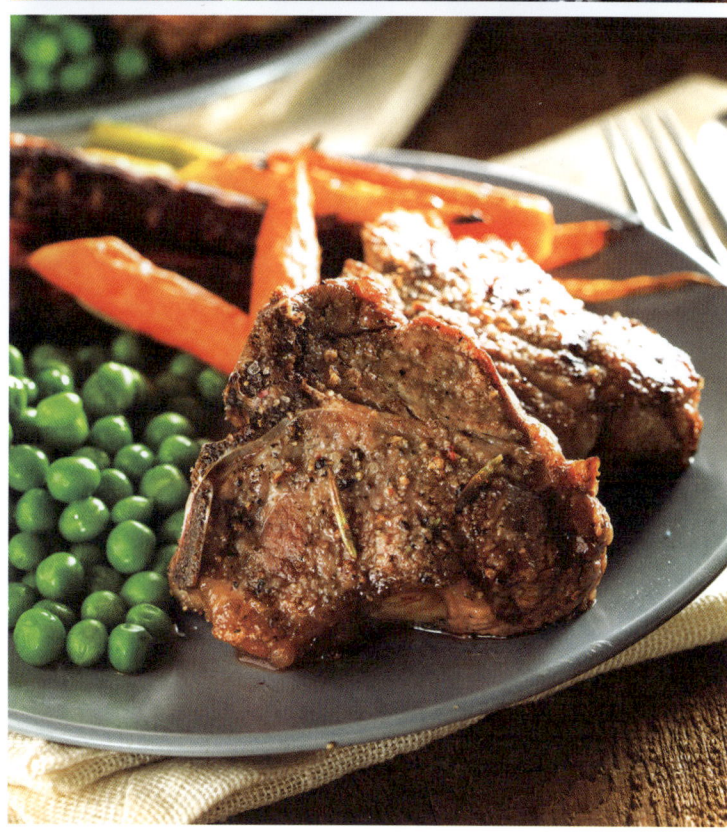

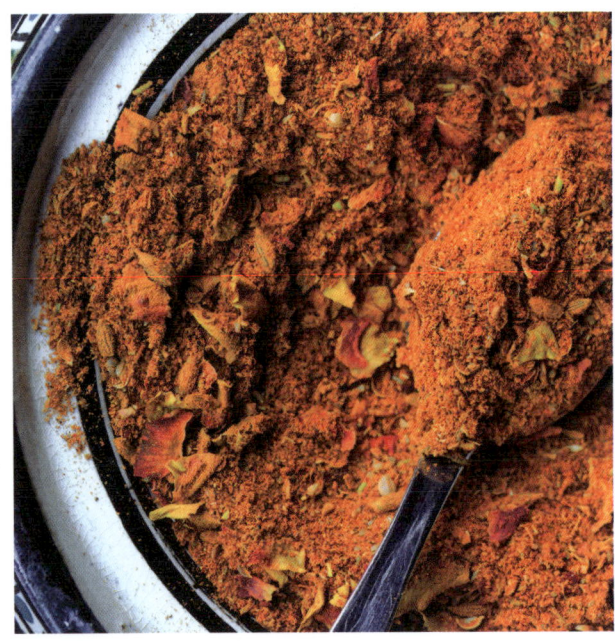

Kofte Spice Mix

1 tsp peppercorns

1 tbsp coriander seeds

1 tbsp cumin seeds

½ tsp cardamom seeds

½ tsp salt

1 tsp allspice

¼ tsp cayenne pepper

½ tsp turmeric

Place all the ingredients in a spice grinder or blender and process until a fine powder forms.

MAKES ¼ CUP

Kofte Kebab

1 tbsp olive oil

450g lamb mince

4 tbsps mint, chopped

2 cloves garlic, minced

2 tbsps kofte spice mix (see opposite)

1 tsp salt

Skewer rack

Combine all the ingredients in a large mixing bowl.

Cover and transfer to the fridge to chill for 30 minutes (or longer if convenient).

Form the kebabs into sausage shapes using your hands. When roughly done insert a skewer in the centre and then gently roll to reshape if needed.

Place kebabs on the skewer rack and spritz with olive oil.

Preheat the air fryer to 190°C. Cook for 10 minutes or to an internal temperature of 71°C with a thermometer.

SERVES 4

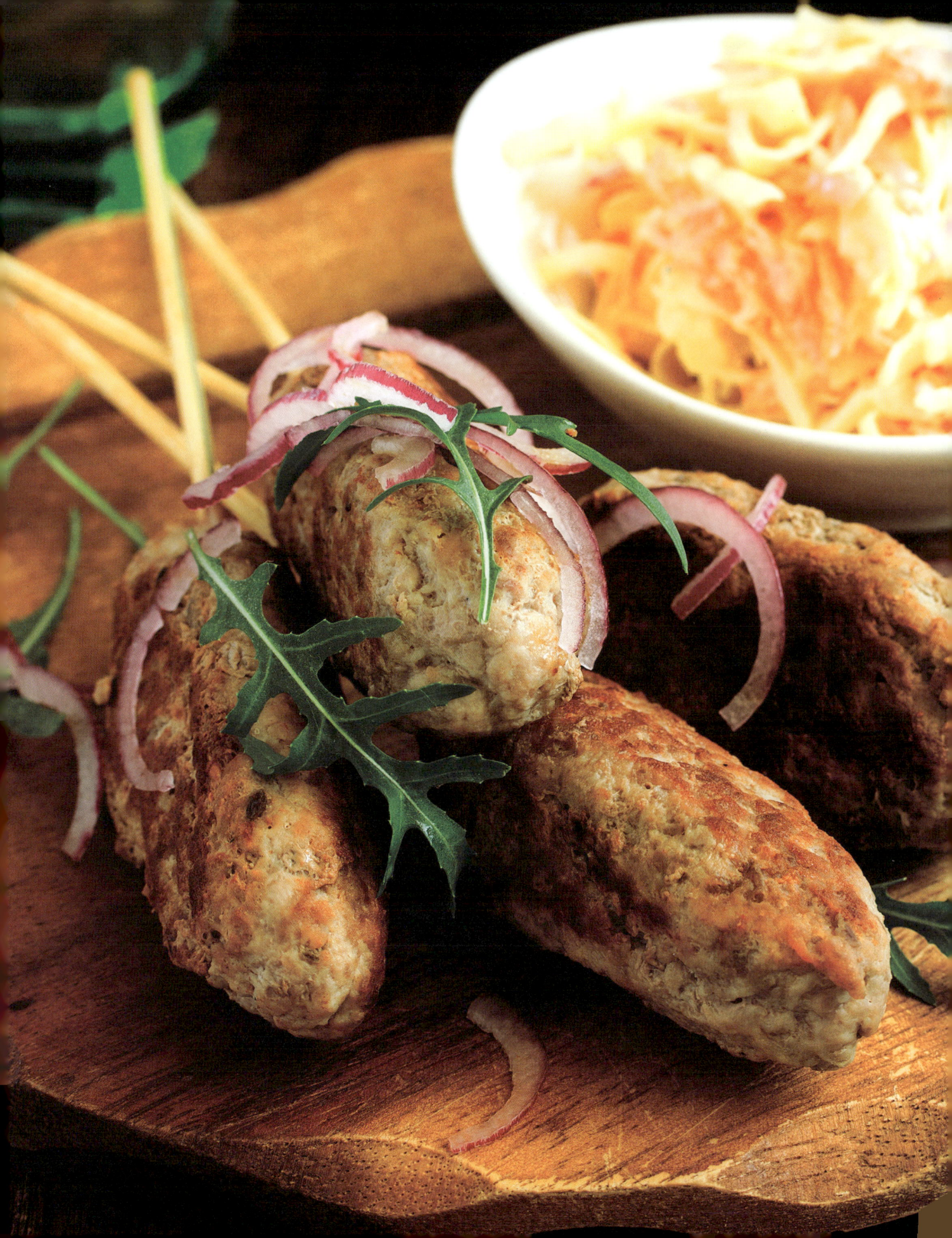

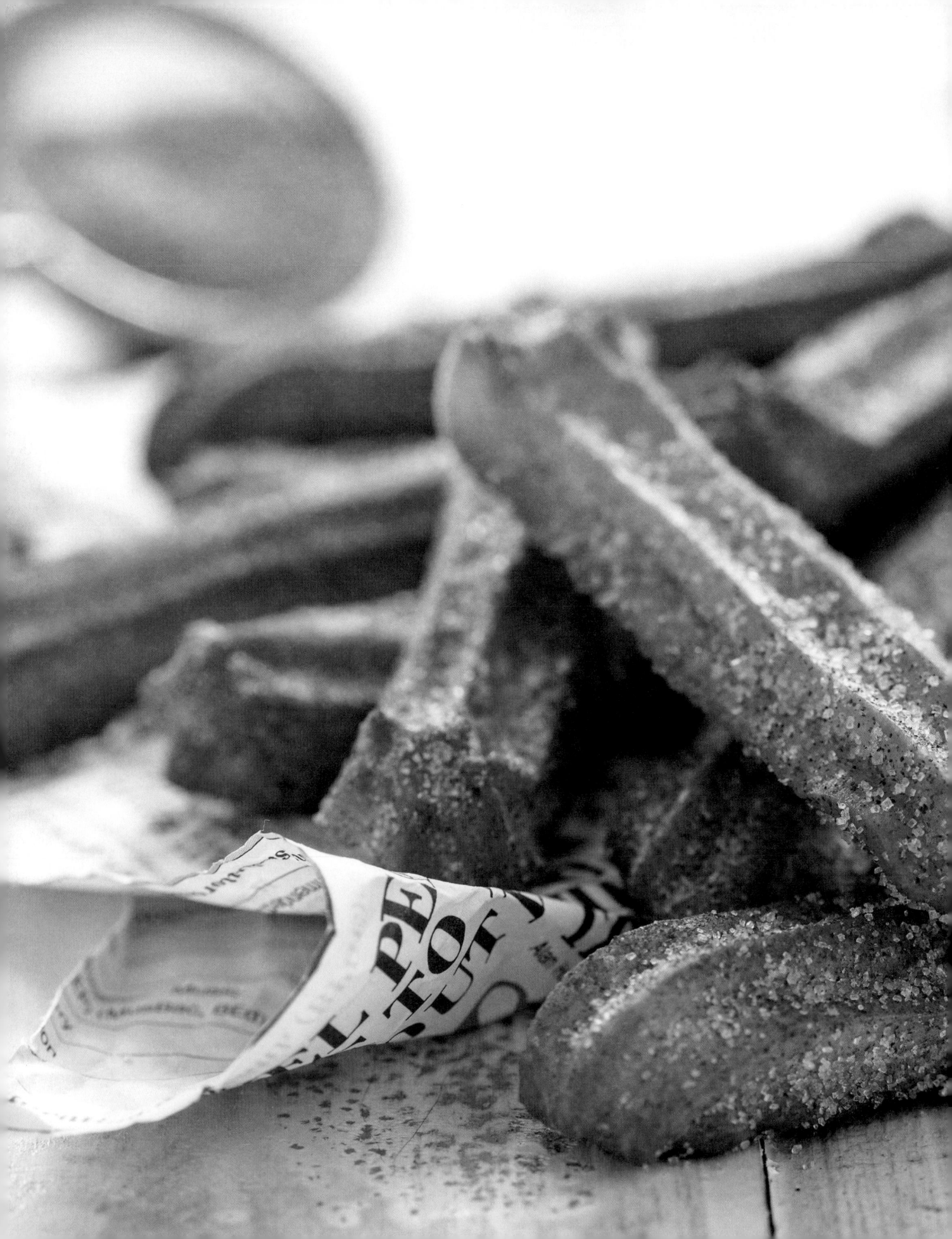

Sweets

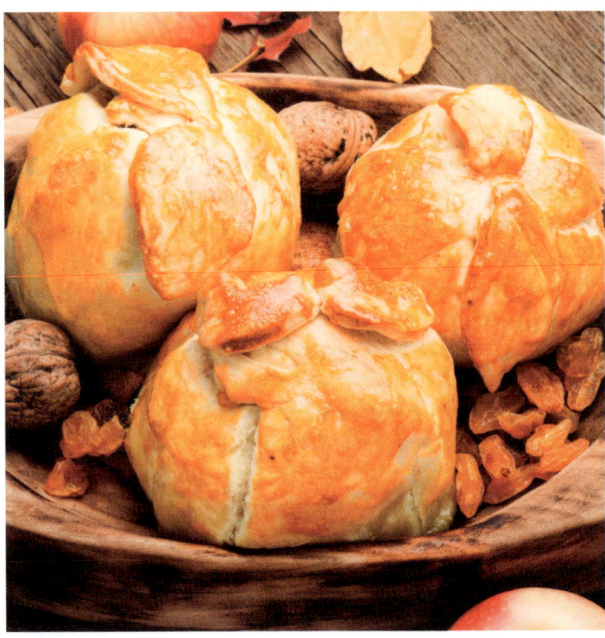

Apple Dumpling

2 apples

1 tbsp brown sugar

1 tsp cinnamon sugar

¼ cup (40g) mixed dried fruit

3 sheets frozen puff pastry, just thawed

2 tbsps butter, melted

Peel and core the apples, using a corer.

Combine the brown sugar, cinnamon sugar and dried fruit and spoon into the centre of each apple.

Lay out one piece of puff pastry and cut out four leaf shapes using a knife or cutter. Set aside.

Lay out remaining two puff pastry sheets on a lightly floured surface. Place one apple bottom-side down onto each sheet and fold the pastry up over the apple to meet at the top. Seal the edges together and cut off any excess. Decorate with the pre-prepared leaves.

Brush the surface of the pastry with melted butter.

Preheat the air fryer to 190°C. Cook for 20 minutes until apple is tender.

SERVES 2

Lemon Butterfly Cakes

150g butter, softened, divided

½ cup (100g) caster sugar

1 tsp vanilla essence

2 eggs

¾ cup (100g) flour

1 tsp baking powder

⅔ cup (100g) icing sugar

½ lemon, juiced and zested

⅔ cup (200g) strawberry jam

Muffin tray

Place 100g of the butter and the caster sugar in a large bowl and beat with an electric mixer until pale and fluffy. Add the vanilla essence and briefly beat to combine.

Add in the eggs, one at a time, beating well after each addition.

Gently fold in the flour and baking powder with a wooden spoon.

Preheat the air fryer to 170°C. Line a muffin tray with patty pans.

Spoon the mixture into the patty pans leaving room for them to rise.

Place the muffin tray into the air fryer. Cook for 8 minutes. Remove and set aside to cool.

Meanwhile, make the buttercream icing. Cream the remaining 50g of butter in the mixer, and gradually add in the icing sugar until softly whipped. Add the lemon juice and zest and mix to combine.

Using a sharp knife, cut out a circle from the top of each of the cupcakes. Cut the circles into halves.

Fill the holes with strawberry jam and then spoon over the buttercream. Place the cut out pieces as 'wings' on top of the cupcakes.

MAKES 6

Note: If you have a small air fryer you could put the patty pans directly into the air fryer basket. Fill the basket with as many as you can and cook in batches.

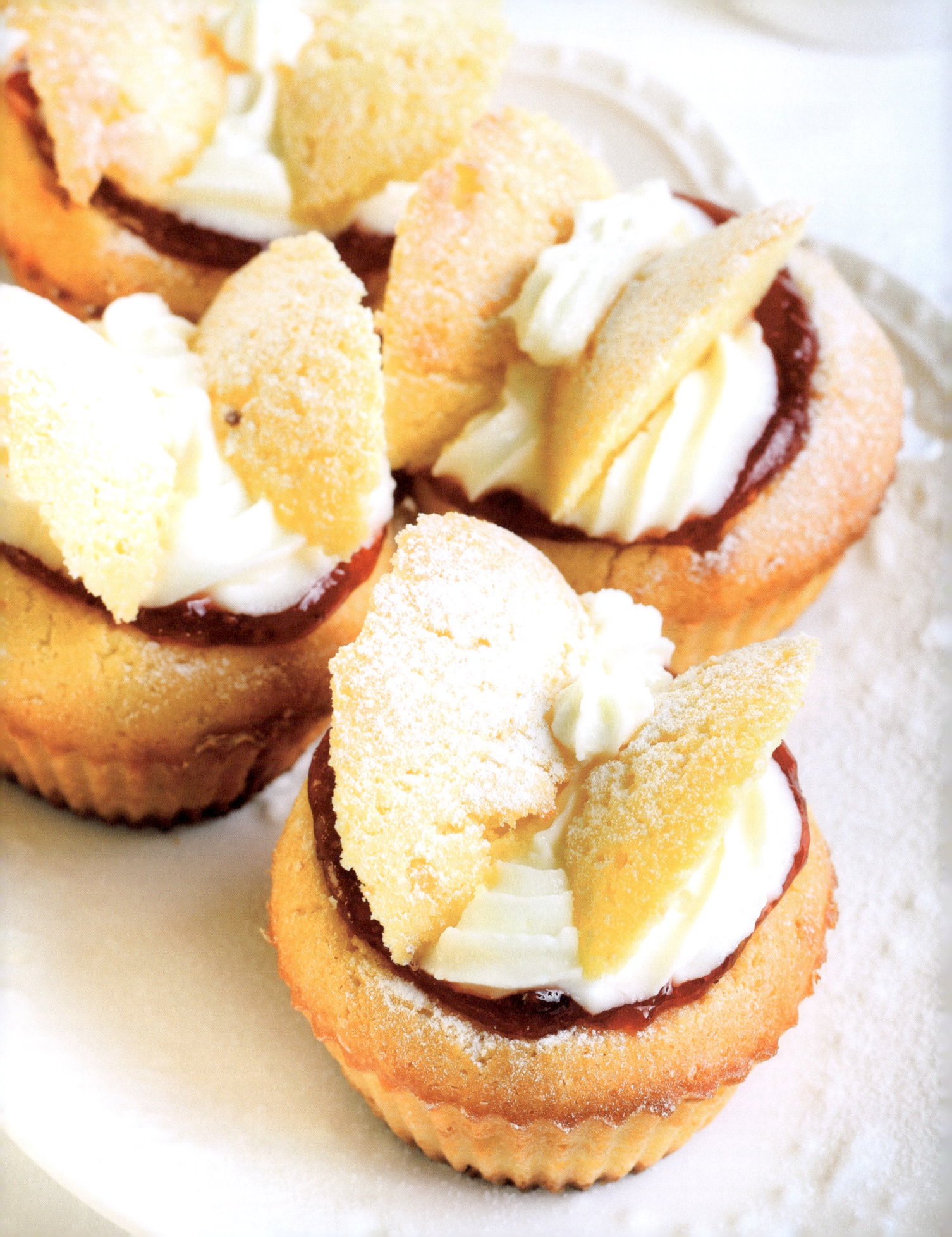

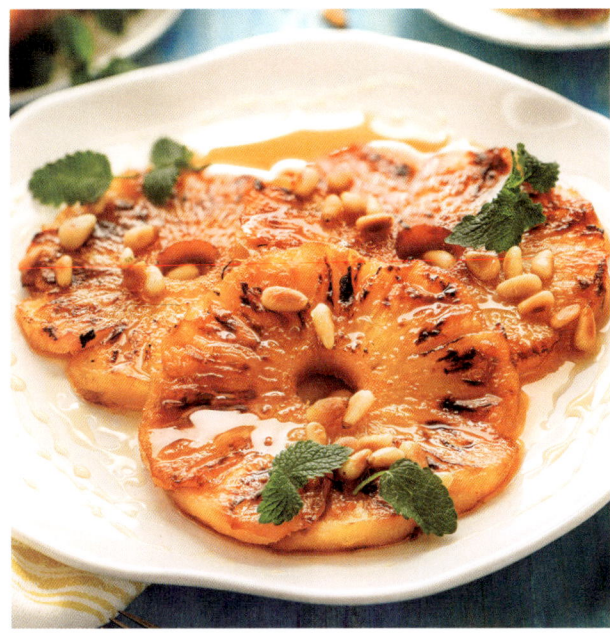

Cinnamon Pineapple Rings

1 x 250g can pineapple slices

3 tbsps butter

½ cup (80g) brown sugar

2 tsps ground cinnamon

1 tbsp pine nuts

Fresh mint, to serve

Drain the pineapple slices.

Preheat the air fryer to 180°C.

Melt the butter in the microwave.

Combine the brown sugar and cinnamon in a bowl.

Brush the pineapple with the melted butter.

Sprinkle cinnamon sugar over the pineapple.

Place into the air fryer basket in a single layer. (Be careful not to overcrowd the basket. Cook in batches or use a double layer accessory if needed.)

Cook for 5 minutes. Remove and flip the pineapple slices over and sprinkle over the pine nuts. Return to cook for a further 5 minutes.

SERVES 2

Note: You can also use fresh pineapple for this recipe. Ensure it is cut thinly.

Pink Glazed Doughnuts

1¾ cups (225g) self-raising flour

1 tsp baking powder

¼ cup (50g) caster sugar

⅓ cup (50g) brown sugar

½ cup (120ml) milk + 3 tbsps milk

70g butter, melted

1 egg

1 cup (155g) icing sugar

½ tsp pink food colouring

Sprinkles, to decorate

Preheat the air fryer to 180°C.

Combine the flour, baking powder, caster sugar and brown sugar in a large mixing bowl.

In a separate bowl whisk together the ½ cup milk, butter and egg.

Pour the wet mixture into the dry ingredients and stir gently until just combined.

Roll dough out onto a floured surface to create a log shape. Slice into disks around 2cm thick. Use a small cookie cutter (or bottle lid) to remove a circle in the centre of the disk. Discard (or see the Doughnut Holes recipe on page 196).

Line the air fryer basket with greaseproof paper. Place the doughnuts inside. (Be careful not to overcrowd the basket. Cook in batches or use a double layer accessory if needed.) Cook for 15 minutes, until they spring back when lightly pressed. Set aside to cool.

Meanwhile, make the icing. Sift the icing sugar over a mixing bowl and whisk in the remaining milk, 1 tablespoon at a time, until the icing reaches a sticky but pourable consistency. Add a couple of drops of pink colouring until the desired colour is achieved.

When the doughnuts have cooled, place the icing over the top, and finish with sprinkles to decorate.

MAKES 4

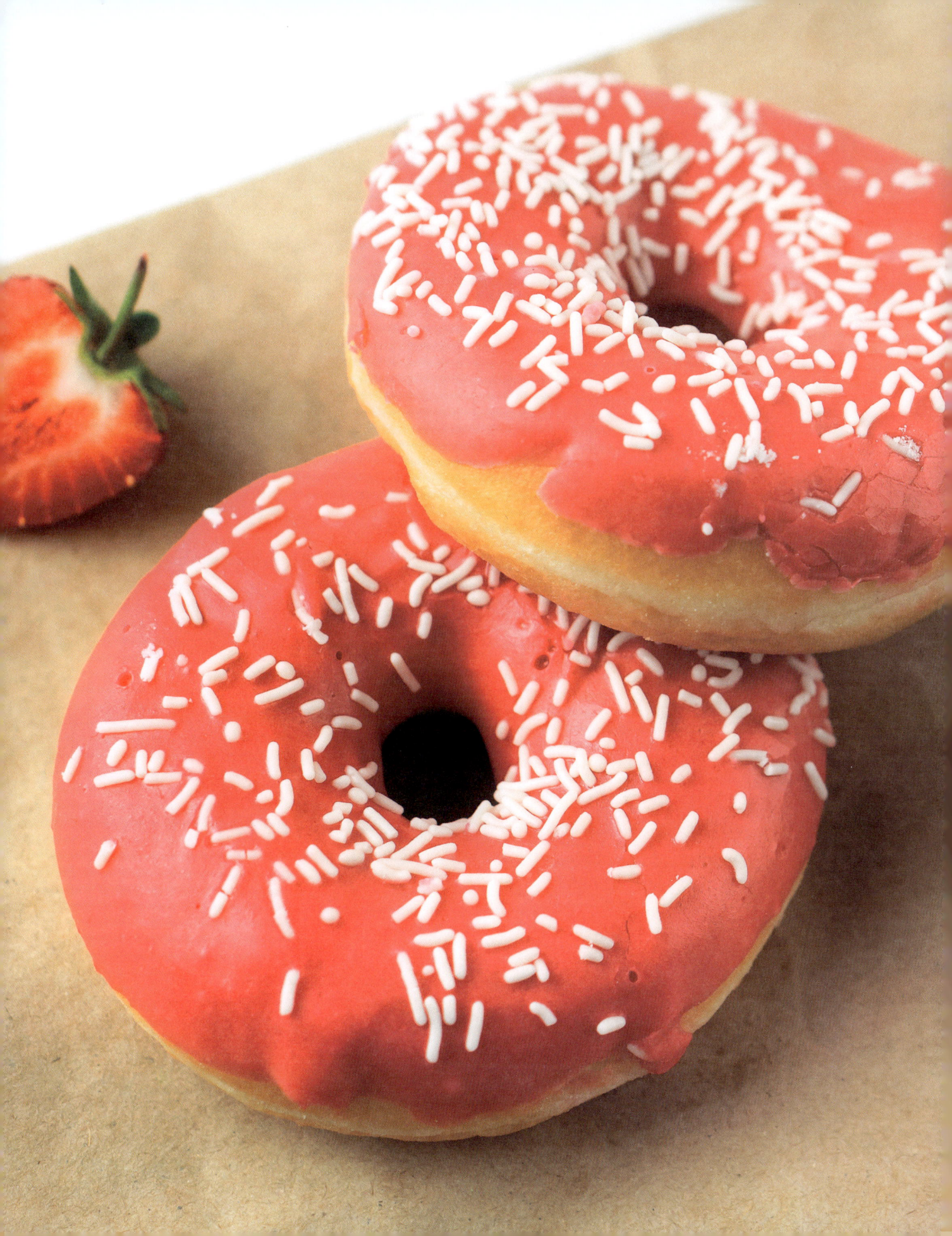

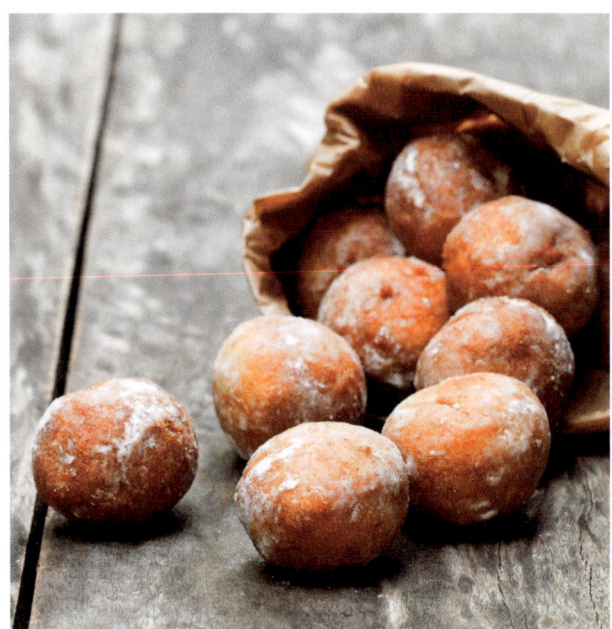

Doughnut Holes

1¼ cups (155g) plain flour

2 tbsps caster sugar

¾ tsp baking powder

¼ tsp salt

100g chilled butter, cut into small pieces

¼ cup (60ml) milk

⅓ cup (70g) sugar

1½ tsps cinnamon

Combine the flour, caster sugar, baking powder and salt in a medium bowl and mix together. Cut in the butter and rub using fingertips until a fine crumble forms. Add the milk and stir until coated.

Transfer the mixture to a floured workbench and knead for approximately a minute until it forms a smooth dough ball. Cut the dough into equal portions and roll each into a ball.

Line the air fryer basket with greaseproof paper and preheat it to 180°C.

Combine cinnamon and the sugar in a medium bowl. Roll the dough balls in the cinnamon sugar and place in the air fryer basket. (Be careful not to overcrowd the basket. Cook in batches or use a double layer accessory if needed.)

Cook for 8 minutes until puffed and golden.

MAKES 12

Homemade Cannoli

4 cups (500g) plain flour, sifted

1 tbsp sugar

Pinch of salt

50g butter, softened

2 egg yolks

¾ cup (185ml) white wine

2 cups (500g) ricotta, thoroughly drained

¾ cup (120g) icing sugar + more for dusting

1 tbsp rosewater

Combine the flour, sugar and salt in a large mixing bowl.

Cut in the butter and rub using fingertips until a fine crumble forms. Add the egg yolks and stir to combine. Gradually add the wine, stirring constantly, until a dough forms. Roll into a ball and cover in plastic wrap. Transfer to the fridge for 30 minutes.

Whip the ricotta, icing sugar and rosewater together in a large bowl until well combined. Spoon the filling into a piping bag (or use a ziplock bag) and chill for 1 hour.

Line the air fryer basket with greaseproof paper and preheat it to 200°C.

Break off a small amount of dough and roll on a floured workbench until very thin but still workable. Cut into circles (use the top of a regular glass for this).

Lightly spritz a cannoli tube (see note) with cooking spray and roll a circle of dough around it. Overlap the ends and press to seal them. Repeat until all the circles have been used.

Place four cannoli in the basket of the air fryer. Cook for 6-7 minutes, turning over halfway through cooking.

Remove and set aside to cool slightly then remove the cannoli by carefully sliding out the tube. Cool on a wire rack or paper towel.

Cut a hole in the piping bag (or snip off the corner of the ziplock bag) and fill each cannoli from both ends. Dust with icing sugar, to serve.

SERVES 4

Note: If you don't have a cannoli tube, you can improvise with something tubular (a dowel or even a stick would do) wrapped in foil.

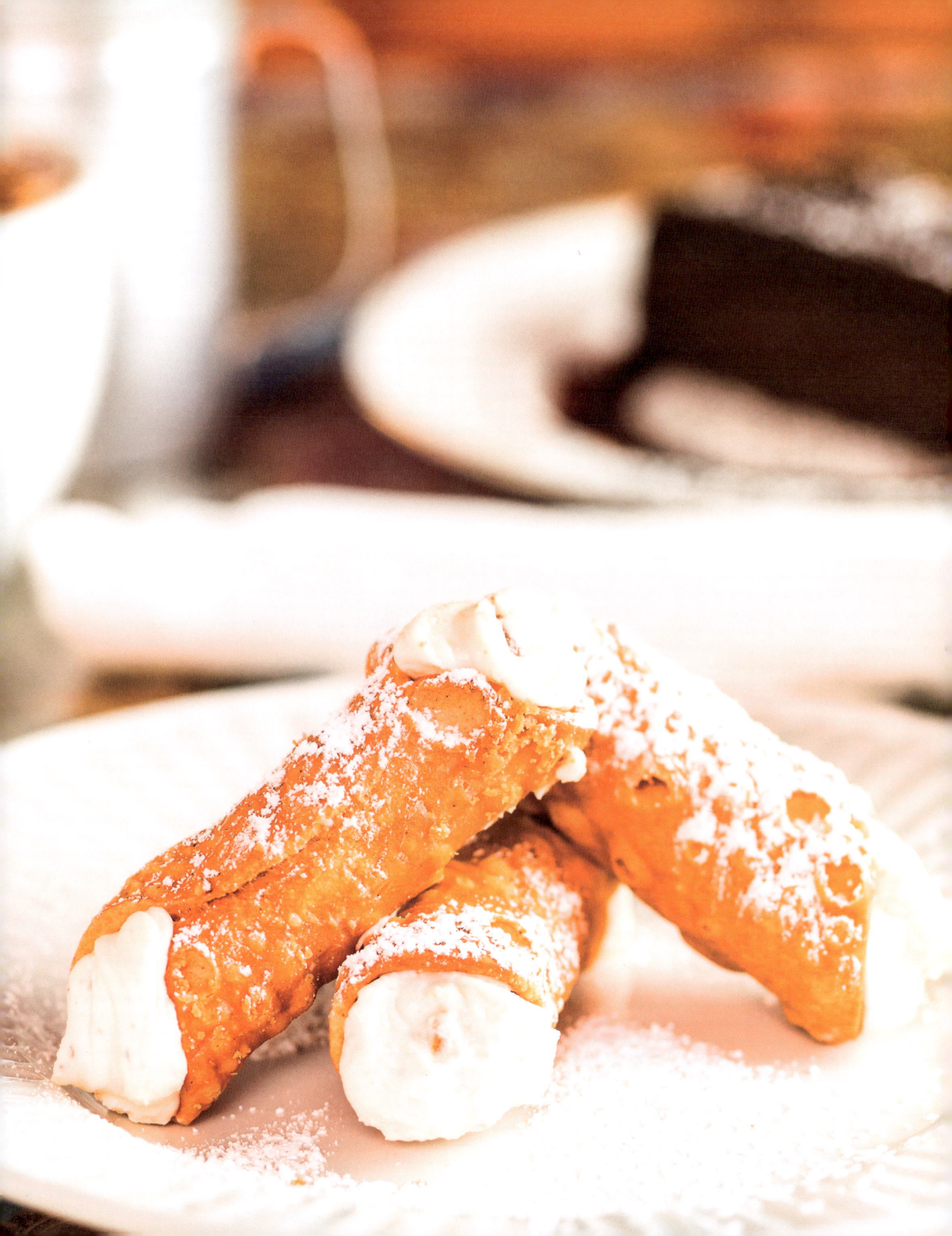

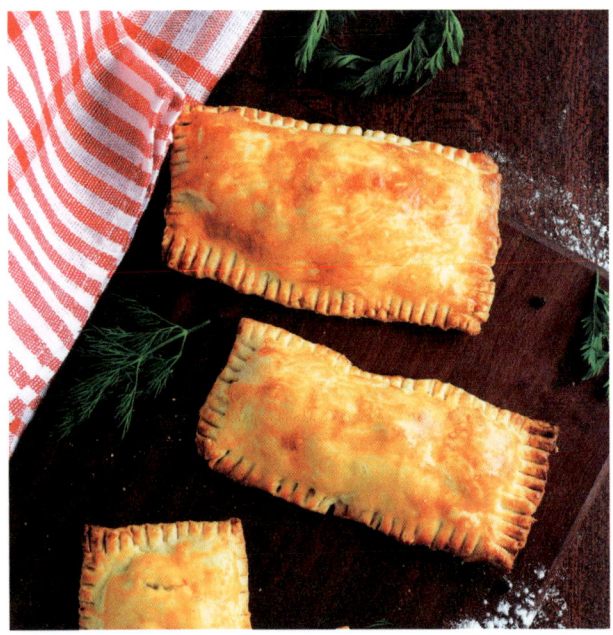

Hand Pies

1 egg

1 tbsp milk

4 sheets shortcrust pastry, just thawed

Filling of choice (see opposite)

Brown or white sugar, to finish (optional)

Beat the egg and milk together in a small bowl to make an egg wash.

Brush one edge of each pastry sheet with egg wash, retaining some for the tops. Place the filling on one side of each sheet. Fold the pastry over and press the two seams together. Use a fork to crimp the edges.

Using the remaining egg wash, brush the tops of the pies and sprinkle with sugar, if desired. Poke holes in the top with a fork.

Preheat the air fryer to 175°C. Transfer one or two pies into the basket (depending on the size of your air fryer) and cook for 12 minutes.

Repeat until all pies are cooked.

MAKES 4 PIES

Notes: Make the pies in whatever shape you prefer. Use a cookie cutter for round pies, which can be cooked in a muffin tray. Or use a different shaped cutter, such as heart-shaped, for a special occasion.

Filling Ideas

BERRY

¼ cup (80g) berry jam

1 cup (150g) berries of choice

1 tsp lemon zest

Spoon jam onto the pastry, then top with fresh berries and lemon zest before sealing.

CHOCOLATE MARSHMALLOW

¼ cup (75g) Nutella

2 tbsps mini marshmallows

Spoon filling onto the pastry before sealing.

CARAMEL APPLE

¼ cup (40g) cooked apple or apple sauce

4 salted butter caramels

Spoon filling onto the pastry and top with a butter caramel before sealing.

VANILLA AND PEACHES

2 fresh peaches, peeled and chopped

1 tbsp lemon juice

3 tbsps sugar

1 tsp vanilla extract

1 tsp cornflour

Place peaches, lemon juice, sugar and vanilla in a mixing bowl and stir well. Drain peaches over a bowl to catch the liquid. Transfer the peaches back into the original mixing bowl. Whisk cornflour into the liquid to create a slurry and then pour this back with the peaches. Spoon filling onto the pastry before sealing.

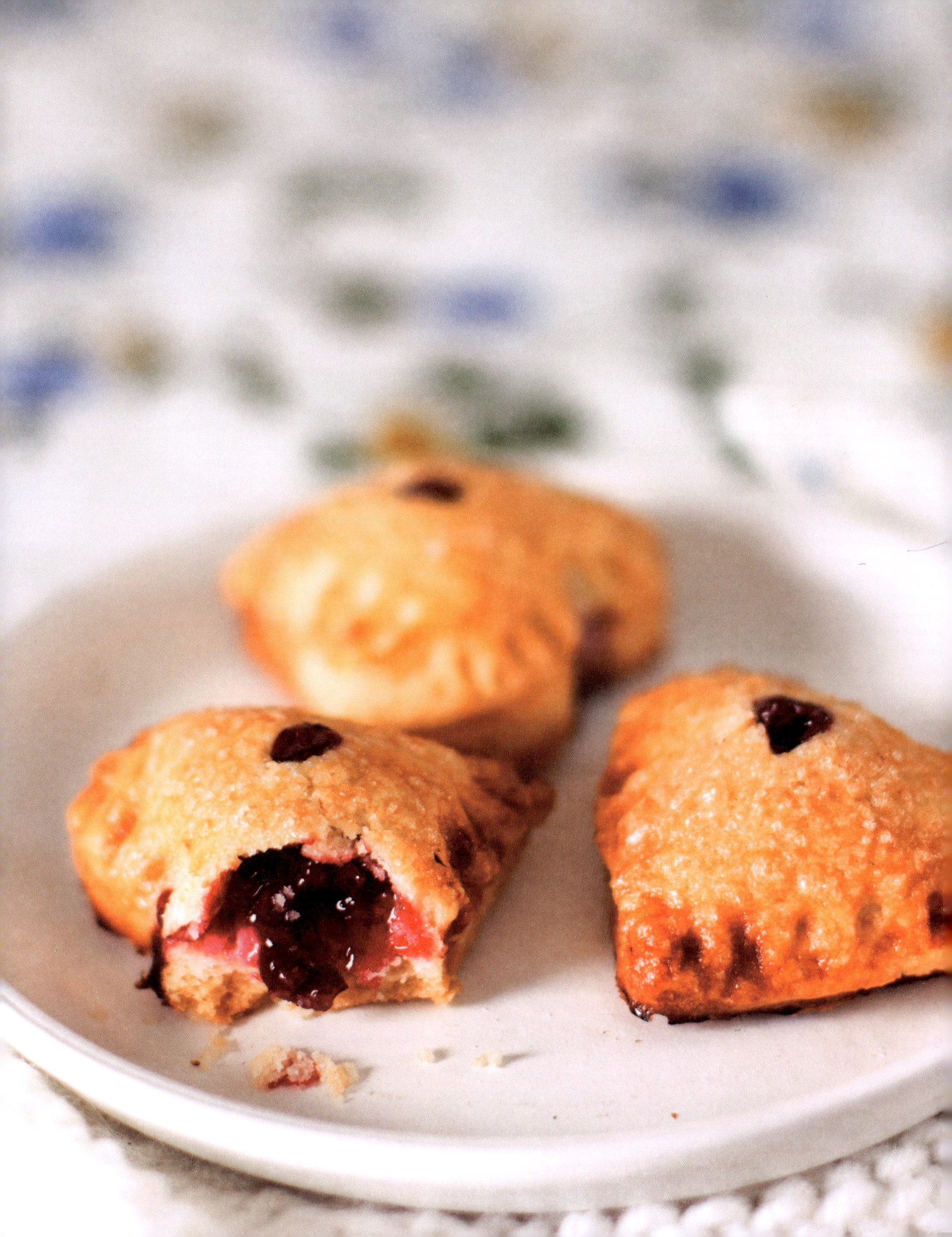

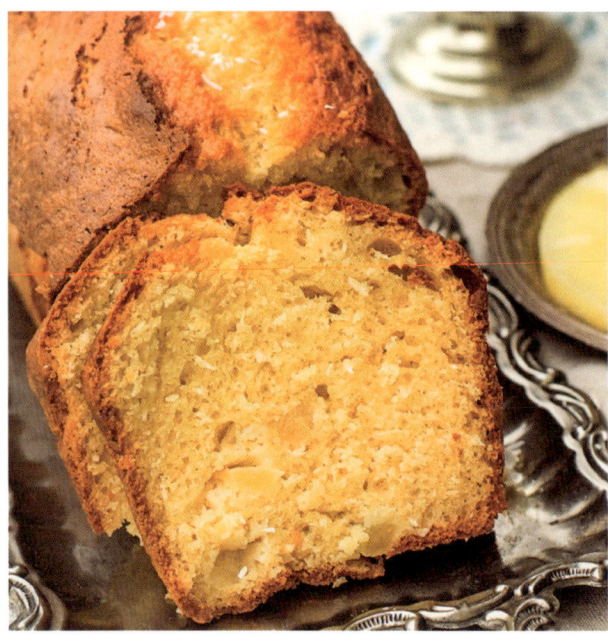

Pineapple Loaf

1¾ cups (225g) self-raising flour

100g butter

½ cup (100g) caster sugar

1 x 230g pineapple chunks in juice

1 egg

2 tbsps milk

Loaf tin

Preheat the air fryer to 200°C and lightly spritz a loaf tin with non-stick spray.

Combine the flour and butter in a large mixing bowl. Rub mixture together with fingertips until it forms a crumble.

Next add the sugar, pineapple chunks and juice and stir well. Set aside.

Whisk the egg and milk together in a separate bowl.

Pour the egg liquid into the bowl with the other ingredients and stir with a wooden spoon until the mixture is fully combined.

Preheat the air fryer to 170°C.

Transfer the mixture to the prepared loaf tin and cook for 40 minutes.

SERVES 6

Banana Cupcakes with Banana Frosting

2 ripe bananas + ½ banana

2 eggs

1¼ cups (310ml) Greek yoghurt, divided

2 cups (180g) oats

Pinch of salt

4 tbsps + 5 tbsps honey

2 tbsps vanilla essence, divided

250g cream cheese, softened

Muffin tray

Preheat air fryer to 200°C. Line muffin tray with patty pans.

Place the two bananas, eggs, 1 cup of the Greek yoghurt, oats, salt, 4 tablespoons honey and 1 tablespoon vanilla essence into a food processor and pulse to create a thick batter.

Spoon batter into patty pans, leaving a little space to the top. Transfer to the basket of the air fryer.

Cook for 10 minutes or until a skewer inserted in the centre comes out clean. Set aside to cool on a wire rack.

Meanwhile, make the frosting. Combine the remaining banana, yoghurt, honey and vanilla essence with the cream cheese in a stand mixer and beat until well combined. Adjust the consistency as you desire by adding more yoghurt to thin the mixture and more banana to thicken it.

Frost the cupcakes when cool.

MAKES 6

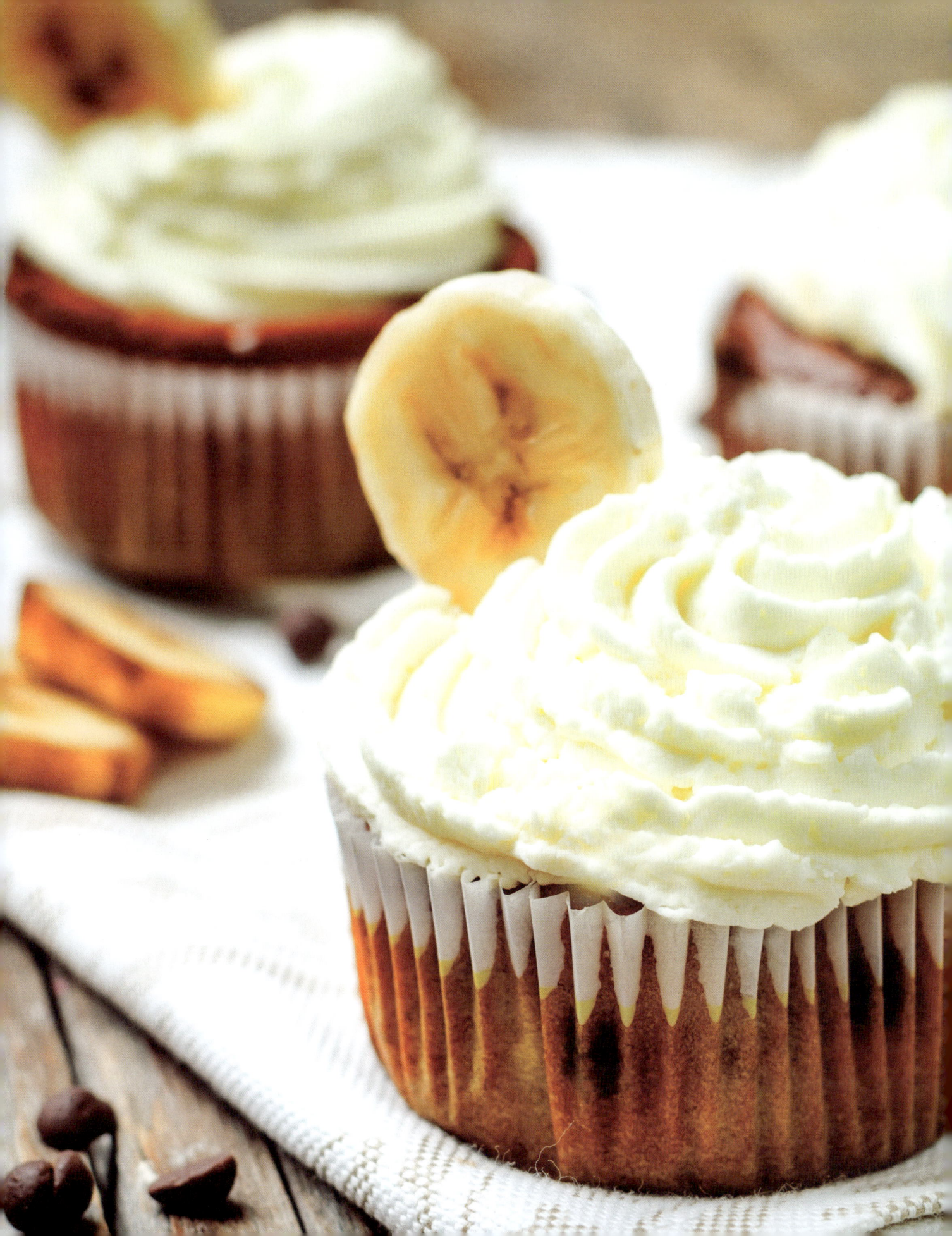

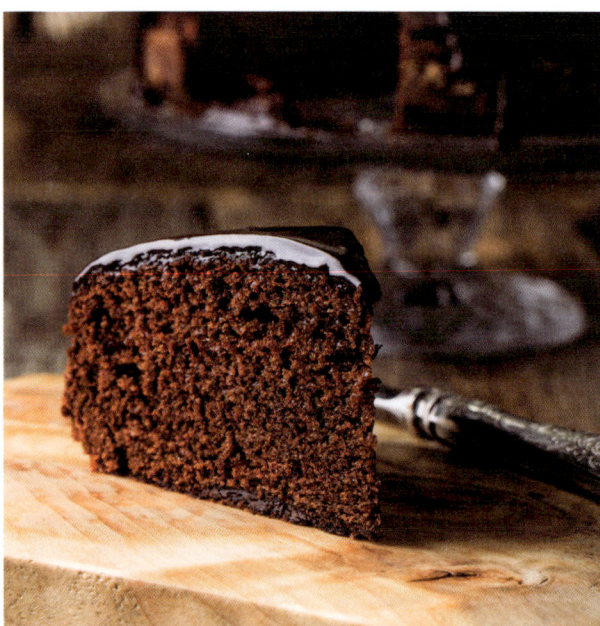

Easy Chocolate Cake

3 eggs

½ cup (125ml) sour cream

1 cup (125g) plain flour

⅔ cup (140g) sugar

Pinch of salt (optional)

115g butter, softened

⅓ cup (35g) cocoa powder

1 tsp baking powder

½ tsp bicarbonate of soda

1 tsp vanilla extract

500g chocolate mirror glaze

Cake tin

Preheat the air fryer to 160°C. Lightly spritz the cake tin with non-stick spray.

Combine all ingredients except the glaze in a large mixing bowl. Stir well.

Scrape the batter into the prepared cake tin and transfer to the air fryer basket.

Cook for 25 minutes. Remove and test with a wooden skewer, which should come out clean when the cake is cooked.

Cool for 5 minutes in the tin then remove and cool on a wire rack. Drizzle with the chocolate mirror glaze.

SERVE 6

Banana Cake with Cream Cheese Icing

2 cups plain (250g) flour

1 tsp baking powder

¾ tsp bicarbonate of soda

½ cup (125ml) vegetable oil

2 eggs

1¼ cups (275g) sugar

½ cup (125ml) buttermilk

1 tsp vanilla extract

4 small, ripe bananas, mashed

250g butter, softened

250g cream cheese, softened

3¼ cups (500g) icing sugar, sifted

Square cake tin

Grease and line the cake tin.

Combine the flour, baking powder and bicarb in a large mixing bowl. Set aside.

Place the oil, eggs, sugar, buttermilk, vanilla and bananas in the large bowl of an electric mixer and beat until just combined. With the setting on low gradually add the flour mixture until fully combined.

Scrape the batter into the prepared tin.

Preheat air fryer to 150°C.

Cook for 30 minutes. Remove and test with a wooden skewer, which should come out clean when the cake is cooked.

Cool for 5 minutes in the tin then remove and cool on a wire rack.

Meanwhile, make the icing. Using the electric mixer, cream the butter and cream cheese until smooth. Add the icing sugar in two separate batches, mixing well after each addition. When well combined, place in the fridge until the cake is cool, then spread carefully using a spatula.

SERVES 6

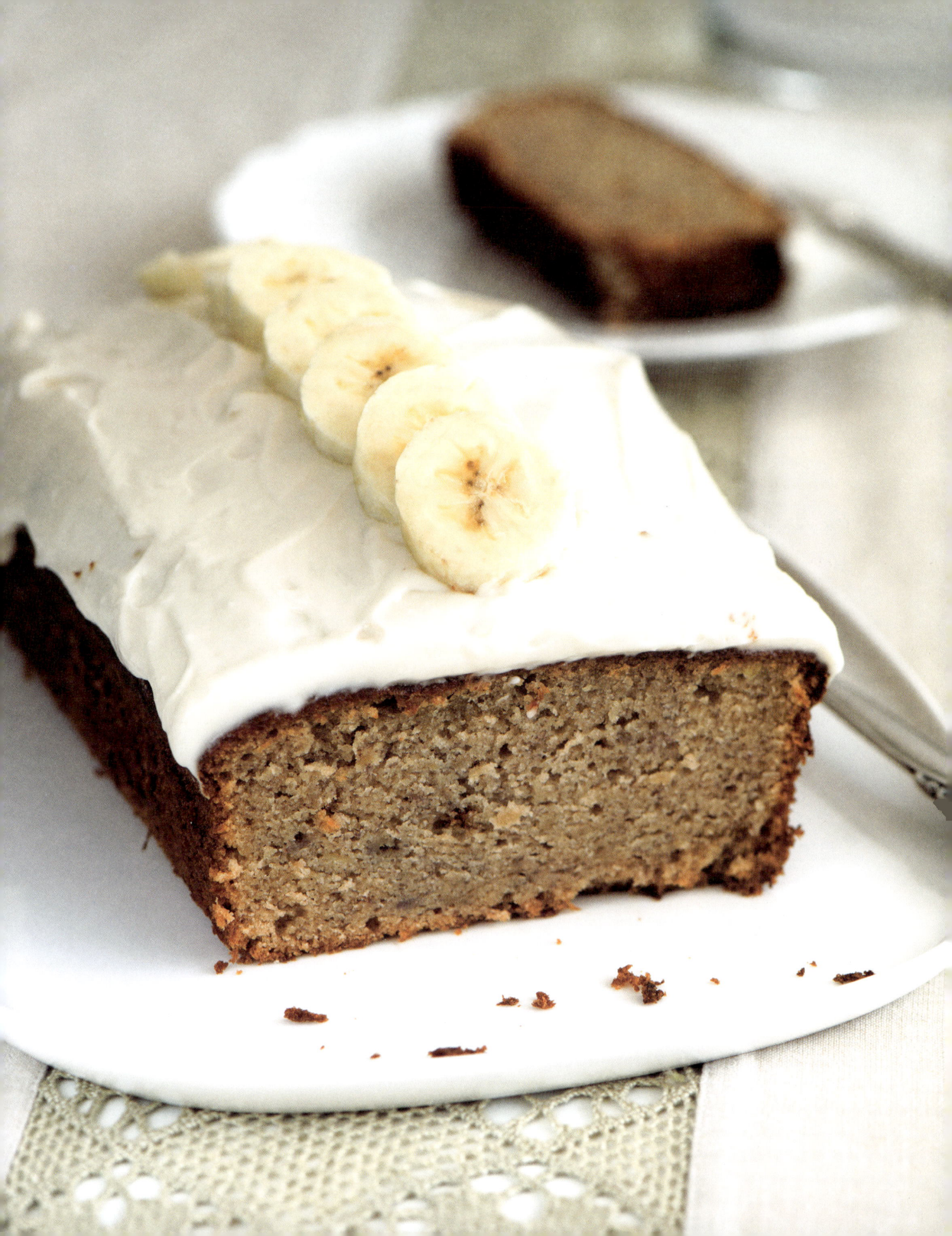

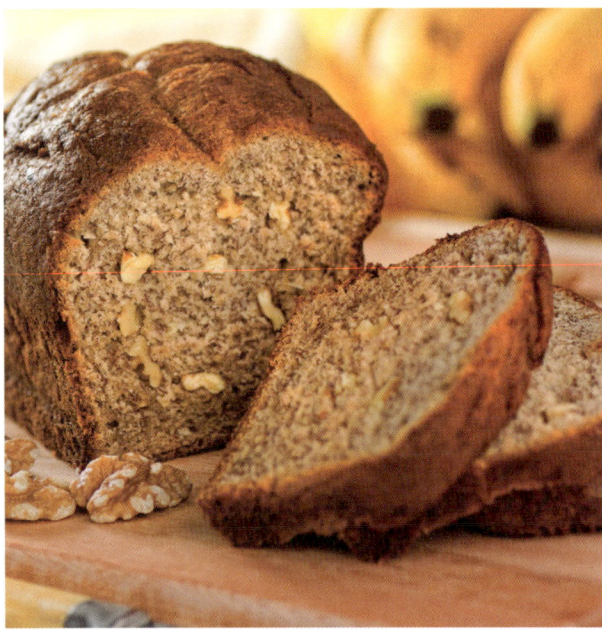

Banana and Walnut Bread

1¾ cups (225g) self-raising flour

½ tsp bicarbonate of soda

¾ cup (180g) caster sugar

75g butter, softened

2 eggs

3 small, ripe bananas, mashed

1¼ cups (150g) walnuts, roughly chopped

Loaf tin

Lightly spritz the loaf tin with non-stick spray.

Combine flour and bicarb in a large mixing bowl.

Place sugar and butter in the bowl of an electric mixer and beat until pale and fluffy. Add the eggs one at a time, beating well after each addition.

Remove bowl from mixer and gently stir in the flour using a wooden spoon. Add banana and walnuts and stir to combine.

Preheat air fryer to 180°C.

Scrape the mixture into the prepared tin and transfer to the air fryer. Cook for 15 minutes. Reduce temperature to 170°C and cook for a further 15 minutes.

Remove and test with a wooden skewer, which should come out clean when the loaf is cooked. Cool for 5 minutes in the tin then remove and cool on a wire rack.

SERVES 6

Blueberry Scones with Vanilla Glaze

2 cups (250g) plain flour

4 tbsps caster sugar

2 tsps baking powder

Pinch of salt

60g butter, melted

1 egg

⅓ cup (80ml) + 2 tbsps milk

1 cup (100g) blueberries (fresh or frozen)

1 cup (155g) icing sugar

1 tsp vanilla extract

Ovenproof dish, lightly greased

Combine the flour, sugar, baking powder and salt in a large mixing bowl.

In a separate bowl, whisk together butter, egg, and ⅓ cup milk.

Pour the wet mixture into the dry ingredients and stir until well combined. Add the blueberries and gently fold them into the mixture.

Transfer the dough onto a floured work surface. Form into a circle and cut into eight wedges.

Preheat the air fryer to 175°C.

Place the wedges into the prepared pan and slide into the air fryer. (Be careful not to overcrowd the basket. Cook in batches or use a double layer accessory if needed.)

Cook for 15 minutes. Remove and test with a wooden skewer, which should come out clean when the scones are cooked. Cool for 5 minutes in the tin then remove and cool on a wire rack.

Meanwhile, make the glaze. In a small bowl, whisk together the icing sugar, vanilla and 2 tablespoons milk until well combined. Drizzle the icing over the scones to serve.

SERVES 6

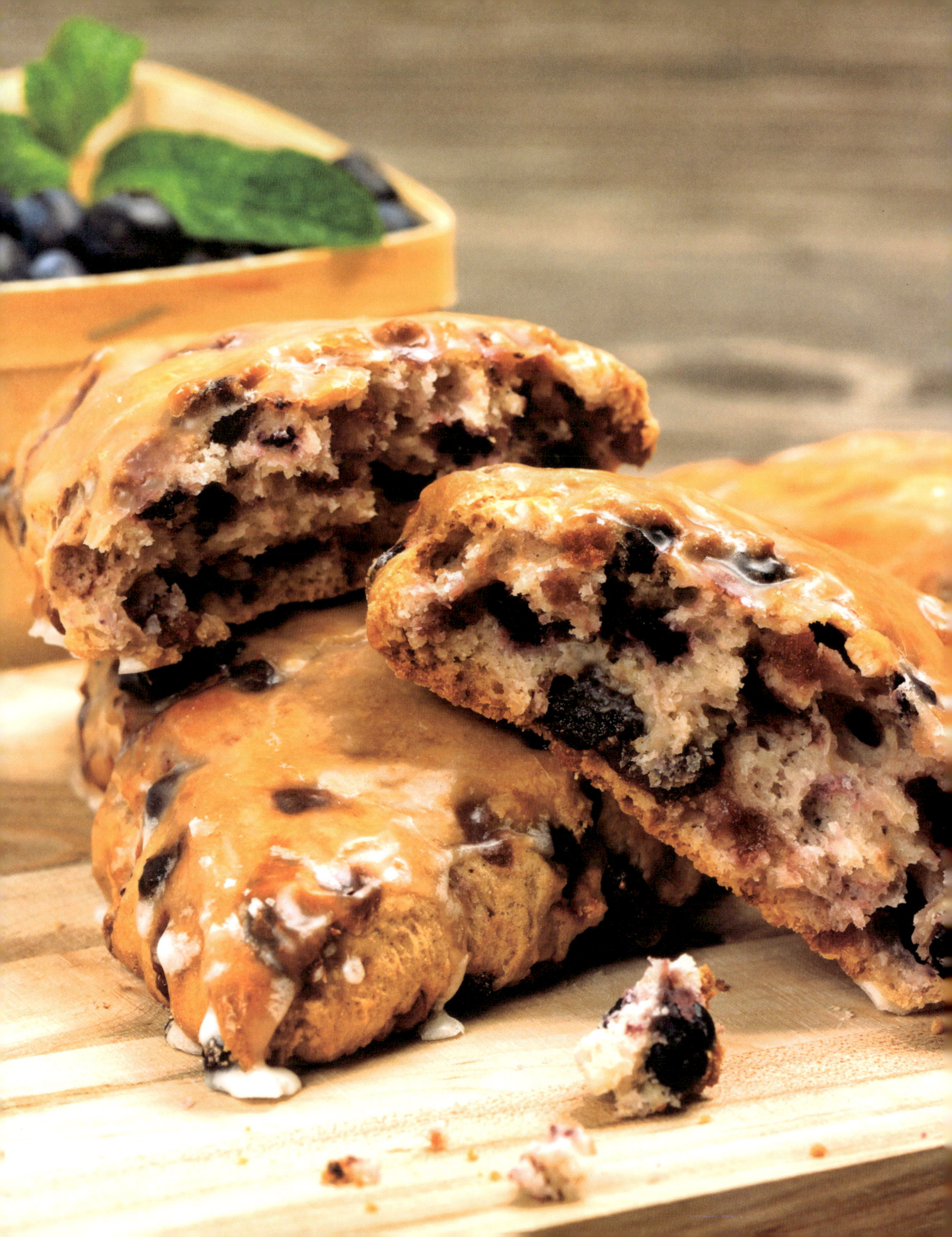

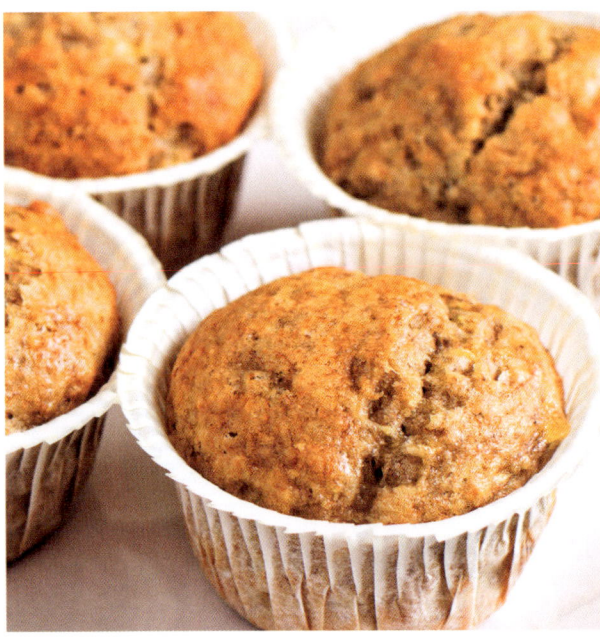

Cheat's Banana Muffins

4 very ripe bananas

2 eggs

½ cup (125g) smooth peanut butter

Muffin tray

Preheat the air fryer to 180°C.

Put all the ingredients into a blender or food processor and process until a thick batter forms.

Line the muffin tray with patty pans. Pour the batter into the patty pans and transfer to the air fryer. (You may need to cook in batches.)

Cook for 10 minutes.

Remove and test with a wooden skewer, which should come out clean when the muffins are cooked.

When cooked, cool for 5 minutes in the tray then remove and cool on a wire rack.

MAKES 12

Banana Choc Chip Muffins

1¾ cups (225g) self-raising flour

1 cup (225g) caster sugar

100g butter, cold, cut into cubes

2 eggs

5 tbsps milk

1 tsp vanilla essence

3 very ripe bananas, mashed

3¼ cups (100g) milk chocolate chips

Muffin tray

Combine the flour and sugar in a large mixing bowl.

Add butter. Rub mixture together with fingertips until it forms a crumble.

Whisk the eggs and milk together in a small bowl.

Pour egg mixture into the crumble mixture and add the vanilla essence. Stir well. Add bananas and chocolate chips and stir to combine thoroughly.

Preheat the air fryer to 180°C.

Line the muffin tray with patty pans. Spoon the batter into the patty pans and place in the basket of the air fryer. (You may need to cook in batches.)

Cook for 10 minutes. Reduce heat to 160°C and cook for a further 5 minutes.

Remove and test with a wooden skewer, which should come out clean when the muffins are cooked.

When cooked, cool for 5 minutes in the tray then remove and cool on a wire rack.

MAKES 12

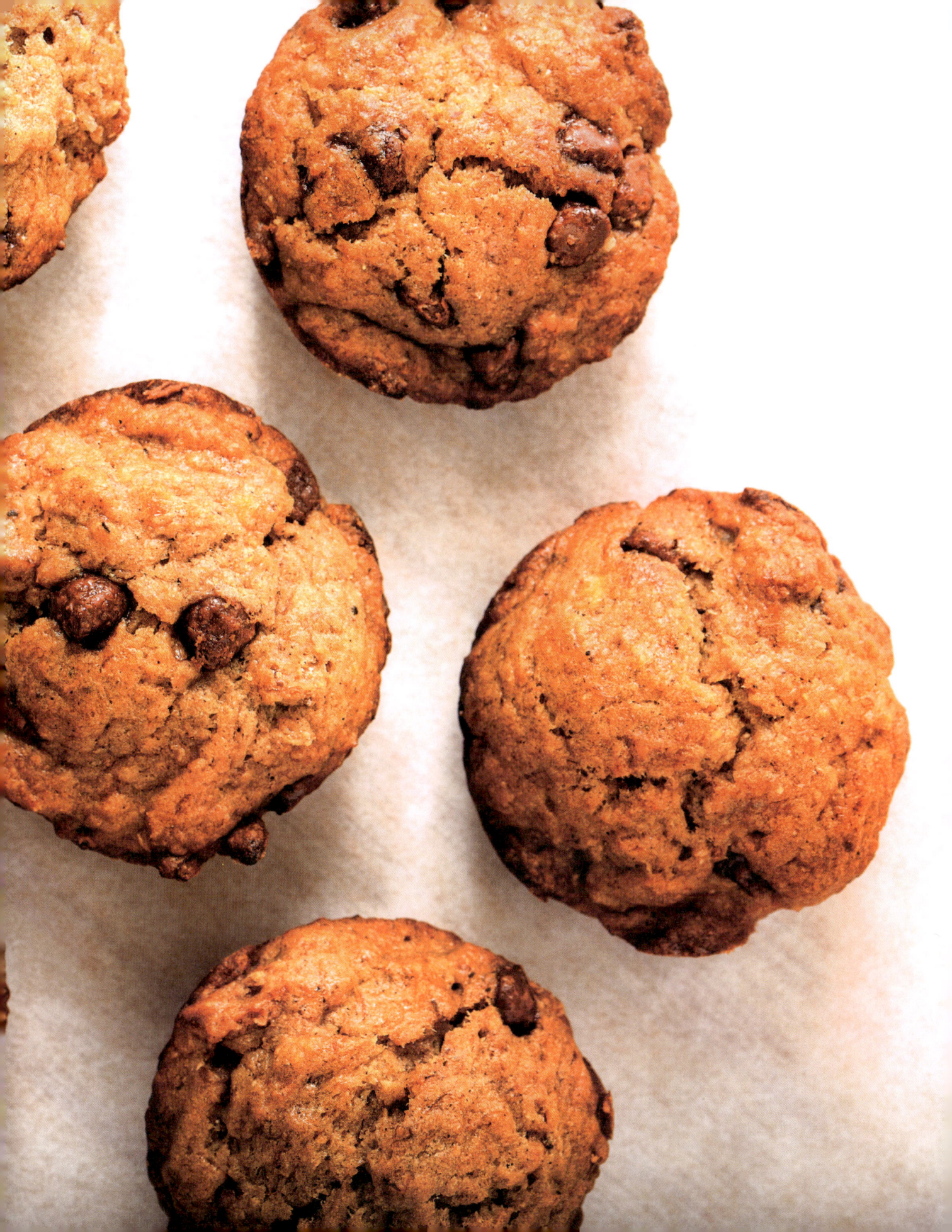

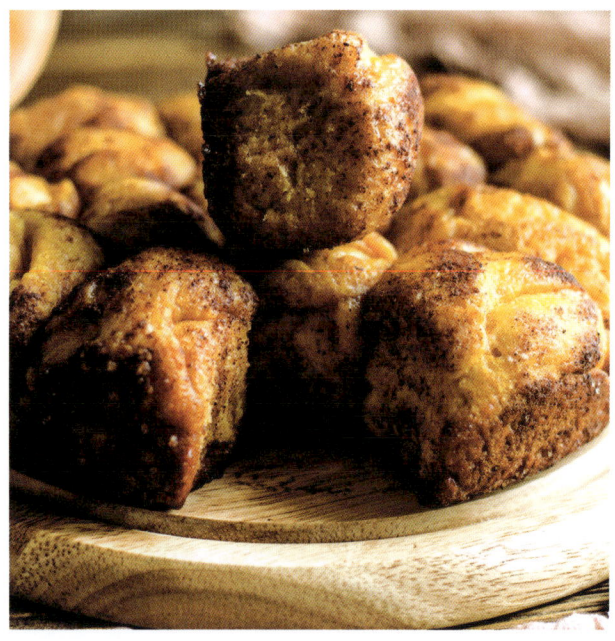

Monkey Bread Balls

1 cup (125g) self-raising flour

1 cup (250ml) Greek yoghurt

1 tbsp cinnamon sugar

115g butter, melted

¾ cup (120g) brown sugar

Cake tin

Place the flour and yoghurt into a mixing bowl and stir to combine until a crumbly mixture forms.

Shape into a round ball. Flatten the ball and cut into pieces to make the process more manageable. Roll each piece into a small ball.

Place dough balls in a large bowl and sprinkle with the cinnamon sugar. Gently toss to coat them thoroughly.

Light spritz the cake tin with non-stick spray. Preheat the air fryer to 190°C.

In small bowl, mix together the melted butter and brown sugar.

Transfer the dough balls into the cake tin, trying not to overcrowd them. Pour the butter and sugar mixture over the top.

Slide pan into the air fryer and cook for 12 minutes.

Remove and test with a wooden skewer, which should come out clean when they are cooked.

SERVES 4

Zebra Cake

125g butter

½ cup (120g) caster sugar

2 tsps vanilla essence

2 eggs

1½ tbsps milk

1 cup (110g) self-raising flour, sifted

2 tbsps cocoa powder, sifted

Cake tin

Preheat air fryer to 160°C. Grease and line the cake tin.

Place the butter and sugar in a large bowl of an electric mixer and beat until pale and fluffy. Add the vanilla essence and briefly beat to combine.

Add in the eggs, one at a time, beating well after each addition. Add in the milk and beat to combine.

Gently fold in the flour with a wooden spoon.

Remove half of the batter from the mixer and set aside.

Add cocoa to the batter remaining in the mixer and beat to incorporate.

Scoop around 2 tablespoons of the cocoa batter and place it in the centre of the cake tin. Add the same amount of the plain batter, gently swirling it around the cocoa batter, and keep alternating the batters until they have been used up and the tin is full.

Place cake tin in the air fryer and bake for 30 minutes.

Remove and test with a wooden skewer, which should come out clean when the cake is cooked.

When cooked, cool for 5 minutes in the tin then remove and cool on a wire rack.

SERVES 6

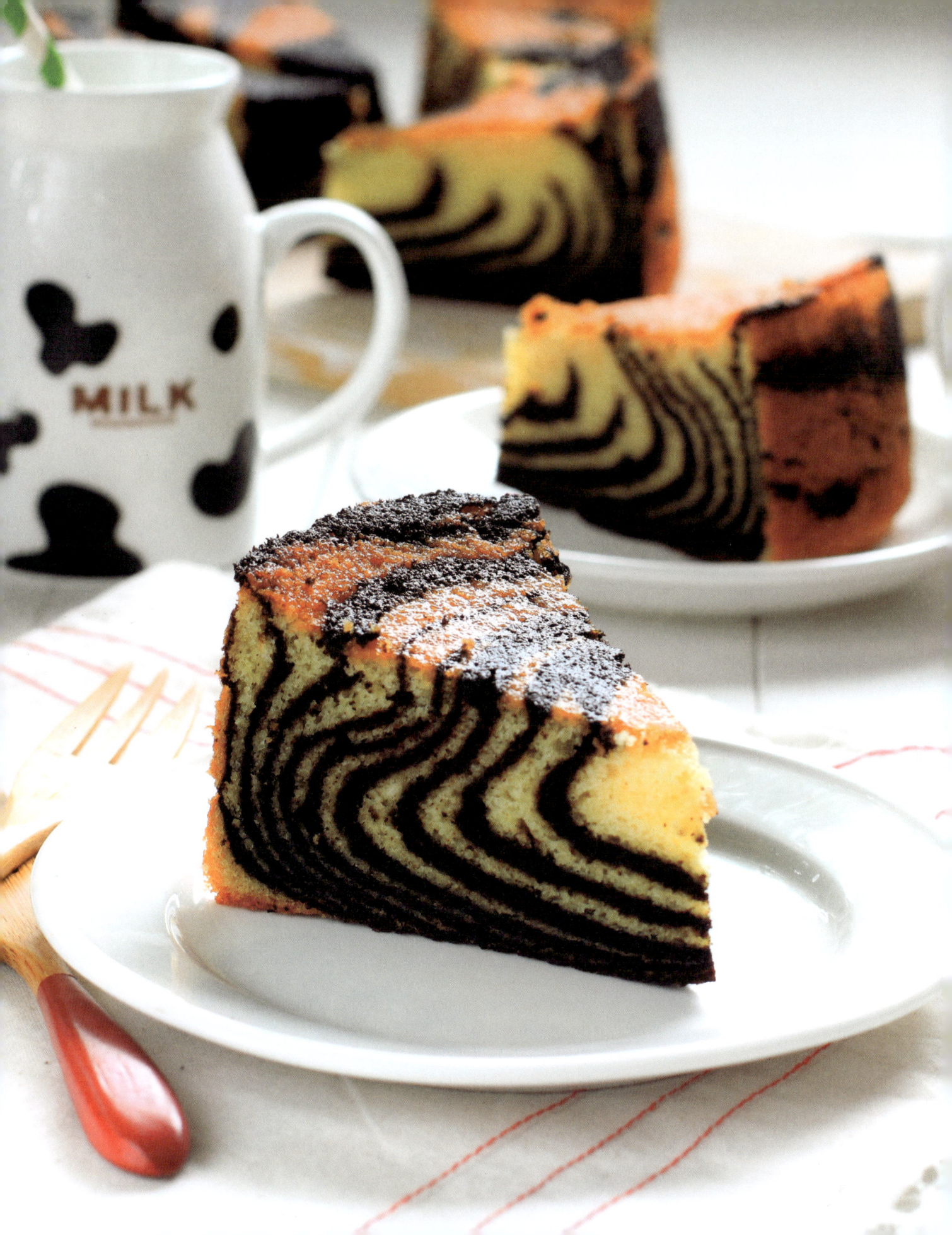

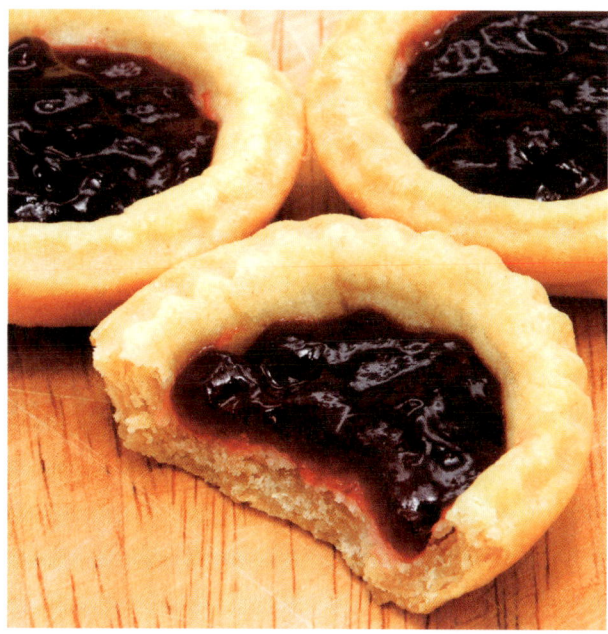

Easy Jam Tarts

1¾ cups (225g) plain flour

2 tbsps caster sugar

110g butter

1 tbsp water (+ more, as needed)

Strawberry jam (approximately 2 tbsps per tart)

Muffin tray, greased

Preheat the air fryer to 180°C.

Combine the flour and sugar in a large mixing bowl.

Add butter. Rub mixture together with fingertips until it forms a crumble.

Add water as needed and mix until a firm dough forms.

Press pastry into the bottom and a little way up around the sides of the muffin tray holes. You may need to cook in batches.

Preheat the air fryer to 180°C.

Spoon the jam onto the centre of the pastry and smooth around with the back of the spoon.

Cook for 10 minutes.

MAKES 10 (APPROXIMATELY)

Sultana Scones

3 cups (375g) self-raising flour

1 tsp salt

1 cup (250ml) thickened cream

1 cup (250ml) cold ginger ale

¾ cup (65g) sultanas

1 egg yolk

1 tsp milk

Extra flour for dusting

Sift the flour and salt into a large mixing bowl.

Combine the cream and ginger ale in a second bowl. Add sultanas and mix.

Pour the wet ingredients into the bowl with the flour and quickly cut through with a knife until a rough, crumbly dough forms. Don't overmix the dough.

Turn out onto a lightly floured surface and form dough into a disc. Roll out the dough to a thickness of 3cm then cut out rounds using a cookie cutter.

Preheat the air fryer to 180°C. Lightly spritz the basket of the air fryer with a non-stick cooking spray.

Transfer the scones to the basket. (Be careful not to overcrowd the basket. Cook in batches or use a double layer accessory if needed.)

Mix the egg yolk and milk in a small bowl to make an egg wash. Brush the tops of the scones with the egg wash.

Cook for 15 minutes until golden.

When cooked, remove from the air fryer and cool for 5 minutes in the basket, then remove and cool on a wire rack.

MAKES 12 (APPROXIMATELY)

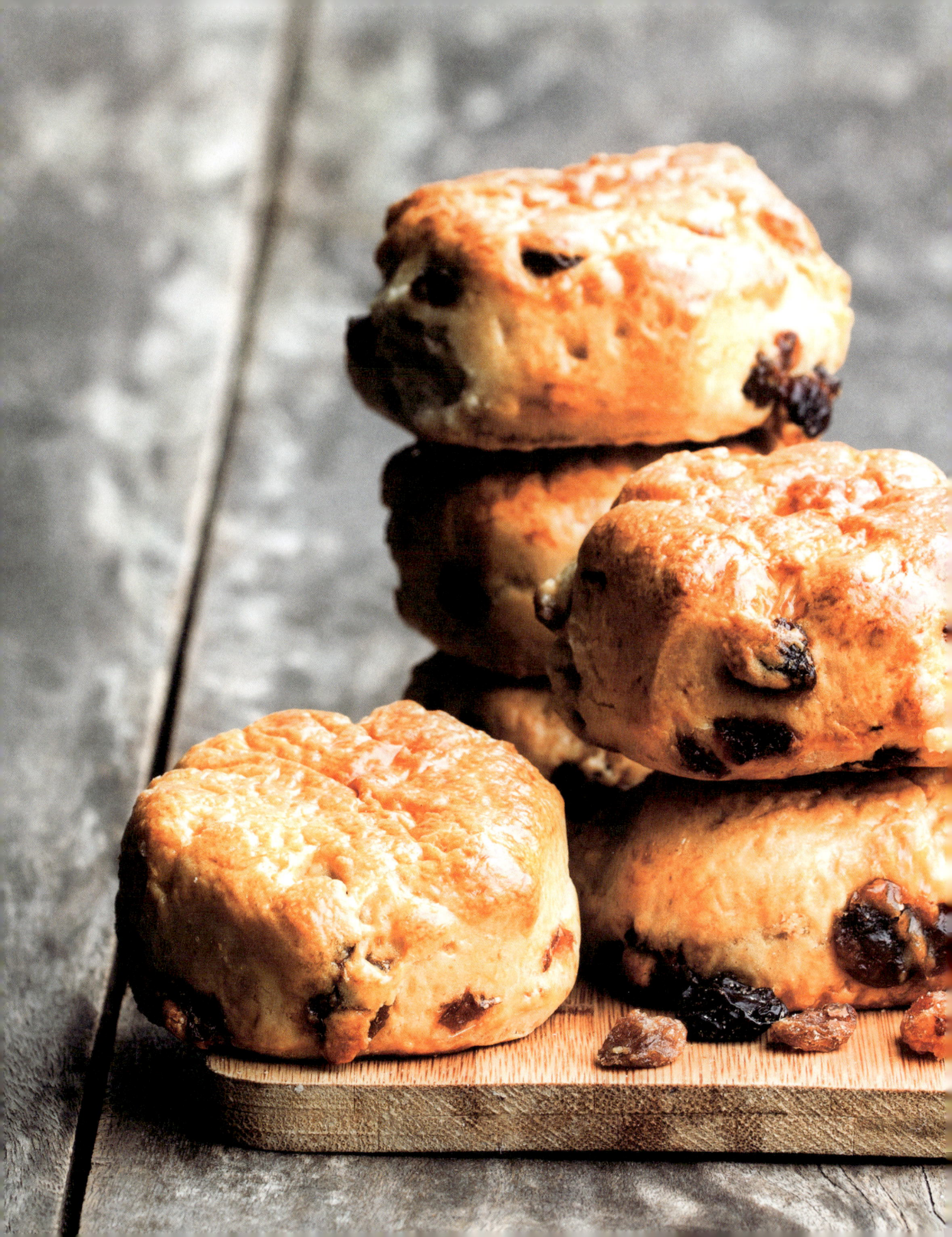

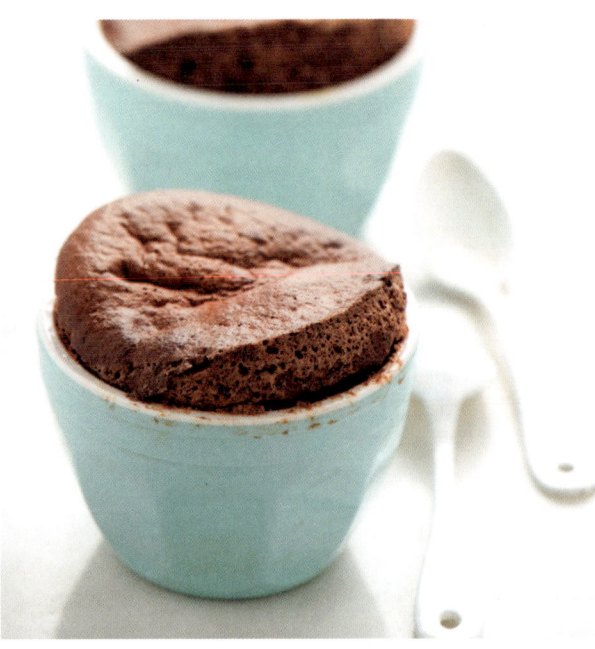

Chocolate Mug Cake

¼ cup (30g) self-raising flour

2 tbsps caster sugar

1 tbsp cocoa powder

3 tbsps milk

2 tsps mild-tasting oil (such as canola)

Ovenproof mug, greased

Combine all the ingredients together in a bowl until well mixed.

Transfer to the prepared mug.

Place the mug in the air fryer and cook for 10 minutes at 200°C.

SERVES 1

Molten Lava Cakes

150g dark chocolate

125g unsalted butter

2 eggs

3½ tbsps caster sugar

½ cup (70g) self-raising flour

Icing sugar, for dusting

4 individual ovenproof ramekins

Grease and flour the ramekins. Place them in the air fryer basket.

Break the chocolate into pieces and place it in a microwave-safe bowl with the butter. Melt in the microwave until the mixture has a smooth, even consistency.

Using an electric mixer, beat the eggs and caster sugar until pale and fluffy.

Remove the bowl and pour the melted chocolate mixture into the egg mixture. Gently stir in the flour using a rubber spatula.

Preheat the air fryer to 190°C.

Fill each ramekin three-quarters full with the cake mixture.

Cook for 10 minutes.

Remove from the air fryer and cool in ramekins for a few minutes. Carefully turn ramekins upside down onto a serving plate. Tap with a knife around the edges and bottom to loosen. Gently slide the cake onto the plate.

Sprinkle with icing sugar to serve.

SERVES 4

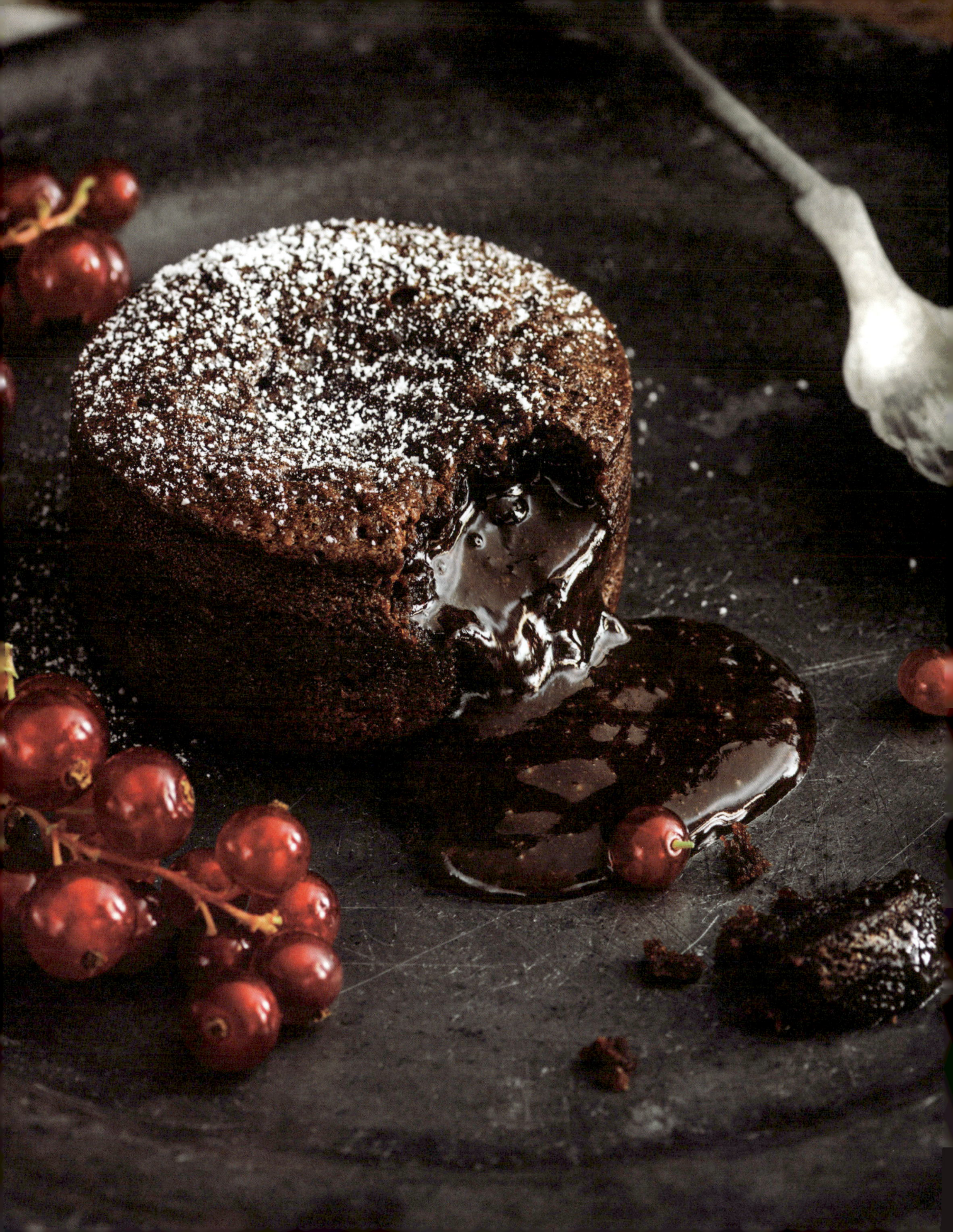

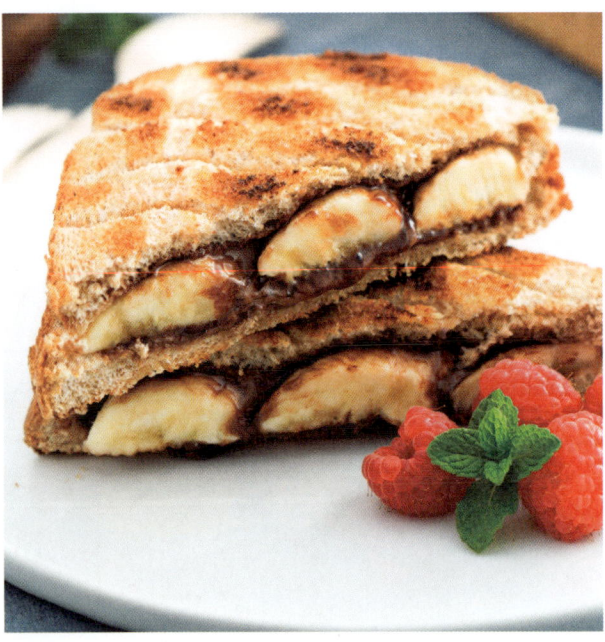

Nutella-Nana Sandwich

1 tbsp butter, softened

4 slices white bread

¼ cup (75g) Nutella

1 banana, halved and sliced

Preheat the air fryer to 190°C.

Spread the butter on one side of each piece of bread. Place buttered-side down on a plate.

Spread the Nutella on the other side of each piece of bread.

Place banana slices on top of Nutella on two slices of bread.

Close the sandwiches and transfer to the basket of the air fryer.

Cook for 8 minutes, turning halfway through cooking.

SERVES 2

Fried Ice-Cream Balls

3 cups (100g) cornflakes

2 tbsps plain flour

1 egg

1L vanilla ice cream

Chocolate sauce, to serve

Cake tin, greased and lined

Place the cornflakes in a ziplock bag and crush using a rolling pin (or you can blitz in the food processor to get the same result). Sprinkle onto a plate or shallow bowl and set aside. Place the flour in another shallow bowl and beat the egg in a third shallow bowl.

Scoop the ice cream into 10 balls. Place the balls into the lined cake tin. Return to the freezer until hard.

Coat the balls in flour. If necessary return to the freezer until hard again.

Coat the balls in egg and then roll through the crushed cornflakes. If necessary return to the freezer until hard again.

Preheat the air fryer to 200°C. Place the balls in the cake tin into the air fryer and cook for 2 minutes.

Drizzle with chocolate sauce and eat immediately.

MAKES 10

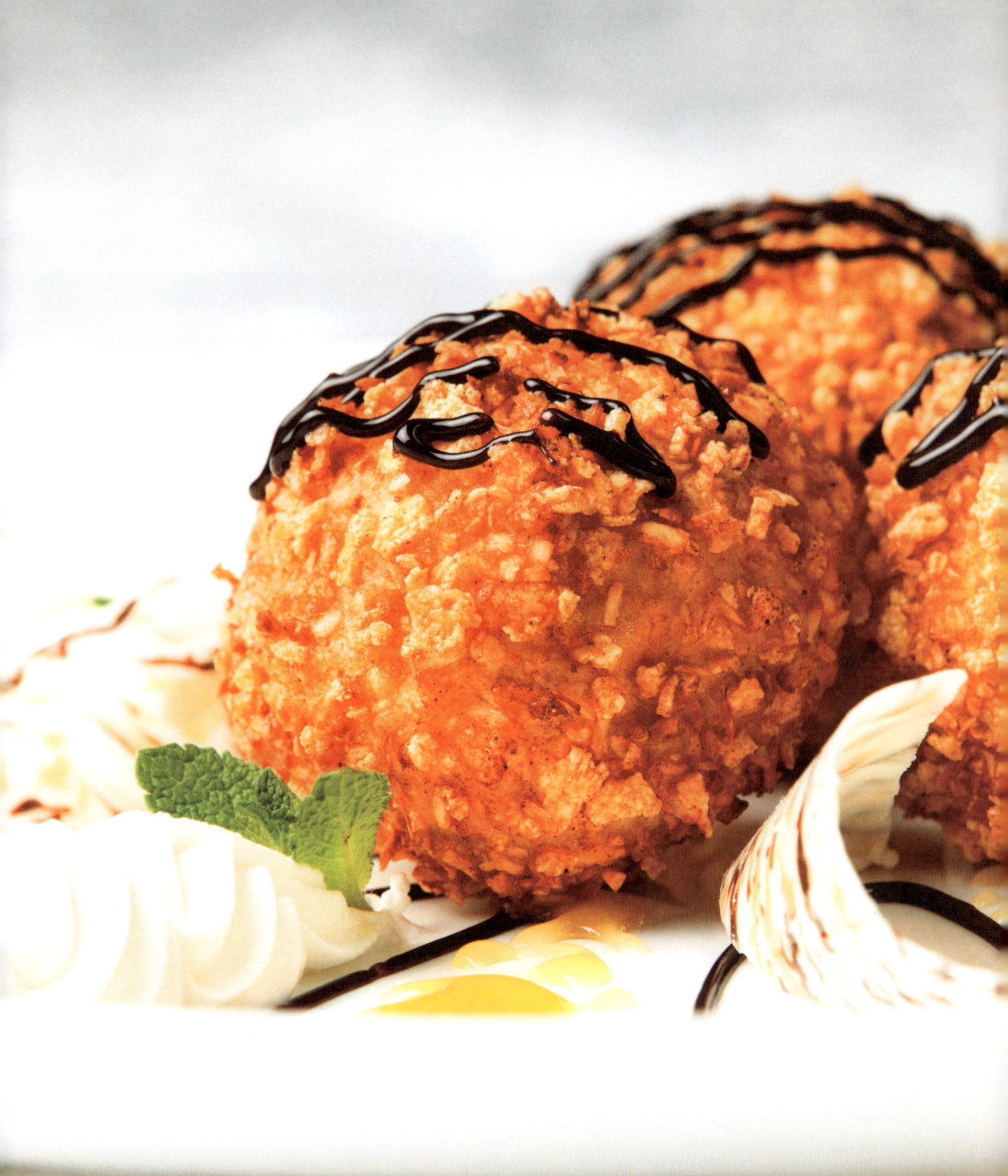

Mini Berry Crumbles

1 apple, peeled, cored and finely chopped

½ cup (75g) frozen mixed berries

¼ cup (30g) plain flour

2 tbsps sugar

2 tbsps butter

2 tbsps cream, to serve

½ tsp cinnamon, to serve

2 ovenproof mini ramekins

Preheat the air fryer to 180°C.

Place the apple and frozen berries in the ramekins.

Combine the flour, sugar and butter in a small bowl. Rub together with fingertips to form a rough crumble. Spoon the crumble over the fruit.

Cook for 15 minutes.

Serve with fresh cream and a sprinkle of cinnamon.

SERVES 2

Note: Replace plain flour with brown rice flour for a gluten-free variation.

Chocolate Brownies

90g butter

¼ cup (30g) cocoa powder + 1 tbsp to garnish

2 eggs

1 tsp vanilla extract

¼ cup (30g) plain flour

1 cup (155g) brown sugar

½ cup (60g) walnuts, roughly chopped

Square cake tin, greased

Combine butter and cocoa in a medium bowl and heat in the microwave until just melted. Set aside to cool for 2 minutes, then whisk in the eggs and vanilla extract.

Sift in the flour and stir to combine. Add the brown sugar and nuts and again stir to combine.

Preheat the air fryer to 165°C. Scrape the mixture into the prepared cake tin and cook for 35 minutes.

Allow to cool before removing from the pan and cutting into eight squares.

MAKES 8

Berry Puffs

4 sheets frozen puff pastry, just thawed

1 egg, beaten

2 cups (250g) frozen mixed berries

Icing sugar, to serve

Preheat the air fryer to 200°C.

Place the pastry sheets on a floured workbench and cut into 8 squares. Place two squares in the air fryer basket, spacing them apart so they do not touch. Brush with eggwash. Place a second pastry square on top of each, and again brush with eggwash. Cook for 10 minutes or until pastry puffs are golden brown.

Remove the basket from the air fryer. Using a spoon, press down in the centre of the pastry to make an indentation. Push berries into each indentation.

Return to the air fryer and cook for a further 6 minutes. Transfer to a wire rack and allow to cool for a few minutes. Dust with icing sugar and serve warm.

Repeat steps with the remaining ingredients until you have made four tarts.

MAKES 4

Fruit Crumble

1 red apple, cored and chopped

4 plums

1 cup (150g) frozen berries

1 tbsp lemon juice

1 tsp cinnamon

⅔ cup (75g) plain flour

2½ tbsps caster sugar

35g butter

2 tbsps oats

Pie dish

Preheat the air fryer to 180°C.

Place the fruit in the pie dish. Squeeze over the lemon juice and sprinkle with cinnamon.

Combine the flour, sugar and butter in a small bowl. Rub together with fingertips to form a rough crumble. Spoon the crumble over the fruit. Sprinkle oats on top.

Cook in the air fryer for 15 minutes.

SERVES 4

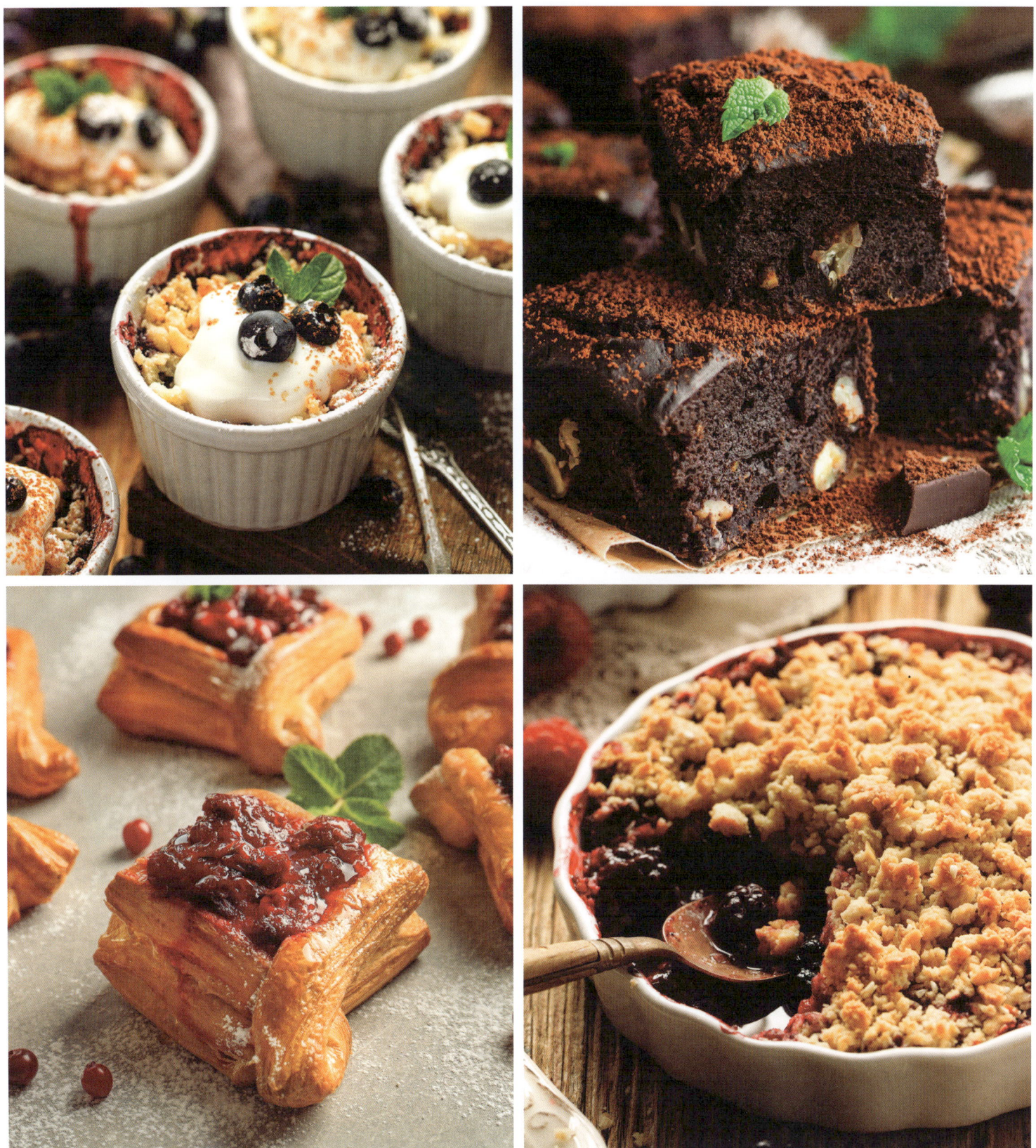

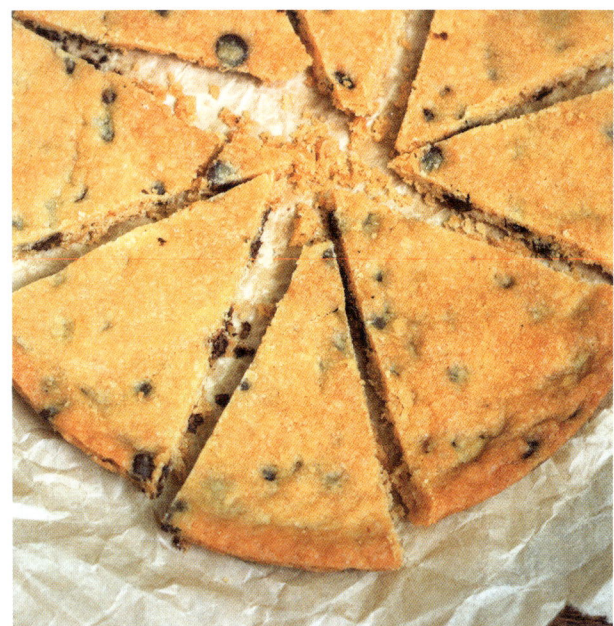

Giant Chocolate Chip Cookie

120g butter

½ cup (110g) sugar

½ cup (80g) light brown sugar

1 egg

1 tsp vanilla essence

1½ cups (185g) plain flour

½ tsp bicarbonate of soda

¼ tsp salt

1 cup (155g) milk chocolate chips

2 cake tins, greased

Preheat the air fryer to 180°C.

Place the butter, sugar and brown sugar in the bowl of an electric beater or stand mixer. Beat until light and fluffy, then add the egg and vanilla. Beat again until combined. Add the flour, bicarb and salt and gently beat to combine. Finally stir in the chocolate chips using a spoon.

Press the dough into the prepared cake tins. Transfer one to the fridge and place the other in the air fryer basket. Cook for 12 minutes until just golden.

Repeat with the other cookie.

SERVES 4

Apple Pie

2 apples

2 sheets frozen shortcrust pastry

1 tbsp lemon juice

1 tbsp ground cinnamon

1 tsp vanilla extract

3 tbsps brown sugar, divided

20g butter, cut into small pieces

1 egg, beaten

Cake tin

Peel and slice the apples.

Preheat the air fryer to 200°C.

Place the pastry sheets on a lightly floured surface and cut around the cake tin to make two circles, one larger than the other to extend up the sides of the tin.

Lightly grease the cake tin. Place the larger circle into the base of the tin, pressing the pastry up the sides. Place the tin into the basket of the air fryer.

Place the sliced apple, lemon juice, cinnamon, vanilla extract and 1 tablespoon brown sugar in a bowl and stir to combine.

Pour the filling into the cake tin on top of the pastry. Top with butter and remaining brown sugar.

Gently lower the second pastry circle on top of the filling. Pinch the edges to seal. Use a sharp knife to make a few slits in the surface of the pastry.

Brush the beaten egg over the top of the pastry and then transfer to the air fryer. Cook for 10 minutes, moving the tin around once or twice during cooking.

SERVES 4

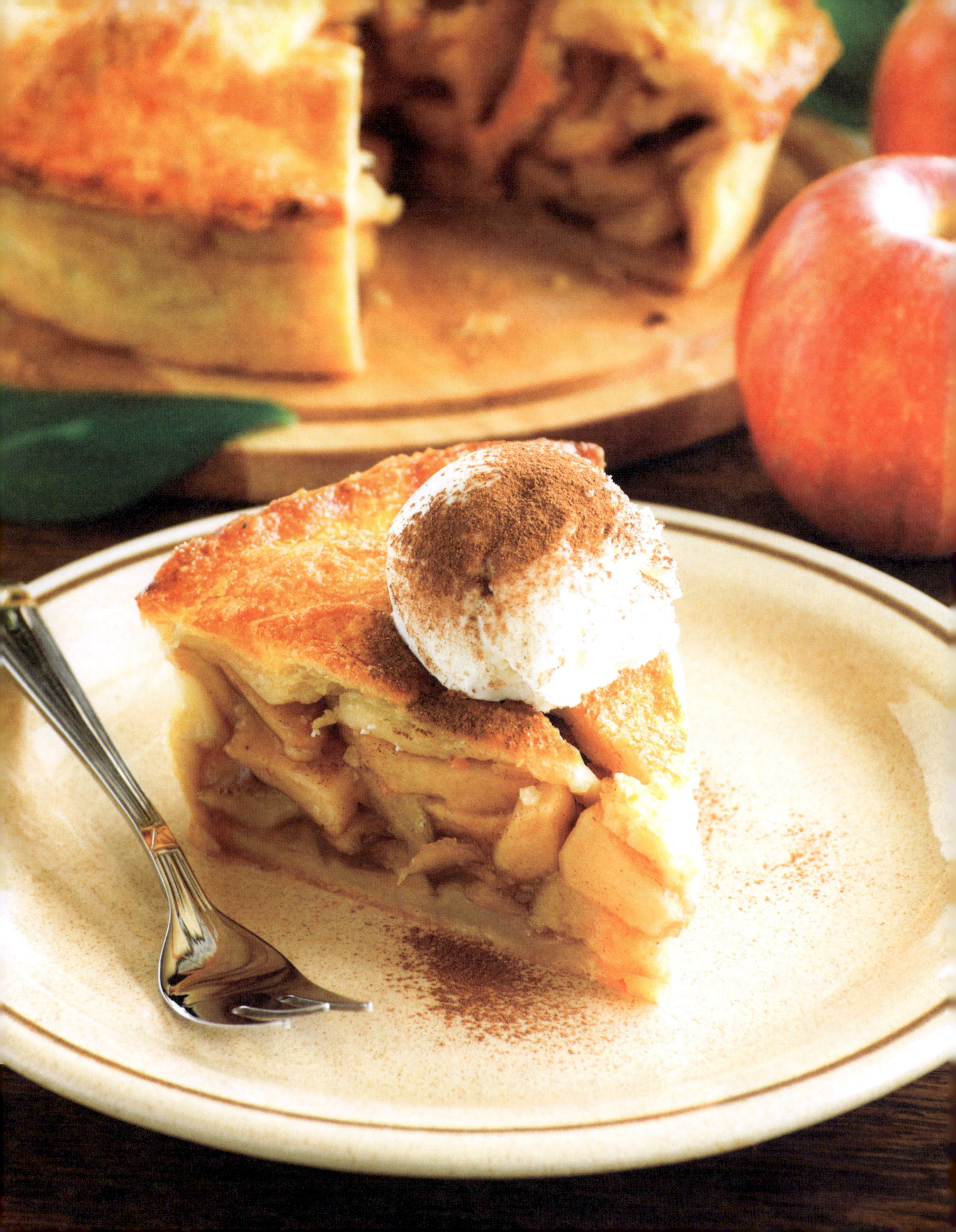

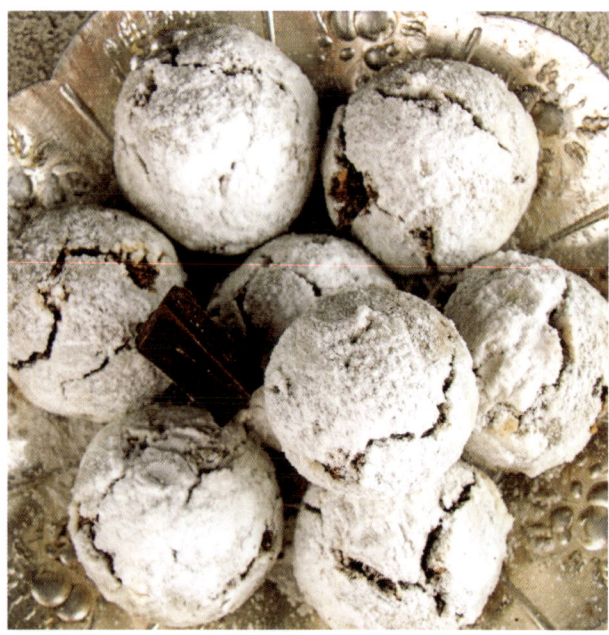

Shortbread Chocolate Balls

¼ cup (25g) plain flour

⅓ cup (75g) caster sugar

2 tbsps cocoa

180g butter, chilled and cut into cubes

½ tsp vanilla extract

10 pieces of good-quality chocolate

Baking pan

Combine the flour, sugar and cocoa in a mixing bowl. Rub in the butter to form a crumble. Continue mixing and then knead to form a smooth dough.

Roll the mixture into 10 balls. Squeeze a piece of chocolate into the centre of each and re-shape the ball around it.

Preheat the air fryer to 180°C.

Place the chocolate shortbread balls onto the baking pan and transfer to the air fryer.

Cook for 12 minutes, turning with tongs halfway through cooking.

MAKES 10

Sweet Potato Pie

1 sweet potato

1 tsp oil

2 sheets frozen shortcrust pastry

2 eggs

¼ cup (60ml) cream

2 tbsps honey

1 tbsp brown sugar

2 tbsps butter, melted

1 tsp vanilla extract

½ tsp ground cinnamon

⅛ tsp ground nutmeg

Whipped cream, to serve

Pie dish, greased

Rub the potato in oil and place in the basket of the air fryer. Cook for 30 minutes at 200°C. Remove and set aside until cool enough to handle. Peel off the skin and transfer the flesh to a mixing bowl.

Line the pie dish with the pastry, trimming off and discarding any overhanging pastry. Place the pie dish in the basket of the air fryer and set aside.

Add the eggs, cream, honey, brown sugar, butter, vanilla, cinnamon and nutmeg to the bowl with the sweet potato and stir well to combine all the ingredients.

Preheat the air fryer to 165°C.

Scrape the sweet potato batter into the pie shell and transfer to the air fryer. Cook for 35 minutes.

Allow to cool in the dish for 10 minutes before removing. Serve with whipped cream, if desired.

SERVES 4

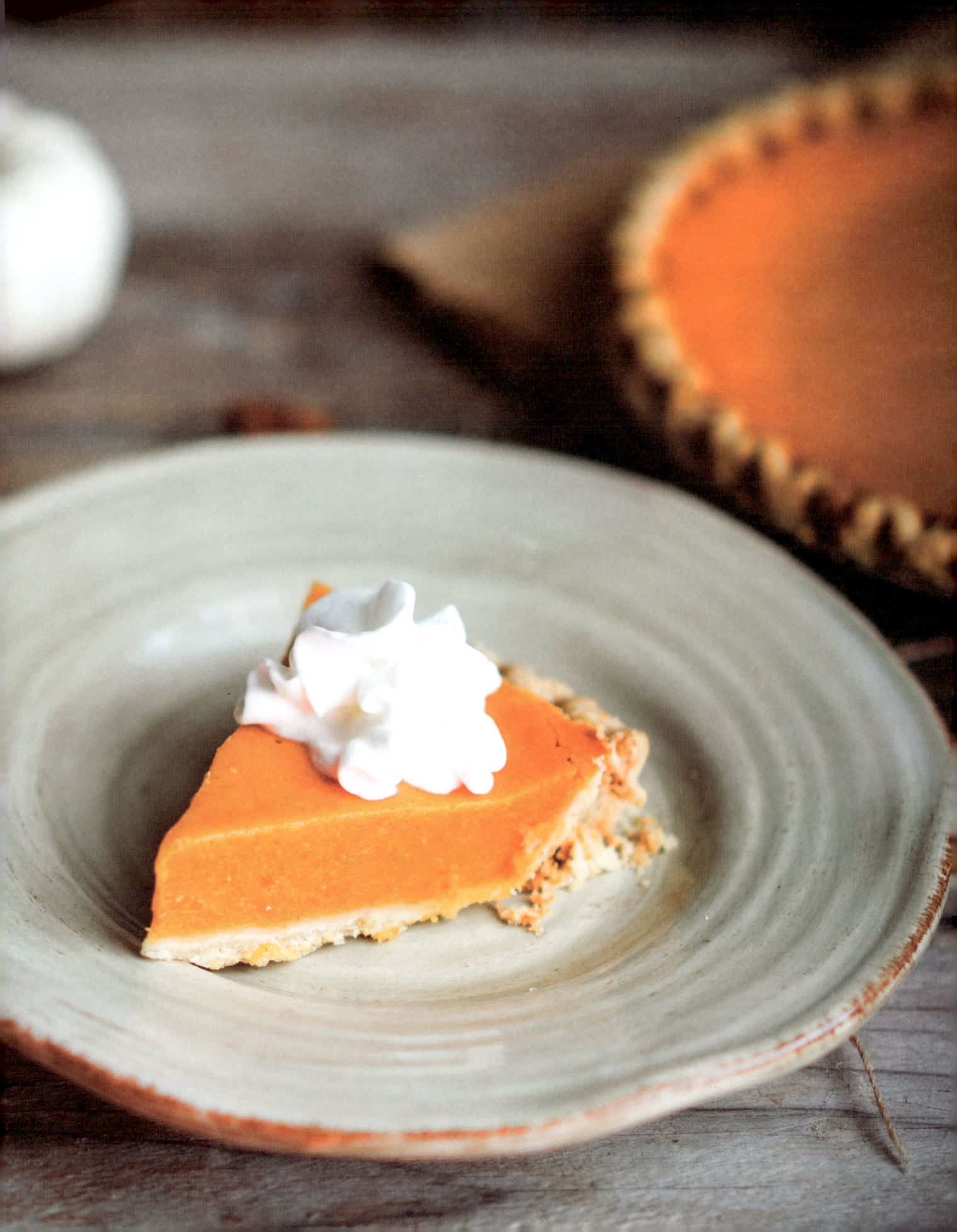

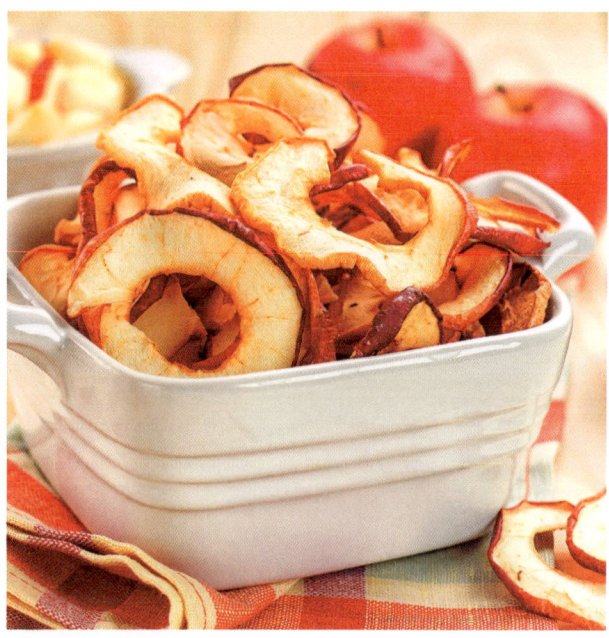

Fruit Chips

2 red apples (such as Pink Lady), thoroughly washed and cored

½ tsp cinnamon

Thinly slice the apples. Sprinkle with cinnamon.

Preheat the air fryer to 200°C.

Arrange the apple slices in the air fryer basket in a single layer. You will need to cook these in batches.

Cook for 8 minutes, flipping halfway through cooking.

Repeat the process until all apples are cooked.

Cool the chips on a wire rack.

SERVES 2

Mini Fruit Pies

⅔ cup (80g) plain flour

1 tbsp caster sugar

35g butter

1 tbsp water (+ more, as needed)

2 apples, peeled, cored and diced

4 tbsps fruit mince mix

Pinch of cinnamon

Mini pie tins, lightly greased

Combine the flour, sugar and butter in a small bowl. Rub together with fingertips to form a rough crumble.

Add the water until the mixture comes together as a dough.

Turn out onto a lightly floured surface and knead until a smooth dough forms. Roll out the pastry.

Drape pastry over the pie tins and cut around the edges. Press pastry into the tins.

Roll out leftover pastry, and make the pastry lids by cutting it into circles the same circumference as the pie tins.

Preheat the air fryer to 180°C.

Spoon the apple and fruit mince evenly into the pastry cases.

Place pastry lids on top and seal the edges with a fork. Cut holes in the surface with a sharp knife.

Cook for 18 minutes.

MAKES 4

Note: Use ramekins if you don't have mini pie tins and don't want to invest in them. Use store-bought pastry to make this recipe even easier.

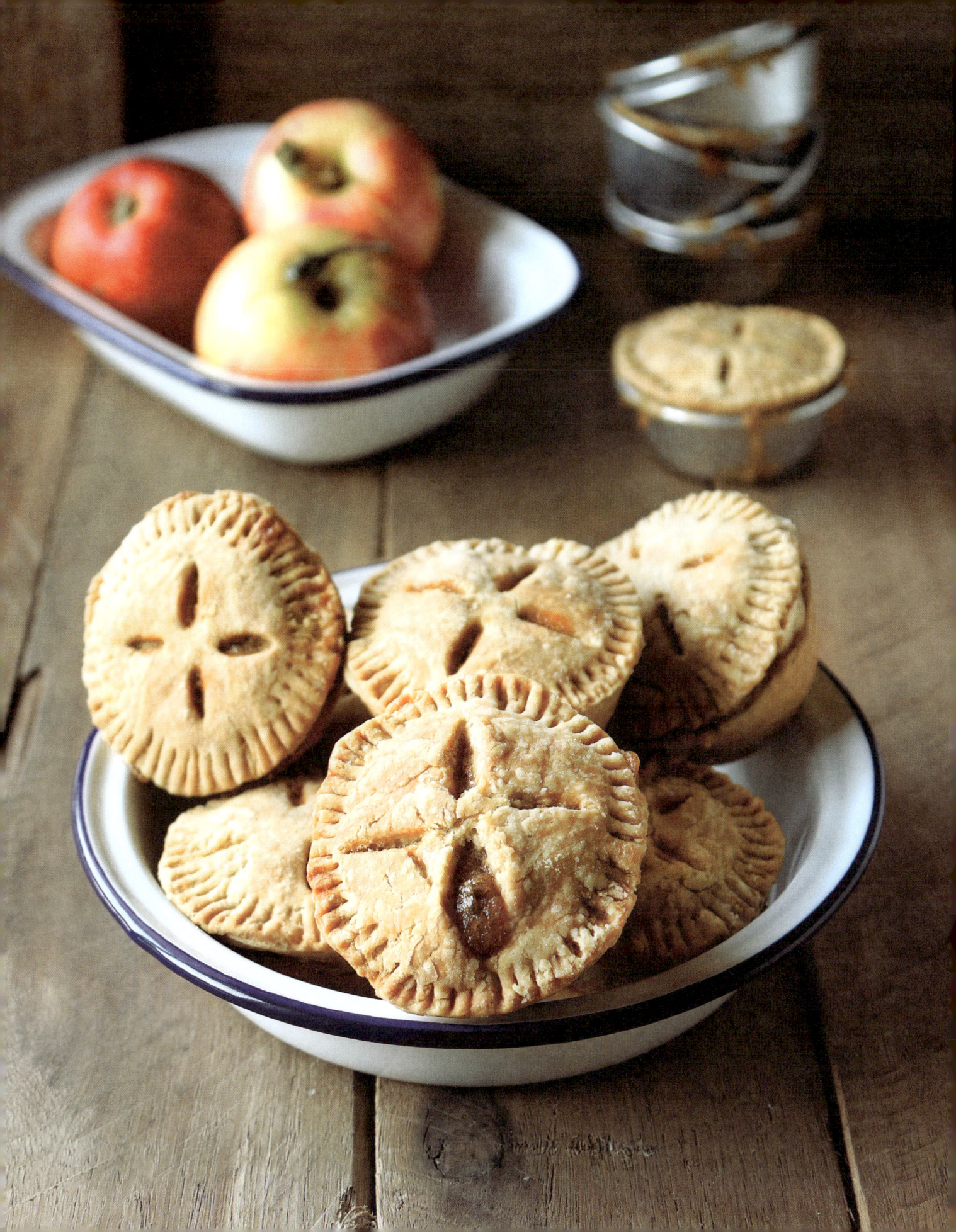

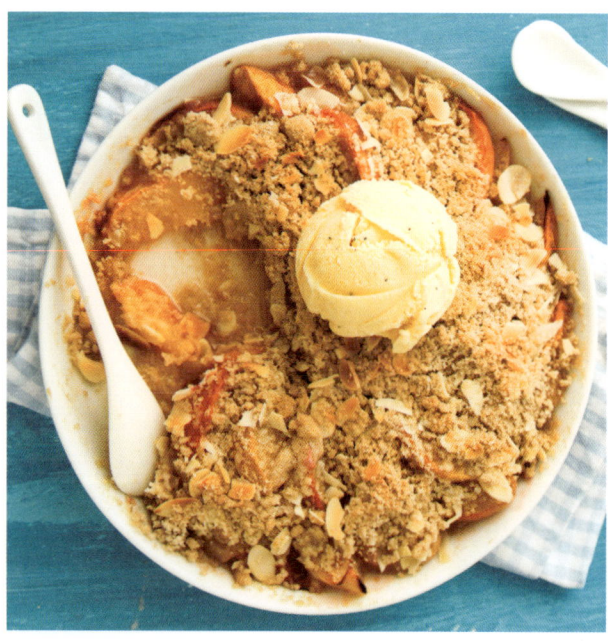

Peach and Apricot Crumble

200g frozen sliced peaches

100g tinned apricots

⅔ cup (75g) plain flour

3 tbsps brown sugar

35g butter

2 tbsps flaked almonds

Vanilla ice-cream, to serve

Pie dish

Preheat the air fryer to 180°C.

Place the fruit in the pie dish.

Combine the flour, brown sugar and butter in a small bowl. Rub together with fingertips to form a rough crumble. Spoon the crumble over the fruit. Sprinkle almonds on top.

Cook for 10 minutes, until golden brown.

Enjoy the crumble with a scoop of vanilla ice-cream.

SERVES 4

Churros

½ cup (125ml) water

45g butter, cut into cubes

1 tbsp + ¼ cup (55g) sugar

Pinch of salt

½ cup (60g) plain flour

1 egg

½ tsp vanilla extract

½ tsp ground cinnamon

Grease and line a baking tray. Set aside.

Place the water, butter, 1 tablespoon sugar and salt into a large saucepan and bring to the boil over medium heat. Reduce heat to low and gradually add the flour stirring continuously until the batter is smooth. Remove from the heat and transfer to the mixing bowl of an electric beater or stand mixer. Let cool for a few minutes.

Next add the egg and vanilla and beat well until a sticky dough forms. Transfer to a piping bag (with a star-shaped tip) using a spatula.

Pipe the churros onto the prepared tray. Transfer to the fridge to chill for 1 hour (no more than that or the dough will become too dry).

Preheat the air fryer to 190°C.

Transfer the churros to the air fryer basket being careful not to overcrowd it. (You may need to cook in batches). Lightly spritz with cooking spray. Cook for 10 minutes until golden.

Meanwhile combine the ¼ cup sugar and the cinnamon in a shallow bowl or plate.

When churros are cooked, immediately roll them in the cinnamon sugar to fully coat.

SERVES 4

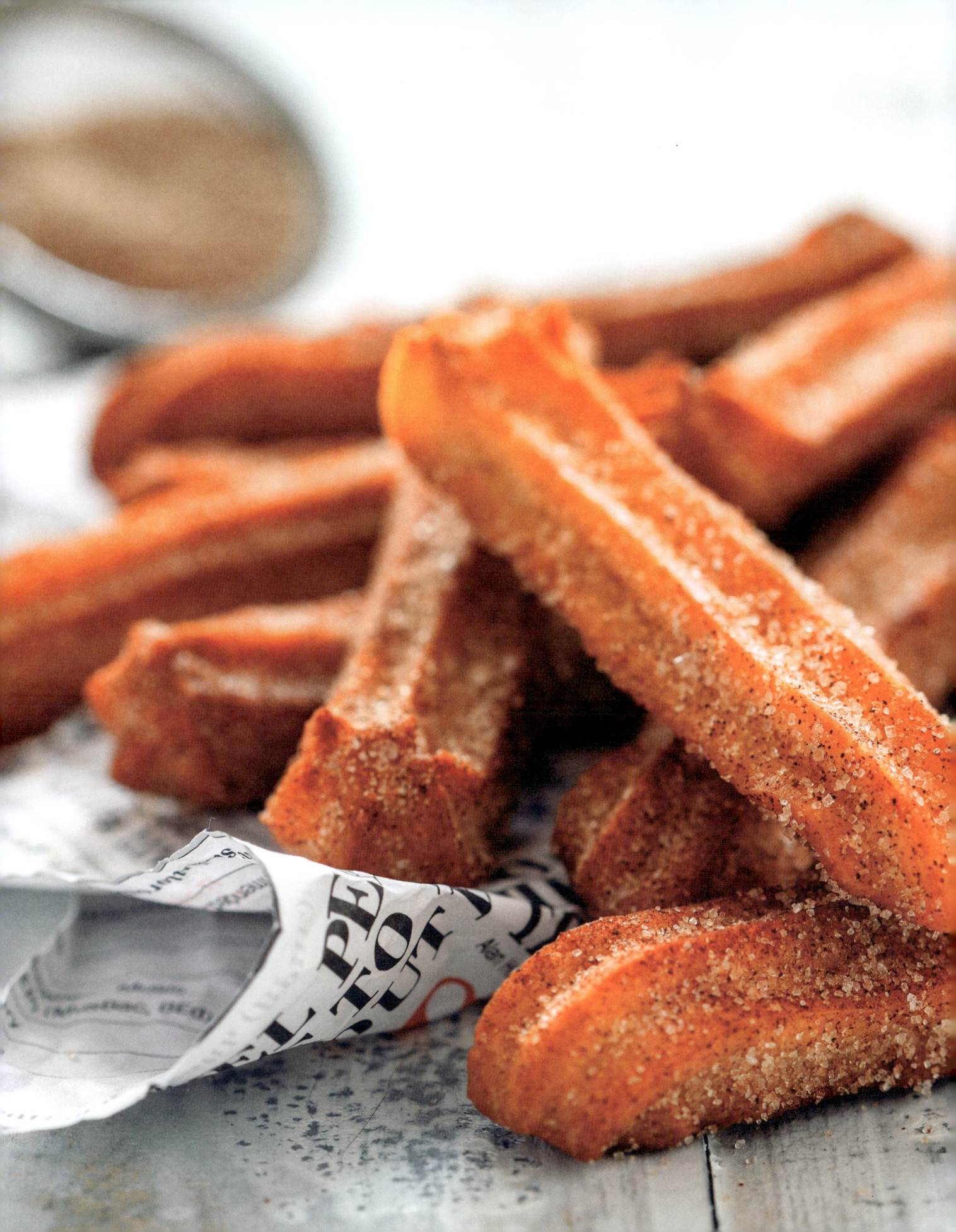

Index

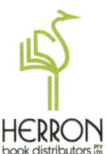

First Published in 2020 by Herron Book Distributors Pty Ltd
14 Manton St
Morningside
QLD 4170
www.herronbooks.com

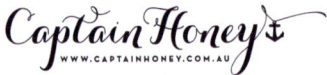

Custom book production by Captain Honey Pty Ltd
12 Station St
Bangalow
NSW 2479
www.captainhoney.com.au

Text copyright © Captain Honey Pty Ltd 2020

The moral right of the author has been asserted.

All rights reserved. No part of this book may be reproduced or transmitted by any persons or entity, including internet search engines or retailers, in any form or by any means, electronic or mechanical, including photocopying (except under the statutory exceptions provisions of the Australian Copyright Act 1968), recording, scanning or by any information storage and retrieval systems without the prior written permission of the author.

Cataloguing-in-Publication. A catalogue record for this book is available from the National Library of Australia

ISBN 978-0-947163-63-1

All images used under license from Shutterstock.com
Printed and bound in China

5 4 3 2 1   20 21 22 23 24

NOTES FOR THE READER

All reasonable efforts have been made to ensure the accuracy of the content in this book. Information in this book is not intended as a substitute for medical advice. The author and publisher cannot and do not accept any legal duty of care or responsibility in relation to the content in this book, and disclaim any liabilities relating to its use.